AF228664

The Healers

The Healers

*Physicians, Spiritualists, and Shamans in
the Search for Holistic Health*

Thomas S. Helling

ROWMAN & LITTLEFIELD
Lanham • Boulder • New York • London

Rowman & Littlefield
Bloomsbury Publishing Inc, 1385 Broadway, New York, NY 10018, USA
Bloomsbury Publishing Plc, 50 Bedford Square, London, WC1B 3DP, UK
Bloomsbury Publishing Ireland, 29 Earlsfort Terrace, Dublin 2, D02 AY28, Ireland
www.rowman.com

British Library Cataloguing in Publication Information available

Library of Congress Cataloging-in-Publication Data

Names: Helling, Thomas, 1947- author.
Title: The healers : physicians, spiritualists, and shamans in the search for holistic
    health / Thomas S. Helling.
Description: Lanham : Rowman & Littlefield, [2025] | Includes bibliographical
    references and index. | Summary: "Celebrated surgeon and medical historian offers
    brief biographies of medical healers through the ages, from the ancient Greeks to the
    present day, illuminating various approaches to healing body and spirit"-- Provided
    by publisher.
Identifiers: LCCN 2024042446 (print) | LCCN 2024042447 (ebook) |
    ISBN 9798881803254 (cloth ; alk. paper) | ISBN 9798881803261 (epub)
Subjects: MESH: Traditional Medicine Practitioners--history | History of Medicine |
    Holistic Health
Classification: LCC R733 (print) | LCC R733 (ebook) | NLM WZ 112.5.T7 |
    DDC 610--dc23/eng/20241118
LC record available at https://lccn.loc.gov/2024042446
LC ebook record available at https://lccn.loc.gov/2024042447

For product safety related questions contact productsafety@bloomsbury.com.

∞™ The paper used in this publication meets the minimum requirements of American
National Standard for Information Sciences—Permanence of Paper for Printed Library
Materials, ANSI/NISO Z39.48-1992.

To the ill of body and spirit

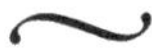# Contents

CHAPTER ONE

How Do We Heal?

Everyone falls victim to sickness. It is no different now than in antiquity. Disease and illness are simply the consequences of nature's imperfections. Their targets are not only the flesh but also the spirit. Ancient man pondered their implications and wondered at solutions that seemed more of heaven than of earth. Only begrudgingly slow revelations of physical science have added a distinctly tangible element to understanding. Yet permeating all is still the intangible, the mysterious, the unexplainable. At times, healing defies reason and defies science. Is it from lack of discovery or lack of comprehension?

So how have we healed? Has it been technological? Pharmaceutical? Societal? Cultural? Or spiritual? Man has pondered those questions since the dawn of time. This book will explore the answers. It is history but also pertinent. It is timely but also timeless. How we heal going forward has indelible roots in the past. In antiquity healing incorporated knowledge of nature and its effects on mankind. The practice of healing, then, would be called *physic*, from the Greek, φυσικη ("phusike," meaning "nature"), the knowledge of *natural things*. "Physic" and "medicine" would be used interchangeably with "healing" for centuries hence.

Man suffers like all animals suffer. Pain, fevers, immobility, weakness, helplessness. "Nature" has seen to that. Yet human beings know they suffer. They understand the implications of suffering. And they understand the existential threats to suffering. Man knows he will die, and he dreads that knowledge. He has developed an entire industry around it: the Healing Arts. He strives to heal; to restore health—that joyous condition abounding in energy, vitality, laughter, companionship, and celebration. It is life itself. Thus, to understand suffering is to understand those conditions that remove health. Disease, injury, afflictions. And with ill health comes illness: that condition of worry, anxiety, depression, frustration, sadness.

It is pain of the body that begets pain of the soul. Both are equally disturbing and threatening. Pain withers the spirit. Relief of suffering in antiquity largely meant relief of pain—and it still may to this day: somatic throbbing or visceral churning. Societies acknowledged that pain can be made so much worse by the spiritual anguish of fear, anxiety, or grief. To quell the painful disturbances of the body often entailed relaxing a frantic mind. Separating one from the other, as modern science is apt to do, may more precisely direct targeting therapy but may fail to untangle the intimate association of mindful factors that, in still unexplained ways, seem to exert a promotional influence on organs and tissues—for better or worse.

As the ancients believed, we must heal both body and spirit. And what is the spirit? It is the essence of an individual, the personality, the complex of inward feelings and tendencies complementary to their outward expression, or what psychiatrist Carl Jung called the "persona." It incorporates unconscious experiences that often conflict with conscious awareness. Regardless of public displays of confidence, optimism, or trust, inward feelings of anxiety, fear, timidity, and dread may consume quiet times of solitude and reflection.[1] In an Aristotelian sense, it is this constellation that defines an individual, the unique aggregate of interactive body and soul. For humans it is the rational essence. "Now the soul is that whereby primarily we live, perceive, and have understanding. . . . It is not body but something belonging to body, and therefore resides in body."[2] In that sense, as a component of humaneness, it is the indwelling spirit.

The ill have always shown their misery. Disease tears at the fabric of health, and the spirit yearns for that joy of living, that vigor which bestows a rich and social existence. Yet ill health ruins everything and subjects the mind—that complex repository of spiritual essence—to the sufferings of despair, uncertainty, and doom. Disease, and the distresses it provokes, become bound one to another in an embrace of fate. The nineteenth-century theologian Søren Kierkegaard had written that despair itself is a sickness, a sickness of the spirit. In fact, Kierkegaard reasoned, despair can become a sickness unto death, but only worse, because despair itself is a living death, a constant reminder of the looming anguish of mortality, a struggle with death that renders its victim disconsolate, that even relief by death will not rescue them.[3]

The healing arts were designed to restore health in all its implications. From antiquity those dedicated to the task labored to understand causes of diseases: unhealthiness. What bodily distresses produced feelings of sickness, debility, and death? And what could be done to reverse them? Even correction of symptoms could not always restore health. The mind would not cease to fret. Depression would not abate. Fear would not subside. The spirit remained ill. So, in history, manners of healing—some more physical, others more metaphysical—proliferated. Some were cultural; some faith-based; some spiritual; some technical. Some lacked hard evidence; others wallowed in it. All hoped to recover for those unfortunate ones total health; the coveted *joie de vivre*, the joy of living. It is with this authority that healers practice. As social historian Paul Starr wrote, "[t]he kind of authority claimed by the [medical] profession, then, involves not only skill in performing a service, but also the capacity to judge the experience and needs of the clients."[4]

The history of these healers and their labors is a fascinating one. They were ruled by passions. None could have such devotion to healing without it. They invoked gods and spirits. They dissected and analyzed. They cut and spliced. They delivered prescription after prescription to hope that one or the other might just provide even temporary respite. And they pondered the essence of humanness. How could they ease the hopelessly complex and worried human mind—literally the spirit of being itself—and at the same time correct disrupted anatomy and physiology?

Because humanness is imperfect.

And humans are of precarious health. The fine harmony of complexities of anatomic and physiologic arrangement, when in balance, produce that unmistakable equanimity, an inner contentment. On the other hand, disharmony is distressful. Unbalanced interior integrity often signals feelings of ill health: sickness, the bane of existence. Disease, illness, and healing: three terms that have guided attempts by mankind to alleviate that most distressing of encounters—human suffering. That man has been crippled by infirmities is a consequence of his environment, both external and internal. Trauma, tumors, epidemics, and the eventual degeneration of biophysical components inflict a status of unhealthiness, often characterized by pain, debility, and mental anguish. Very often the victim fears an existential threat adding to their agony. It is simply a matter of humaneness. In its innate benevolence, mankind has also sought ways to relieve suffering and to restore health. Without an understanding of anatomy, physiology, or pathology, healers have of necessity turned to the invisible world, the world of spirits and gods and superhuman abilities. Priest-healers, anointed to discourse with the invisible, pleaded for intercession and reversal of perceived divine inflictions. History has validated that. Physician Bernie Segal remarked "in traditional tribal medicine and in Western practice from its beginning in the work of Hippocrates, the need to operate through the patient's mind has always been recognized." And with some success. The intricate human mind and its interaction with physical workings could, in fact, alleviate pain, suffering, and even physical infirmities. In fact, physician Bernie Segal remarked "in traditional tribal medicine and in Western practice from its beginning in the work of Hippocrates, the need to operate through the patient's mind has always been recognized."[5] The Asclepian temples of ancient Greece were prime examples, fully designed to influence that interminable spirit of hope. Pilgrims with their ailments were pampered, catered to, and subjected to inspirational rituals of their priests so that the healing god, Asclepius, might come in a dream and rid them of their disease. But it was only available to the rich, prestigious, and noble. Common man was allowed to fester by the roadside, begging for sustenance or any relief of their sicknesses.

By no means was the desire to heal universal or equitable.

Individual worth had no basis in antiquity. *Αρετη*, meaning "virtue," was a quality possessed by one who manifested the desired behavior of the patrician class. "Virtue" *Humanitas*, Latin for humanitarian qualities, were not extended to all people but only the upper crust who need not bestow empathy on the less deserving. Therefore, human "worth" was a factor of societal virtue rather than intrinsic value. Human dignity and human rights were not intrinsic in classical cultures, but only defined judicially. Inequality, on the other hand, was expected, and even desirable. Those of lesser stature, including slaves, were a necessary component of an aristocracy which thrived on the subjugation of designated inferior types. Those infirmed, deformed, or defective were not thought deserving of attention, much less sympathy and were too often marginalized as impediments to a dignified civilization. As a consequence, care of the ill took on a particularly specific mission—treatment of those deemed "worthy" of such attention. Inferior subjects were very often ignored and even shunned. Healing, for ancient cultures, was attempted only for those able to demonstrate evidence of "virtue" and "value." The sanctuaries of Asclepius were magnificent edifices, but available only to those of a status to afford such rituals and attention. Diseased and leprous victims very often were dismissed from their household and peppered the streets and alleyways in desperate attempts to subsist. They did not hold value or dignity, and society gave them no quarter. What impact Hippocratic teachings had on care of the underprivileged is largely unknown, although Hippocrates did not emphasize compassion for all as part of the honorable physician's practice.

The worker of wonders, Jesus of Nazareth, changed all that. He cured by human touch but also by healing of spiritual suffering. His message was twofold: heal the body through healing the spirit. And he instructed his followers to do the same. So impressive were his teachings that fellow Jews acknowledged him as the long-awaited Messiah, the Anointed One. History would call him Jesus the Christ.

His followers were called Christians; their religion, Christianity. This new Christianity, then, radicalized healthcare. The teachings of the charismatic Jesus of Nazareth, called the Anointed One, held that every man and woman had intrinsic worth and deserved equal consideration for empathy and charity. Every individual was created in *imago Dei*, in the image of God.[6] Christianity absorbed the Hebrew concept of *imago Dei* as part of their philanthropy, their love of neighbor. Healing extended to everyone, particularly to those traditionally deprived of such attention:

> "Lord, when did we see you hungry and feed you, or thirsty and give you something to drink? When did we see you a stranger and invite you in, or needing clothes and clothe you? When did we see you sick or in prison and go to visit you?" The King will reply, "Truly I tell you, whatever you did for one of the least of these brothers and sisters of mine, you did for me."[7]

Christians also subscribed to the Jewish belief that *bāśār*, flesh, and *nephesh*, life, are integral. To destroy the flesh was to destroy God-infused life and, therefore, insult the will of God. Those Christians intent on healing—formally educated or not—first, understood the intimate union of body and spirit and, second, might extend their talents to anyone suffering from injury or ailments. Of course, in the first centuries after Christ, most Christian healthcare was done in monasteries where attention to the spirit was likely given priority over attention to the flesh. But their comforts to the suffering were as satisfying as in the temples of Asclepius.

But healing practices remained rudimentary. The first-century philosopher and physician, Galen, attempted to provide some evidentiary basis for theoretical concepts of disease and suffering. His anatomic portrayals, while imperfect, were at least an attempt to give reality to supposition. It provided a framework in which to implant the Hippocratic teachings of inner harmony, and disease. His physiology, like much of his anatomy, was flawed but so convincing that his teachings lasted centuries. They were the first inkling of natural explanations for the heretofore conviction of supernatural causation. Even more, Galen was a pragmatist and a principled practitioner, in accord with the Hippocratic school. He strongly advocated an ethical approach to healing, considering all aspects of the person, not just the disease. Knowledge and experience were his preconditions. Later, philosopher Thomas Aquinas echoed his principles by remarking:

> If anyone has the theoretical knowledge of an art but lacks experience, he will be perfect insofar as he knows the universal; but since he does not know

the singular, because he lacks experience, he will very often make mistakes in healing. For healing belongs to the realm of the singular rather than to that of the universal, because it belongs to the former essentially and to the later accidentally.[8]

It was not until well into the second millennium that curiosity opened a new pursuit of knowledge—the medievalists called it *sciencia*—of the human machinery. Focus then turned away from the spirit to reassess the body. Theories of Hippocrates began to pale in favor of identifiable organs and tissues as the sites of disease. The effects of body on spirit, disease on illness, was put aside with the fascination of a new anatomy and a new physiology. Only a few continued to insist on the interference of godly designs on the corruptness of man. The outspoken German theologian and physician Hildegard of Bingen promoted a healthy soul (being an impregnation of the image of God from within) on a healthy constitution. Woe to the sinner, she wrote, punishment was sure to follow.

Yet others were promoting a new skill of the hands—surgery. While the conventional pharmacopoeia of the day proved largely ineffectual and the ruminations of educated physicians did little to offset the pain and anguish of their patients, surgery oftentimes provided miraculous relief. Disease could be extirpated and, with it, the mental agony that accompanied. Regarded as base butchery at first, surgery slowly acquired the respectability of academia through careful and thorough scientific explorations of human anatomy and physiology. Besides the dexterity necessary to slice through human flesh, surgeons strived to learned literacy: the classics, philosophy, pharmacology, and even the refined art of physic. Two pivotal figures in medieval surgery, Henri de Mondeville and Guy de Chauliac, launched educated surgery into the ranks of university scholars, and provided written bases for their artistry. And what of the spiritual? God indeed remains the supreme physician but uses the hands of men, in their physicality, to correct the misfortunes of nature.

Still, the impact of such pragmatism was slow. Rather, medical orthodoxy still held sway. Even by the so-called Age of Reason, European science advanced by glacial proportions, and Hippocratic humoral theory still dominated medical thinking. No wonder, then, that the religiously educated—the preacher-physicians of colonial America—were convinced in an angelical conjunction: the union of the "angelic" spirit world with earth. God and his cohorts determined corporal penalties. Convinced that mankind's ills were punishment for sinful wickedness, preachers demanded repentance as a prerequisite for corporal healing. With few worthy physicians available in the early New England days, preachers often participated in bodily healing as well, frequently better versed than their professed medical counterparts. With the sweeping epidemics of the day, particularly smallpox, few concoctions provided any relief, and any true respite was spiritual, at the behest of the clergy. Long on compassion, in many cases a soulful peace was all that could be expected as the plagues relentlessly took their victims. Suffering and death were constant companions, and little could man do to forestall the inevitable. Little, that is, except pray.

In many other cultures the supernatural reigned. For Native Americans, the universe was rich with the spirit world. Spirits inhabited all things: the earth, plants, animals, man, and the sky. Proper acknowledgment and appeasement might promote health, but aberrations of nature happened. Minor ailments were best treated by standard folk remedies, but for those that did not improve, tribal healers were called. These men, deigned and blessed by the spirit world—the forefathers of all points of the compass— were the *wakȟáŋ wičháša*, the holy ones. They practiced the fundamentals of herbal remedies but, in refractory cases, embarked on the sacred healing ceremonies. For the Lakota tribes of the Dakotas, these were carefully orchestrated and ritualized rites performed with preordained songs, smoke, dances, and proper acknowledgment to the spirits that oversaw earthly activity. They were much like the Greek Asclepian rituals and were equally valued by tribal members. Many illnesses were cured by these rituals. Probably more healing of the spirit happened than healing of the body. But peace of mind was often preferred over complete cure. Would it not be in all cultures?

And what about incurable disease? How has mankind coped with the looming prospect of death? Despite hopes in complex technology that healers are bound to offer, so often the supernatural and unexplainable are invoked. Miracles. Divine intercession. The spirit world. Surgeon Alexis Carrel witnessed it. Father Damien promoted it. Churches fill for it. Families gather because of it. Incurability, too, becomes a healing process—the spirit over the flesh. A tendency to believe in other worlds invisible to the senses, but draped in the prospect of life continued.

The burst of scientific experimentalism of the late nineteenth and early twentieth centuries overtook spirituality as the remedy for disease. The burgeoning art of surgery brought into focus repairs of the body so sophisticated that they were truly miraculous works in their own right. Was man inching toward the divinities?

By the twenty-first century many scientists have subscribed to the model of disease as one of purely biomedical proportions, with molecular biology as its fundamental science. If true, disease, then, can be fully explained by deviations from normative biological variables. Less tangible elements of social, psychological, and behavioral dimensions of illness could be largely ignored. Not so, noted psychiatrist George Engel maintained. Such "reductionistic" pursuits of disease do not fit with the inescapable integration of the biosphere—environmental, societal, and psychological elements—into shaping human response to afflictions. These "systems" methodologies, Engle argued, "provides a conceptual approach suitable not only for the proposed biopsychosocial concept of disease but also for studying disease and medical care as interrelated processes." It was time for a new biomedical model, one that incorporated social, psychological, and behavioral elements into analyses of disease and its incumbent illness on the human person.[9] At times, still, the physicality of healing has to dominate. Intense surgery or medicinal therapeutics must at least temporarily take precedence over spiritual concerns, although the very human nature within persists and, on some level, must still be recognized. In fact, the more egregious the treatment, the more fearful the mind. And history is replete with examples of this as well. Foremost might be the stark mutilation necessary for some forms of cancer.

In all cases though, anthropologist Margaret Mead observed that "in the sciences of living things we find the greatest confusion but also the clearest demonstration of the ways in which the two kinds of observations—the observation of human beings by human beings and of physical nature by human beings—meet." She promoted the concept of "macroscopy" instead of "microscopy" in the analysis of the interaction of land, sea, air, and life as pure integration and not segregation.[10]

Yet health has implications far exceeding exacting biological phenomena. Environmental, societal, cultural, and psychological factors almost certainly play into the alteration of biological function or susceptibility to internal and external pathological stressors. The "spirit," then—that amalgamation of intangible psychic influences—is a vital and, very often, underappreciated factor in maintenance or restoration of health—thus in *healing*. Scientifically, such "epigenetic" processes—those behavioral and ecological catalysts on gene function—"can affect the expression of genes associated with regulatory pathways throughout life. . . . A developmental perspective to the origins of cardiovascular and metabolic disease has widespread sociological, economic, and ethical implications." There likely are any number of external triggers on internal molecular pathways pertaining to homeostasis. It would seem rational, then, that rising rates of certain conditions such as cardiovascular disease, have a developmental component.[11] Sociologists John Brooke and Clark Larsen have realized a looming influence of external forces on internal milieus.

"The genetic and physiological relationship between humanity past and present has become a pressing issue with the recent decoding of the human genome, one that will inexorably link biology and culture, science and the humanities . . . the boundary between biology and culture, nature and nurture . . . is an open question."[12]

Then, with science in the forefront, what have our ancestral healers taught us? Perhaps a great deal. That disease plays havoc on the human mind is unarguable. Knowing little else about pathological nuances, it was the ill spirit with which they contended. Is it so far-fetched that we do still today? Certainly, the human psyche in all its joys and fears and sorrows has remained unchanged and unfathomable in its complexity, even while the physique encasing it has now been scrutinized by scalpel and microscope and measurement. Biology sizzles in its analytical juices while psychology remains a wandering vapor poorly contained and largely invisible. Whether scientists will ever be able to dissect, disassemble, or define the impossibly intricate patterns of neural networks to explain the biologic basis for human emotions, fears, and hopes that, in the aggregate, constitute the spirit is arguable. Even then, in all their biotechnical acumen, physicians are still left with the human constitution and its reaction to suffering and mortality.

In any event, as the ancients well knew, do not ignore the intangible sickness for the tangible ailments. Notable medical pioneers in history have tried to integrate the two. And does that not form the foundations of holistic healing? Care of the disease and care of the illness.

Both will always remain essential.

Yet and still, the most common response among health care providers when a family member brought up religion or spirituality in critical, life-threatening situations was to change the subject.[13]

Can it all be ignored? Doubtful. Perhaps author John Steinbeck said it well in his travels throughout America. "A sad soul can kill you quicker, far quicker, than a germ."[14]

CHAPTER TWO

~

Between Gods and Men

The Asclepiads

In the earliest of times, the mythical gods of ancient civilizations were har-
bingers of suffering and diviners of healing. They appealed to intelligent but
desperate human beings hungry for relief. For people of that age the uncer-
tainties of nature were distressing and hopelessly perplexing. Surely there
must be *supernatural* powers at play. American philosopher William James
remarked that "gods are conceived to be first things in the way of being and
power. They overarch, and from them there is no escape. What relates to
them is the first and last word in the way of truth."[1]

For the uninterpretable—the blights and hardships of common man—
omnipotent (but terribly fallible) gods were a perfect explanation. Invisible.
Imaginative. Assigned by man as lords of the universe. Their illusory power
was awe inspiring but their conjured foibles as human as any of mankind—at
once godlike and human-like. Fickle wills fit seamlessly with the chaotic
happenings of nature. How better to decipher the malignant fevers, malicious rashes, and maleficent exhalations of the sick? Treat what may, healers
advised, but look to the gods for final relief. Could the spirit accommodate
that? Much more so than the mysterious and distinctly godless internal torment of disease; such misery that could ruin men and seemed impervious
to remedies of the most educated. Gods would know. Surely their celestial
prowess would strike down even the most stubborn of illnesses.

In times of implacable suffering those wishing to heal turned heavenward,
and no better example of them was the Classical Period of Grecian culture.

The Greek historian Thucydides reported that in the days of the Peloponnesian War, a peculiar plague descended on Athens. During the second
year of conflict with Sparta, 430 BCE, terrible sicknesses suddenly appeared
across the fortified city. Men, women, and children, strong and weak, were

stricken by violent fevers, redness and inflammation of the eyes, and putrid, fetid throats. There soon followed nasal discharges, hoarseness, chest pain, and fitful coughing. Before long, violent spasms of the gut started, with vomiting and diarrhea. The victim literally burned from within and could not get relief. Eruptions of the skin occurred, covering hands, feet, and genitalia. Within a week, the sufferer collapsed, bloody diarrhea now almost continuous, and death quickly came. Victims succumbed in such numbers that no one could remember a plague equal in its viciousness. So rotten were the corpses that not even birds or beasts of prey, it was said, would feast on them. Most distressing was the fate of physicians tending to the afflicted—the first to respond. They could do nothing to relieve their anguish, and they themselves were felled by contagion after visits, dying one after another. The great Athenian military strategist Pericles would succumb, already having witnessed the deaths of his two sons from the illness. Worse, too, the city was packed with refugees of the war, which flamed the sickness further. Streets, homes, and even public places became clogged with bodies of the afflicted and stained with their excrement. Thucydides wrote:

> When they arrived at Athens though a few had houses of their own to go to, or could find an asylum with friends or relatives, by far the greater number had to take up their dwelling in the parts of the city that were not built over and in the temples and chapels of the heroes.[2]

An odor so foul hung over the metropolis and its sanctuaries that even the gods themselves must have choked. Miserable with suffering, the populace wondered why. Was the mighty god Apollo, master of disease, the author? Had he been slighted and now unleashed his wrath? Athenians, fearful of Apollo's anger, turned to his son, the god-man Asclepius, the merciful healer. Until now, he had been ignored. No more. Restored health was of utmost concern. During the fragile peace of Nicias in 420 BC and in proper ceremony, the statue of Asclepius, with his slithering, coiled snake, was brought from Epidaurus across the Saronic Gulf, paraded along the walled corridor from the port of Piraeus, through the marbled city, and placed in a wooden shrine at the foot of the Acropolis. Asclepius' healing sanctuary was in place. Now the public hoped the epidemic would vanish. Athenians prayed the gods had been appeased.

And so they were. The plague abated, not to return. Asclepius and his followers had begun a redemptive social movement and helped renew religious healing practices in Athens. In fact, in a larger sense, the legend of Asclepius, the Greek god-healer, sparked a healing transformation throughout antiquity. Largely fanciful, his legend was profound. Even in the abstract, his energies and imagined presence stilled anxieties, restored hope, and promoted inner peace. If not the body, he mended damaged minds. The spinoff would be the genuine skill and ethos of his ordained practitioners who accompanied folklore.

For Greeks, such fiction made sense. Sickness and pestilence came from an arbitrary nature in conflict. Celestial phenomena—cold, heat, and restless winds—collided with forces of an earthly world: air and water. Yet the many gods of Greek mythology had influence on all of nature, so the Greeks believed. Even the influential fourth-century BCE Greek philosopher Plato (c427–348 BCE) marveled:

> [T]hink of the earth, and sun, and planets, and everything! And the wonderful and beautiful order of seasons with its distinctions of years and months! Besides, there is the fact that all mankind, Greeks and non-Greeks alike, believe in the existence of gods.

"All things are full of gods," Plato went on to declare.[3] The gods could stir, calm, and stoke the proclivities of heavenly and earthly forces. The turbulence they created struck through flesh and into the percolating substances of life. Illness, suffering, and misery followed. In antiquity, these were the beliefs of the common man. Yes, certain progressive healers of the time promoted renegade bodily fluids as cause. Yet even the most erudite respected the gods. "I too think that these diseases are divine, and so are all others, no one being more divine or more human than any other; all are alike, and all divine," the great Hippocrates would later write.[4]

Sufferers already knew that in their hearts. These afflictions were from above—a play of natural and supernatural, as the stricken would feel for millennia to come. Divine meddling in tragic events was too tempting to deny. To Greeks of the day, human wrongdoings must bring down divine retribution. Corruption. Greed. Promiscuity. Shame on mortals. No better way to rebuke in godly fashion than hurl grief and suffering. Health, in those times, seemed fleeting anyway. It could be dispensed with in the blink of an eye: at the mercy of climate, seasons, and will of the gods. City dwellers and countrymen alike sought local folk remedies and professed healers, but, in the end, they pilgrimaged to temples and shrines. They turned to the gods. The priestly physicians there might petition and, if pleasing to the deities, alter fate. All would plead for intercession.

Above all gods, was the great healer Asclepius.

Who was Asclepius, represented by this majestic manly statue with staff and snake that Athenians carried through their city? It was the image of the merciful one. The One Who Healed. By fable, he was mortal but divine as well. Only with his godlike ability could he return the ailing to health. But the wise Asclepius—with his messages of tranquility—could probe deeper, to restore peace to the intangible spirit as well. So prominent was his following that one cannot understand his centrality to ancient healing without understanding his legend.

In Greek mythology, before Asclepius there was the handsome god Phoebus Apollo. Son of Zeus and his concubine Leto. To Apollo were attributed the powers of curing afflictions and comforting the unwell. Apollo was magnanimous among his godly peers. Sculpted as strikingly handsome with chiseled features and muscled proportions, he offered the epitome of masculine gallantry. "How, then, shall I sing of you who in all ways are a worthy theme of song," the Homeric hymn went. "For everywhere O Phoebus [Apollo] the whole range of song is fallen to you."[5]

From the loins of Apollo came the legend of Asclepius, the great physician. Perhaps he was no more than a fanciful; perhaps even predating the Greeks. Some say long before Mycenaean culture, the wandering Phoenicians considered that a phantom god named Asclepius was air itself, bringing health to man and animal alike. His father, called Apollo, as well was the sun god and, as the sun, through the changing seasons, he imparted to the air its healthfulness—father to son. It was the course of the sun, they believed, that brought health to mankind.[6]

Or, if he really lived, he may have come from the city of Tricca, on the broad plains of Thessaly. Tricca was located on the left bank of the river Peneus. The country of Thessaly was home to fertile fields, and its kingdoms were ruled by aristocratic Thesprotians, original settlers of the region and, perhaps, all of the Greek mainland. The poet Homer called Tricca's expansive meadows the "pastureland of horses." Hesiod's Greek theogony described the gentle plain between Mount Oeta and Mount Olympus as hallowed ground, the battlefield of Titans and Olympians.[7] With such distinguished heritage, the area, in mythology, gave rise to Mycenaean heroes such as the noble warriors Achilles, Odysseus, and Jason. And by legend it gave rise to Asclepius.

Asclepius most certainly was not of strictly human lineage. If truly ever mortal, legend cocooned him in elaborate tales and supernatural abilities. By story, he was the product of divine intrigues. Only the rich fabrications of Greek mythology could provide such a compelling fable. Asclepius came from the womb of the tempting Thessalian princess Coronis. She could not resist the seduction of handsome Apollo, who was one of extreme beauty and versed in worldly arts—music, poetry, and healing. Lovely Coronis lay with Apollo, and their carnal passions led to divine impregnation. Apollo treasured her and pledged his betrothal, so enamored was he with her love-making. Yet the insatiable Coronis, even with child, could not restrain her promiscuity. She then copulated in secret with a stranger, Ischys, from the distant highlands of Peloponnesian Arcadia. But her illicit affair was discovered. An errant raven spoke of the deed to Apollo, and in a vengeful fit, he sent his sister Artemis to find her. Artemis obliged and found the fornicator in Epidaurus. Without hesitation she killed Coronis with a volley of arrows. Apollo himself slew the hated suitor Ischys with his own hands. As the lifeless Coronis was placed on the funeral pyre, Apollo could not bear that his child would perish as well and quickly snatched the fetus from her belly. This child he named Asclepius and sought that he be raised by the centaur Chiron.

Yet more fabrication.

Legend said that Chiron was foremost among the centaurs, those half-man and half-horse beasts of mythology—upper body, man; lower body and legs, horse. As opposed to the barbarous tendencies of other centaurs, the mythical Chiron was described as gentle and wise. He had been himself wounded by an arrow from the bow of Herakles, so he knew well agony and was one of compassion. Apollo instructed Chiron to teach Asclepius how to heal mortal men of their afflictions. In fact, Apollo himself had taught Chiron, and both shared in the knowledge of magical herbs. Chiron, in turn, was a capable teacher for Asclepius. He had already patiently taught many healers, it was said. Young Asclepius learned quickly. Even as a child, he knew well the powers of healing the sick and raising the dead. From his mentor, Chiron, Asclepius studied the many prescriptions of healing and valued, as Chiron had taught, the virtue of compassion—*to suffer with*. Poets wrote about him:

> [T]hose whosoever came suffering from the sores of nature, or with their limbs wounded either by gray bronze or by far-hurled stone, or with bodies wasting away with summer's heat or winter's cold, he loosed and delivered divers of them from diverse pains, tending some of them with kindly incantations, giving to others a soothing potion, or happily, swathing their limbs with simples or restoring other with the knife.[8]

Asclepius delighted in his newfound skills, and Chiron marveled at his dexterity. He had become a cutter of the flesh and mender of humans. So renown was he that Asclepius attracted the admiration of the warrior-goddess Athena, who, as a gift, smeared him with the blood of the Gorgon, Medusa, whose locks, it was said, coiled with venomous snakes and whose eyes turned men to stone. With that blood Asclepius could call out disease and pestilence and even, it was claimed, raise the dead. Those serpents of

Medusa would accompany him, crawling up his walking staff, and hiss their cures to him. In poetry he was proclaimed as the healer of sicknesses and a soother of great suffering.

This dashing miracle-worker attained such notoriety that his place of birth became sacred ground. Despite some who claimed Asclepius hailed from Tricca, the pious would forever more call his home Epidaurus where, in mythology, he had been snatched from the womb. "In the country of the Epidaurians she [Coronis] bore a son [Asclepius] . . . over every land and sea Asclepius was discovering everything he wished to heal the sick." Epidaurians declared preeminence among Greek towns as the residence of Asclepius and his wondrous remedies.[9]

But the myth continues: Asclepius had angered mighty Zeus with his powers over the dead. Zeus feared that Asclepius would, in turn, teach all men how to restore life. Immortality was the realm only of the gods. "Seek not my soul, the life of the immortals; but enjoy to the full the resources that are within thy reach," Zeus declared.[10] Zeus had an ally in Hades, god of the underworld and those lifeless forms who inhabited it. Asclepius, in bringing the dead to life, might depopulate Hades' coveted dominion—he was stealing jealous Hades' subjects. In his fury at it all, Zeus then slew Asclepius with a thunderbolt. This created rebellion on Olympus. Father Apollo was incensed at the killing of his prized son. In retaliation he killed the Cyclops who had given Zeus the lethal thunderbolt. For that, Zeus banned Apollo from Olympus for a year. He sulked, serving a minor god in Thessaly. Only after that was his position on Olympus returned and Asclepius himself restored to life—the great healer *resurrected*.[11]

Once again among the gods, Asclepius would marry and sire five daughters and three sons. Two of his sons, Podalirius and Machaon, would follow in his footsteps. Homer wrote of them in his epic *Iliad*. In that well-known saga of war, Mycenean-era Greeks besieged the Asia Minor citadel of Troy. Among the Greek armies were Podalirius and Machaon, the sons of Asclepius and now healers themselves. While each were chieftains of their own contingent of countrymen, they were also called by Homer ιητροι ("iatroi"), healers—synonymous with physicians—offspring of Asclepius, whom Homer referred to as *ἀμύμονος ἰητρος*, "the distinguished healer." As for Podalirius and Machaon, the two knew well the course of sinews, veins, bellies, and breasts: how they could be staunched of blood, stitched together, or treated with simple salves and potions. On fields of battle, it would be they who were called to the fallen, the many victims of weaponry of the times: razor-edged swords, pointed lances, and barbed arrows.[12]

As part of the Asclepiad epic, Podalirius and Machaon would feature in mythology of their own—or perhaps there were fragments of truth in their stories, who is to know? Homer told of the astounding deeds of the two on the plains of Troy. How Machaon, summoned to the aid of the great Greek prince Menelaus, deftly pulled an impaled arrow from his torso and sucked dark blood from the wound. Then fearing deeper trouble, Machaon drew from his pouch a magical salve that he smeared over the wound just as Chiron, the benevolent centaur had instructed. These simple salves Chiron himself had given to the father and so, the father to the sons. So skillful was Machaon that Menelaus rallied soon and returned to the fray. Like many military healers, Machaon, as physician, was invaluable; so much so that, at one point during combat, the Greeks worried for his safety. Fearful he would be wounded, they snatched him away from the battlefield so that no harm would come to him. Homer then delivered the famous line "[f]or a physician is of the worth of many other men for the cutting out of arrows and the spreading of soothing simples [poultices]."[13]

Machaon was to be another victim of this bitter siege, killed by an incensed Trojan warrior. His brother Podalirius might have fallen also in those vicious struggles had he not been near the Greek ships, repairing the stricken. After the sack of Troy, Podalirius endured an odyssey of his own. In time he settled in Caria, in Asia Minor not far from the island of Kos. There, he married Syrna, the daughter of King Damathos, to whom he had tended after a fall. Damathos blessed the union, and Podalirius built a town, which he named after his bride. Then, Podalirius taught his progeny the art of healing as his father had taught him. In rich mythology, then, these talented ιητροι dispersed among the Aegean islands and gave rise to the cult of their ancestor, Asclepius. They were called the Asclepiads.[14]

Was there ever such a man named Asclepius, father of Machaon and Podalirius and so gifted as to be a godlike figure? Did he reside in Tricca, as many believed? Was he a healer? Like much of Greek mythology, snippets of truth weaved through fanciful imaginings. There very possibly could have been a renowned healer of that name. Nothing of hard evidence supports his existence, but tradition likely had some factual basis. By reputation he would have been a wise, caring individual, well-versed in remedies of the day, maybe even surgical skills. Paramount among those would have been his discernment in treatment and his compassion for the suffering. Even Plato, centuries after Homer's *Iliad*, acknowledged Asclepius in glowing terms as one whose remedies relieved ailments and who "revealed the art of medicine [for] driving out their disease by drugs and surgery."[15] In dreams he would visit the sick, bringing his coiling serpents who, with flickers of their tongues, licked infirmities away. He would touch, even kiss them. They knew it was he. Their spirit was instantly comforted.

Asclepius—god or man—was to become the nexus of a sanctified cult of healers. They would be called "Asclepiads," ones who blended the natural with the supernatural. They would heal both disease and illness—body and mind. But his followers were not priestly shamans. They also aimed to add logic to healing. They wanted to understand disease in terms of nature and natural things. If it be nature that the gods toy with to bring sickness, then they must rectify it. Of course, even scholarly Asclepiads could not shun the divinities—horrors that they would earn disfavor on Olympus—but they would also learn the tangible. Blending theory and pragmatism, Asclepiads developed a method they called τεχνη ("techne"). Τέχνη was "the doing" in the most literal sense, the art of healing. Τέχνη steered nature's imbalances to proper symmetry, restoring health. It was no hack work, not for drones, daw-dlers, or rogues of the day. As part of their τεχνη Asclepiads studied philosophy and theology. They understood the interplay of the mortal and immortal. Healers schooled in τέχνη commanded respect. "Whoever is going to attain a true understanding of medicine must have the following: natural ability, a suit-able place [for learning], education beginning in childhood, love of toil and time." Eventually, if deemed worthy, pupils would be inducted into the mysti-cal rites of the profession. They would become Asclepiads. "To mortals must be assigned the medical art resulting from theory and experience by means of which some master the divine art of healing to a greater . . . degree."[16]

Yet in the fifth century BCE, Asclepiads shared the Hellenic landscape with any number of proclaimed healers. Many were illiterate craftsmen or midwives. Their handiwork was particular—lancing boils, bloodletting, or birthing. Some had been captured in war and become household slaves responsible for the minor maladies of everyday life. The philosopher Plato knew them well. He also knew they were not Asclepiads, the true artists of medicine:

> There are physicians, and again there are physicians' assistants, whom we also speak of as physicians. . . . All bear the name whether freemen or slaves who gain their professional knowledge by watching their masters and obeying their directions in empiric [observational] fashion, *not in the way in which freemen learn their art and teach it to their pupils.*[17]

Only Asclepiads could discern the subtleties of illness, the waxing and waning of internal milieus corrected only by the proper mixture of diet, exercise, and nostrums—and occasionally, the judicious use of the knife. The Asclepiads drew upon their favor with the god Asclepius. In the method of incense, songs, and sacrifices, they sent their petitions aloft. Pilgrims waited patiently that in slumber Asclepius would visit. Priests gave soothing potions for sleep and dreams. It was in those dreams Asclepius would speak. Upon awakening the patient felt unburdened, relieved of anguish, fortified—maybe even cured.

These Asclepieia—shrines of Asclepius—were magnificent sanctuaries. Roughly five hundred were built in all of Greece. Those on Epidaurus and the island of Kos were particularly noteworthy, as impressive and revered in the day as the medical centers of Boston or Baltimore or the Mayo Clinic are today. Their setting was purposely bucolic, often near natural springs and away from cities. A complex of buildings housed staff, patients, and families. There were private quarters for patients and dining halls where pilgrims could consume the meat offered to the gods, and bathe for ritualistic purification before entering treatment. There could even be found symposium halls for educational sessions. Centrally located was a domed edifice called the *Abaton-Enkoimeterion*, restricted to only staff and patients where the main treatment was rendered, usually to a narcotized and sleepy subject, a ritual known as *ενκοιμεσις*, literally, "you are sleeping." That was where the Asclepiads emerged to perform their healing rituals or even surgery. Other rooms contained snakes and dogs that were used in certain therapeutic procedures. The personnel included Asclepiads, of course, the priests-healers, but also trained assistants, special therapists, *hieromnemones* (administrative record keepers), and vergers, usually women, as escorts. Those who could afford the travel and stay came with a variety of chronic infirmities: neuropsychiatric disorders, skin problems, lung conditions, paralyses, dropsy (mostly congestive heart failure), arthritis, and rheumatism.[18]

Accounts of wondrous healings in Asclepieia abounded. Etched on the limestone and marble walls were testimonies describing deeds the god performed. A woman miscarrying for five years finally, after her temple visit, delivered a healthy active child. Another, bearing a three-year pregnancy (no explanation given), had a much-desired daughter. A mute youth suddenly spoke. An ugly forehead blemish disappeared. Lame men walked. The priests even dabbled in surgery. One inscription read, "Euhippus had for six years the point of a spear in his jaw. As he was sleeping in the temple the god extracted the spearhead and gave it to him into his hands." And another inscription told:

A man with an abscess within his abdomen, when asleep in the temple he saw a dream. It seemed to him that the god ordered the servants who accompanied him to grip him and hold him tightly so that he could cut open his abdomen. . . . Thereupon Asclepius cut his belly open, removed the abscess, and, after having stitched him up again, released him from his bonds. Whereupon he walked out sound, but the floor of the Abaton was covered with blood.

And yet another: Gorgias of Heracleia had been wounded by an arrow in the lung, and would drain pus to fill "sixty-seven basins." "While sleeping in the temple, he saw a vision. It seemed to him the god extracted the arrow head from his lung. When day came, he walked out well, holding the arrow in his hands."[19]

Some were skeptical about the Asclepiad business. It smacked of commercialism. Asclepiads demanded payment, and such rituals were lucrative. There were practitioners of healing most assuredly interested in marketing and self-promoting if for no other reason than offering a competitive edge to the "business" of healthcare rather than the profession of healing. Certainly, in that unregulated and uncensored environment of medicine, reputation was key. Ostentatious methods of cure might have been instrumental in attracting patients, although the scrupulous healer probably abhorred such behavior. Presumably, healers of the sanctuaries of Asclepius and assiduous followers of Hippocrates were the more conscientious of the craftsmen, even though there was opportunity for a bit of the dramatic and spectacular, particularly in Asclepiad dream therapy.[20]

From one of these sanctuaries came a man simply called Hippocrates, one of the Asclepiiad priests of Kos. Kos, an island of the Dodecanese in the southeastern Aegean, was the mythical birthplace of Leto, mother of Apollo. It was first settled by Carians from Asia Minor, the same people with whom Asclepius' son Podilarius took refuge. By Homer's account, Kos had furnished a contingent of warriors for the Greeks besieging Troy. Perhaps, in storied mythology, Podilarius knew well the Corian men from Kos and fled to their safety in his troubled journeys from Troy. Like Asclepius himself, this Hippocrates—principal among his peers—professed a union of body and soul, and proclaimed a strong ethic for the healing profession. Could one understand flesh without knowledge of spirit? No, Hippocrates taught. He stressed that the nature of the body is grounded in the soul. One must embrace both in efforts to heal both, and healing commanded both.[21] Hippocrates, Asclepius' greatest disciple, even dreamed of visits by his mentor and the parade of soothing therapies accompanying him:

> Aesculapius [Asclepius] showed himself, not as images usually represent, gentle and tranquil, but animated in his walk, and with an air which did not fail to inspire fear; he was followed by serpents, enormous reptiles, also slithering in their long coils, and making heard, as in the deserts and the hollow valleys, a formidable hissing sound. His companions, holding tightly

fastened medicine boxes, came behind. The god held out his hand to me; and I, seizing it with ardor, begged him to join me and not abandon me in the treatment.[22]

In truth, Hippocrates may have been as much of a myth as Asclepius. Of the man Hippocrates, details of his life are scarce. It is said that he was born of a long line of physicians, around 460 BCE. He was thought to be the son of Herclides by the woman Phinerata. He learned his healing skills from his father and grandfather (who was also named Hippocrates—Hippocrates I and II) probably among the Asclepiads at Kos. He claimed to be, in that sense, of the lineage of Asclepaidae (in Greek, $A\sigma\kappa\lambda\eta\pi\iota\alpha\delta\alpha\iota$), those who professed descendancy from Asclepius himself, the eighteenth of progeny from the god-man.[23] Hippocrates, by reputation, far surpassed his ancestors and teachers, not only in his natural ability but in his labors to perfect the $\tau\varepsilon\chi\nu\eta$, of healing. His period of greatest activity was around 400 BCE. His was apparently an itinerant practice. He traveled to Thrace, Abdera, Delos, the Propontis, Thasos, Thessaly, Athens, and elsewhere performing exceptional feats of cure and comfort. Two of his sons, Thessalus and Draco, were both his students as was a son-in-law, Polybus. In legend, he represented the perfect physician: learned, observant, humane, and with a profound reverence for the petitions of his patients. He was an author, but it is difficult to pinpoint his authorship. In the Hippocratic *Corpus*, a collection of more than sixty separate works, only a very small proportion can be directly attributed to the man Hippocrates. Most were "of his school and his spirit," but very well could have represented his teachings passed down from generation to generation and dutifully recorded by his disciples.[24]

Medicinal remedies were human inventions, Hippocrates proclaimed.[25] It was not that he renounced the gods. Quite the contrary. He attributed much of nature to divinities. And it was the gods, Hippocrates believed, who graciously gave mankind knowledge of the healing arts; "the art is the grace of god." But he did denounce purely contrived ceremonies invoking these spirits—those odd rituals passed down by the Egyptians perhaps.[26] While Hippocrates gave proper homage to the divinities, they worked through interplay with the physical—with nature. He used the so-called Sacred Disease (epilepsy), the affliction of fits and convulsions that was said of divine origin, whether a blessing or a curse, as an example:

It is not, in my opinion, any more divine or more sacred than other diseases, but has a natural cause, and its supposed divine origin is due to men's inexperience, and to their wonder at its peculiar character. . . . But if it is to be considered divine just because it is wonderful, there will be not one sacred disease but many.[27]

In so reasoning, Hippocratic rejected the notion that disease was punishment from the gods. Often foibles of mankind caused sickness—living conditions, diet, and the various human follies which damaged the senses. And there was an unavoidable interaction of body and spirit, Hippocrates contended. The body, in reference to Plato's *Phaedo*, might be thought of as a lyre and strings and harmony the melodies that issue forth—a mixture of bodily elements.[28]

As for the body, a central Hippocratic doctrine was that:

> The body of man has in itself blood, phlegm, yellow bile and black bile; these make up the nature of his body, and through these he feels pain or enjoys health . . . he enjoys the most perfect health when these elements are duly proportioned to one another . . . and when they are perfectly mingled.[29]

And so was popularized the concept of χυμός, "chumos"—in Greek, meaning juice, soon translated as "humor." Blood, phlegm, black bile, and yellow bile would be the "juices"—humors—responsible for health—balance and imbalance would be key principles of sickness and wellness.

Hippocrates (or his followers) also rejected imposters who prescribed worthless measures to treat the sick. Their preparations were malevolent. What was more, these quacks lacked an understanding of the mystical, the knowledge of disease, divinity, and the practice of τεχνη that Asclepiads professed. In that sense, they violated sacred oaths. Without proper supplication, they only angered the gods:

> In making use, too, of purifications and incantations they do what I think is a very unholy and irreligious thing. For the sufferers from the disease, they purify with blood and such like, as though they [sufferers] were polluted, blood-guilty, bewitched by men, or had committed some unholy act. All such they ought to have treated in the opposite way; they should have brought them to the sanctuaries, with sacrifices and prayers, in supplication to the gods.[30]

The Hippocratic sect of Kos swept across the Mediterranean as an embellishment of Asclepiad tradition. More focusing on humanism and less on deities, followers pronounced attention to body and mind, one a manifestation of the other, but allowed a larger role for disturbances of the body itself. Yet their therapy was holistic. In the Hippocratic *Corpus*, the authors—in the name of Hippocrates—promoted their healing philosophy by three methods: eliminating suffering; mitigating disease; and wisely using τεχνη (skill).[31] Paramount, however, was *eliminating suffering*. The art of medicine required a complexity of talents: empathy, patience, knowledge, and discernment. Treatments were imperfect, and failures invariably occurred, Hippocrates (or his followers) asserted, but this did not take away from the value of the art or the training necessary. "Those who are masters of their profession care neither for the praise nor reproof of such people [skeptics]— they esteem those only who know how to discriminate and discern when and wherein the operation of art are prefect or imperfect."[32]

But do not forget the supernatural, Hippocrates stressed. Healing is honored by the gods, he said. "Though physicians may be the means, the gods are the cause of cures in medicine and surgery," as has been interpreted by scholars. [33] Gods are the real overseers of nature. As their surrogate, healers—ιατρόι—must respect their divine obligations. In the fashion of the gods, then, in all manner of behavior with his patient, healers should exhibit confidence and preparedness. They were to be exemplary among peers; ones of integrity and decency, ones of gentleness and humanity. Their demeanor must not convey confusion or disorganization. As Asclepiads believed, healing must also place hope in patients even though the disease cannot be cured:

> Perform all this calmly and adroitly, concealing most things from the patient while you are attending to him. Give necessary orders with cheerfulness and serenity, turning his attention away from what is being done to him; sometimes reprove sharply and emphatically, and sometimes comfort with solicitude and attention, revealing nothing of the patient's future or present condition, for many patients through this cause have taken a turn for the worse.[34]

It was a demanding vocation. As representatives of Asclepius himself, healers must act as the gentle god would. Their advice and prescriptions were to be thoughtful, wise, and compassionate. If not healing the body, they must heal the spirit. They must be Asclepius incarnate. This was as critical as the medicine itself, because disease was ugly, and suffering was heartrending.

> For the medical man sees terrible sights, touches unpleasant things, and the misfortunes of others bring a harvest of sorrows that are peculiarly his; but the sick by means of the art rid themselves of the worst of evils, disease, suffering, pain and death. For medicine proves for all these evils a manifest cure.[35]

When his τεχνη no longer worked, the healer must reach inside to the worried spirit and begin healing there, as Asclepius in his dream visions would. "The intimacy also between physician and patient is close. Patients in fact put themselves into the hands of their physician," the Hippocratic creed read.[36] It was such a mission upon which followers of Hippocrates pledged their oath. Swear by Apollo the Healer, by Asclepius, and other gods and goddesses to carry out this promise, their oath demanded. Seek faultless behavior and hold hallowed the affairs of man. Be as Asclepius himself, Hippocrates had urged.

CHAPTER THREE

~

Yēšūa the Nazarene and His Followers

He would be called the Great Healer. He would teach mankind renewal.

In fact, his beginnings were much less auspicious. He was a simple man from Nazareth in the Lower Galilee of first-century Palestine. They called him יֵשׁוּעַ, Yēšūa də-naṣəraya in Aramaic—Yēšūa of Nazareth. His reputed hometown, Nazareth, was a sleepy hamlet in the arid country of Galilee. Yēšūa was likely what the Greeks called a τέκτων, a stone mason, woodworker, or handyman—certainly of the lowly peasant class. His home village of Nazareth was so small and inconsequential that he and others like him would travel to neighboring towns to earn their living, such as the up-and-coming Galilean city of Sepphoris, some four miles distant from Nazareth. His clothing reflected a peasant status, the dusty, worn garments of a common laborer. He was a muscular individual—as one might expect of such a physical laborer—slightly taller than average at five feet ten and weighing a hefty 175 pounds. He had hair that extended well below his shoulders in a single braid, as was often the custom of Jewish men. He maintained a full but trimmed beard. An attractive man in full adulthood, now in his thirties, considered the prime of life, he moved comfortably among the crowds of small-town Galilee, and offered a welcoming face and piercing eyes of one with that quality of engagement that quickly put passersby at ease. Women were drawn to him. He had that masculine demeanor that projected strength, confidence, and yet a definite aura of compassion. His gaze on them was one of understanding and harmony as if he immediately knew his role with them and the desires of their heart. Younger men looked to him as one whose easy movements massaged their notions of male behavior desirable for vision and tribal leadership.

This menial worker would gather crowds not by expectation, but by his alluring draw. At times, he spoke nothing at all, but his stride instilled curiosity and his gaze, magnetism. One might fully expect his speech to be plebian, the fumbling base language of illiterate field hands, men whose livelihood did not depend on insight or schooling but on the force of their limbs in moving the earth and stone and timber of their remote pastures and dwellings. One might expect, then, the language of men whose life unfolded directly in front of them, in compact intervals measured in yards and minutes. Yet he uttered pure perception and wisdom, and spoke as if he saw far ahead and his line of sight was not straight but brought in all the bearings of the compass. Yes, he talked in peasant words, but his message was otherworldly—piercing them not from without but within, as if he unraveled mysteries of heart and mind most feared to confront, lest the danger those feelings might pose to their subservient lives rise up in ugliness. It is as if the mythical spirits of their Jewish heritage came alive and prattled as if they had jumped from the scrolls of the Torah and were breathing their providence.

He sought the neglected, the ill, the shunned, the sinful. This strange figure firmly ignored the stifling Roman rule and the rigid inflexibility of Jewish Law. Polite to his Roman overlords, he still talked a different talk, one of respect but insistence in the ways of Elāhā, his God, spoken in Aramaic—the everyday Hebrew patois of Palestine. He argued well with the most learned Jews, and refused their chastising, as if he were immune to the perils of this dangerous land and its threatening customs. He did not preach violence or insurrection. His world was not of earth but in the supernatural. The heavens, he said, engulfed the earth as a blanket of love and caring. The Master Healer preached *Selichah* and *Mechilah* at once. Forgiveness for sins and wiping away of all transgressions with appeal to the almighty יהוה—the Hebrew theonym YHWH—Yahweh, for mercy. He energized faith as dynamism, as a living Yahweh.

The Palestine of the first century was an unhealthy place. Chaotic sicknesses of unbridled contagion leveled many and filled the streets and alleyways with pitiful beggars, the maimed, and dying. There was no respite for them but the kindness of strangers and the inevitability of death. Did passersby care? Not often. They were oppressed with poverty and hunger of their own. Besides, fitting punishment for these wretches whose wrongdoings of the soul and corruption of the spirit led to their dire conditions. Yahweh promised rewards in this life, so went Jewish teachings. Afflictions were a sign of punishment, of wickedness, of offenses against the Covenant. Such people were to be condemned. Friends and neighbors left them, families put them out. The penniless sick. They were not meant for the elaborate and expensive healing rituals of priest-physicians. Too expensive. Do not let them enter the rabbinic temples. They were unclean. Priests had little time for these dregs of society. Let nature take its course, the temple healers might say. Soon they would be dead and tossed on the offal heaps of Gehenna—removed from the earth. This is the way of nature such priests might suggest.

But Yēšūa was different. He did not ignore them. He sought them out. He was at home with the dirty, abandoned, deformed, and festering. Not only those, but also the immoral, corrupt, and criminal he engaged. He would walk toward them. At first the afflicted were hesitant. They knew their place and held back—filthy, ashamed, mad with hallucinations and imaginings. But with his attention, they would slowly approach, even just to touch his garments, so quickly his wonders spread. "Do you have faith—do you believe?" he would ask. They filled with hope and suddenly brightened as if body and soul were impacted by his healing power. They were cured, now convinced of supernatural caring this man offered. Yahweh was suddenly real. This man's Yahweh was present in him.

Those knowing scripture would say, "did not our rabbis talk of such deeds? Did not the prophet man Isaiah who prodded Hezekiah, King of Judah, to resist the Assyrians centuries before, speak of such compassion and the duty of each Jew?" Isaiah said":

> Is not this the kind of fasting I have chosen: to loose the chains of injustice and untie the cords of the yoke, to set the oppressed free and break every yoke? Is it not to share your food with the hungry and to provide the poor wanderer with shelter—when you see the naked, to clothe them, and not to turn away from your own flesh and blood? Then your light will break forth like the dawn, and your healing will quickly appear; then your righteousness will go before you, and the glory of the LORD will be your rear guard.[1]

And is this sinewy, dusty Nazarene telling us the same? We must heal the spirit first, in the name of Elāhā, then our inflamed flesh would calm, quieted by a tranquil soul.

Yēšūa breathed the breath of the divine, yet he truly was just a man—he ate and drank, laughed and angered, slept and woke. Still, he possessed inner temperaments not totally natural, as if a force beyond nature was part of him, a force that inspires and bonds and heals the disordered spirit. He was a worker of wonders and then went further. For those of faith, he promised to rid them, even, of death. It must be so, they reasoned, when he ordered—as if he were the Master of Life and Death—the dead to live. And they did so, whole and uncorrupt, as if they had only been asleep. He saw what no others could—the meshing of seen and unseen, the union of Elāhā and man.

He would be the True Healer, one who knows body and soul are one. Both must be healed for salvation—not just earthly reward, but preparation for a greater life beyond. He was master of τὰ φυσικά, as the Greeks called it—the master of natural things.

The nature of man was one of decay; the smell of decomposition was never far from Jewish noses. No, little did onlookers care to even glance at the dying. They dreaded the evil sure to reach them if they approached the infirmed. These were the untouchables. For Jews, venture too close and suffer the wrath of Yahweh. Any healing came only from Yahweh, the Jewish *Tanakh* had written. Only Yahweh could heal, not the blasphemous chants of so-called healers of the day. "Wherefore thus saith the Lord God, 'Behold, I am against your cushions wherewith ye hunt the souls as birds, and I will tear them from your arms, and I will let the souls go, even the souls ye hunt as birds'."[2] In fact, such shamans were perceived as evil and should be put to death.[3] Only when directly ordered by Yahweh were their charms allowed.[4] Healing practices, then, were the domain of rabbis, who, when they were called upon, subscribed to the medicinal prescriptions of the Greeks.

But Yēšūa would not shun them. He reached for them. Nor did he seem to honor the written word of the *Tanakh*. What was this new order of which Yēšūa insisted? He spoke of caring and love as if with the same fondness of parents, spouse, or children. The same devotion must extend to neighbors, the pushed aside, the unprincipled, the sick, the sinful even, he commanded. It seemed shocking advice in an impersonal world of brutality, marginalization, and castoffs. Elāhā—his God—willed it, he spoke, as if Elāhā Himself was a father to children. He referred Elāhā as a living God, an Elāhā who was immediate, involved, and concerned—not one of anger, laws, and punishment. Yēšūa addressed each person in terms of their spirit. He soothed and understood. He comforted, he reassured. His were all the castaways. He looked through them, into the inner reaches of their hearts. He saw their sins and selfishness—and forgave. And they saw in him a path to acceptance. They trusted his living God.

His miracles were proof.

Yēšūa began his enigmatic ministry by healing the mother-in-law of one of his first followers in the village of Capernaum. She burned with fever and had taken to her bed. Yēšūa entered her home, took her hand and helped her up. The fever broke, never to return. She had been restored to health. Renewed. Word of his powers spread and by evening the house was surrounded by the sick and infirmed. Yēšūa touched many of them and healed those he touched.[5] No one had done what he had done, not even the great god-like Asclepius to whom many pilgrimaged with sacrifices and supplication.

He radiated mystery. His fingers seemed magical; sometimes even his glance. Crowds pressed to be near him. So imbued with healing power was he that the rabble simply vied to tap his garments as he passed, as if they too held special authority over evil. One such woman, who had been suffering from hemorrhages for twelve years, worked her way through throngs and simply brushed his cloak. "If I just touch his clothes, I will be healed," she hoped. Amazingly, witnesses said, in that instant her bleeding stopped. She fell at Yēšūa's feet, admitting to her insolence in approaching him. "Daughter, your faith has healed you. Go in peace and be freed from your suffering," he spoke.[6] And even more, sheer belief would cure. A Roman centurion, in all his authority, humbled himself for the sake of his ill servant. He beseeched Yēšūa to "say the word" and heal. The centurion feared his pagan house would befoul the goodness of this God-like man. "I do not deserve to have you come under my roof," the centurion mumbled. *But say the word and let my servant be healed,*" he finished. "I tell you, I have not found such great faith even in Israel," Yēšūa responded. And indeed, upon returning home, the centurion found his servant well.[7] Maybe it was just that: faith that healed. This Nazarene wonder-worker healed the body through the spirit.

He embraced the vilest—lepers. Such a disease that the oozing ulcers, deformed faces, and missing limbs drove people from them, if not by covenant then by the pure stink of their presence. Yet not this Yēšūa. Instead, he approached them. They stood at a distance, as the Law demanded, but called out, "Yēšūa, Master, have pity on us!" They had heard of his powers and waited for him to cross their paths. Yēšūa addressed them face to face, unafraid of their afflictions. "Go show yourselves to the priests." They did so and, to the amazement of the priests, ἐκαθαρίσθησαν, they were cleansed of disease—purified of body. As if divine vapors had scoured their skin and washed their infirmities from them. Only one returned to thank him. Yēšūa then explained to the healed leper. "Ἀναστὰς πορεύου ἡ πίστις σου σέσωκέν σε," Yēšūa had said. "Get up and go your way; your faith has saved you."[8]

The Nazarene would do more than that. Sometimes he would examine their ulcered skin, deformed faces, and missing limbs. He would unwrap their dirty bandages, maybe even wipe clean their pus-filled infections. Onlookers shrank in horror. To contact a leper was a violation of Rabbinic Law. The Tōrā had said of them:

And the leper in whom the plague is, his clothes shall be rent, and the hair of his head shall go loose, and he shall cover his upper lip, and shall cry: "Unclean, unclean." All the days wherein the plague is in him he shall be unclean; he is unclean; he shall dwell alone, without the camp shall his dwelling be.[9]

The covenant with Yahweh would be broken. On one occasion, "[a] man with leprosy came and begged him [Yēšūa] on his knees, 'if you are willing, you can make me clean'," Jesus reached out his hand and touched the man. "I am willing",' Yēšūa said. "'Be clean!' Immediately the leprosy left him and he was cleaned."[10] *He simply touched the man!* A few educated men, seeing this, recalled a passage from the Talmud about the son of David, to be called the Anointed One who was to save Israel. One clue was that this son of David, they had read, would walk among lepers. "And by what sign may I recognize him [the son of David]? He is sitting among the poor lepers . . . he unties and rebandages each separately."[11]

Yēšūa then did the unthinkable. He brought the dead to life. His dear friend Lazarus had died and was put away in his tomb. When Yēšūa, hearing of the loss, arrived, Lazarus had been dead for four days. "Our friend Lazarus has fallen asleep, but I am going there to wake him up," Yēšūa said. Few believed him, thinking he was delusional in his sadness. He ordered the stone sealing the tomb to be removed. Oh, the stench, his followers thought. This is madness. Yēšūa, sensing what they were thinking, belittled their skepticism. "Did I not tell you that if you believed, you would see the glory of God?" "Lazarus, come out," Yēšūa called, as if beckoning the man from his home. Lazarus came forth, still wrapped in his shroud. "Take off the grave clothes and let him go," Yēšūa ordered. The shroud came off, and Lazarus walked among them, not a hint of putrefaction, clearly now restored to life.[12]

The Nazarene was like Asclepius, who had raised the dead, some said. Even the Jewish historian Flavius Josephus spoke of his talents, writing: "for he [Yēšūa, Ιησούς in Greek] was a man of extraordinary works."[13] But remembering the legend of the Greek god, they worried that Yēšūa's God would retaliate like Zeus, who struck Asclepius dead for toying with natural things.

He was not the only Jewish healer wandering Palestine, but this Yēšūa developed an avid following. [14] Scores of people would accompany him around the countryside and listen to his sermons and parables. But he had broader plans. He soon had collected a cadre of young companions, mostly fishermen or, like him, common laborers. Eventually they numbered twelve, and contained hardly a learned one among the bunch, although one, Matthew, was a tax collector for the Romans. These would be called αποστολείς (apostoleis), roughly translated as "those who were sent," or "ambassadors," to crisscross the countryside and preach his unique brand of Judaism and even perform miraculous events on his behalf.

They were simple peasants, skilled mostly in the casting of nets or the hoeing of the dirt. But they saw in him purpose, meaning, and a passionate gentleness. Maybe they saw something of themselves in him; that they could make a difference in the grueling times in which they lived. As they traveled with him through the many hamlets and villages of Galilee, Samaria, and Judea, they watched him speak, listened to his unorthodox teachings, and marveled at his cures. They saw him know no stranger and comfort man, woman, and child without hesitation—even the despised heretics of Samaria. Before long, their "Master," Yēšūa, told them to do the same, even heal the ill. This they found totally baffling, but they did so and were shocked to see they had the same powers as he. "They drove out many demons and anointed many sick people with oil and healed them," chroniclers wrote later.[15] When questioned about wasting energy on the discarded, these followers simply quoted Yēšūa by responding that it was not the well who needed a physician but the sick. How they healed was even to them a mystery. They were not *ιατροί*, traditional Greek healers. They were mere *χειρουργίοι* ("chirurgoi"): hand-workers. Yet invoking the name of a living Yahweh wiped away horrible scourges.

But Yēšūa, like Asclepius, would suffer the anger of the gods—but his would be at the hands of mortal men. He was a blasphemous figure, working his magic and charms like that forbidden by the Tanakh. Those of Jewish nobility—Pharisees and Sadducees—feared not only for the wrath of Yahweh but also the wrath of their Roman governor, Pontius Pilate. Yēšūa had proclaimed a new kingdom and, in so doing, had become a threat to them and all Jews. He was a rebel, an insurgent to Roman rule. Pilate would ruthlessly put down any revolt—he had done so in the past. With information provided by one of his followers, Yēšūa was arrested and brought to trial. While many Jews admired him, those in authority did not. They gave Pilate every reason to execute him, and the procurator did so. For non-Romans, the standard punishment for treason and rebellion was crucifixion. Yēšūa was beaten, whipped, and taken outside Jerusalem's city gates. There, in a familiar execution spot, he was stripped, pinned to timber, and strung up. That it all occurred was indisputable. Even a historian in faraway Rome, Cornelius Tacitus, mentioned it in his *Annals*: "Christus [Yēšūa, by then called 'Christus'] who was put to death in the reign of Tiberius by the Procurator Pontius Pilate."[16] To let Jews know their fate if they imitated this criminal, Pilate ordered a mocking sign posted above his head identifying his crime, written in Latin, Hebrew, and Greek:

Iēsus Nazarēnus, Rēx Iūdaeōrum

ישו מנצרת מלך היהודים

Iησούς από τη Ναζαρέτ, Βασιλιάς των Εβραίων

It read: Yēšūa *də-naṣəraya*—Yēšūa of Nazareth—King of the Jews

An ugly spectacle—this naked prophet nailed to a tree, gasping for breath. Not quite the King imagined by the Jews. He hung on the wood six hours before he gave up his spirit. "*Elāhā, Elāhā, Lama Sabachthani?*" (which means "My God, my God, why have you forsaken me?") he muttered at one point.[17] A few brave companions stood near and wondered at all this. Was he after all just a clever magician, an imposter, a charlatan? Why did not his Elāhā appear and save him? Now he was quite ordinary. Yēšūa died a choking death, his lungs burning with suffocation. No longer could he lift his chest with limbs nailed to the tree. His face turned blue. Gasping stopped. Death was complete. The centurions saw to that, a spear into his side. Purple fluid gushed, a dead man's fluid. Some followers of his lowered him before he stiffened and violated the Sabbath and, like Lazarus, wrapped him and put him in a tomb. Decaying would begin.

But no. Sources said that on the third day of his entombment, his women attendants found his tomb empty. There was no smell of decay; only his blood-stained shroud left behind. Then he appeared alive, walking as if never troubled. He was full of life—his face animated, his limbs suffused with pink. He ate with them, talked to them, and preached again just like before his crucifixion. He had altered his own *φὔσῐκός*, his own "nature." The Jewish chronicler Josephus remarked that "Yēšūa appeared to them on the third day, alive" after Pilate had condemned him to a cross.[18]

Some weeks later the revitalized Yēšūa summoned his eleven followers (minus the one who had betrayed him to the Romans and hung himself in disgrace) and, in their midst, faded like a phantom, as if he was absorbed into the firmament, just as his Father, Elāhā, might have done. The scribe Luke wrote of the story as told to him, many years later: "While he was blessing them, he left them and was taken up into heaven. Then they worshiped him and returned to Jerusalem with great joy."[19] Yēšūa became part of the unseen, the eternal, the essence of Elāhā, the essence of *χαριτας* (charitas), grace. Those who remembered teachings of Yēšūa, who heard it from his mouth, now proclaimed a new covenant with Yahweh. "Love God with all your heart and with all your soul and with all your mind and with all your strength," Yēšūa said. He added, "[t]he second is this: 'Love your neighbor as yourself.' There is no commandment greater than these." It was that simple.[20]

Before he disappeared, he told his disciples to do what he had done. Go among the people, teach, forgive, heal. His followers did just that, energized by some equally unexplainable confidence. Their travels and miracles became legendary. Two of them, Peter and John, were particularly prolific in their proselytizing. On one occasion the pair had gone to temple to pray and came upon a lame beggar, derisible in his rags and ignored by most, hoping to receive scattered coins tossed at him by passersby. The wretched beggar could not even look at the two; he simply held out his withered hand as if to ask for money. Peter said, "Look at us." The beggar timidly did, afraid of insults and curses. Not money did Peter offer but said, instead, "In the name of Jesus Christ of Nazareth, walk!" He was referring to his Master, Yēšūa, whom he now called Māshīah, the Anointed One. Helped upright by the two, the man's feet and ankles became strong. "*Hallelu Yah!*" the beggar might have said, "Praise to Yahweh!" The vagabond was so delighted that he stayed by their side, skipping and dancing all the way to temple. His new faith consumed him. This god-man Yēšūa and his friends had healed him. He could not be quieted and soon told anyone who would listen.[21]

The same miracle worker Peter also met a man named Aeneas, a bedridden unfortunate who lived in Judea. Aeneas was so debilitated that he could barely raise his head from the pillow. Clearly, he was close to death. As the story went, Peter, struck by compassion, said to him, "Aeneas, Jesus Christ [he would have used the Aramaic "Māshīah" instead of "Christ"] heals you. Get up and roll up your mat."[22] This was no physician speaking, Aeneas knew. He was a commoner, his language coarse, his manners earthy. But he was insistent. *Iātaí!* Heal! Aeneas suddenly found his strength and rose from his mat. He instinctively knew something inside him had changed. He felt the vitality of youth. Then Peter told him about Yēšūa, the long-promised son of David, the Anointed One.

There were more cures that Peter, John, and other companions of the mysterious Nazarene performed. These miraculous happenings bedazzled spectators. Crowds began to gather whenever they heard this Yēšūa's companions were coming. They brought with them the miserable sick and suffering and all those thought to be possessed by demons. They hauled them in carts, helped them limp along, or bound them tight to keep their madness under control. The disciple Peter prayed with them, implored their faith in the Māshīah, Yēšūa, and then, in the name of Yēšūa, healed their bodies and minds. Even in offensive places like Samaria, companions sought out the ailing, spoke of Yēšūa the Māshīah, and healed.[23]

Revelations seemed almost everyday occurrence in those times following Yēšūa's departure. The story of Saul was especially poignant. Saul was a Jewish enforcer, a vicious persecutor of this new Yēšūa cult. On his way to Damascus to track down more of the cult followers, he was struck from his horse and blinded. "Saul, Saul, why do you persecute me?" he heard a voice say. "Who are you, Lord?" Saul asked. "I am Jesus [Yēšūa], whom you are persecuting."[24] That was enough to convince about anyone, and so, his vision soon restored, Saul changed his name to Paul and became a fervent

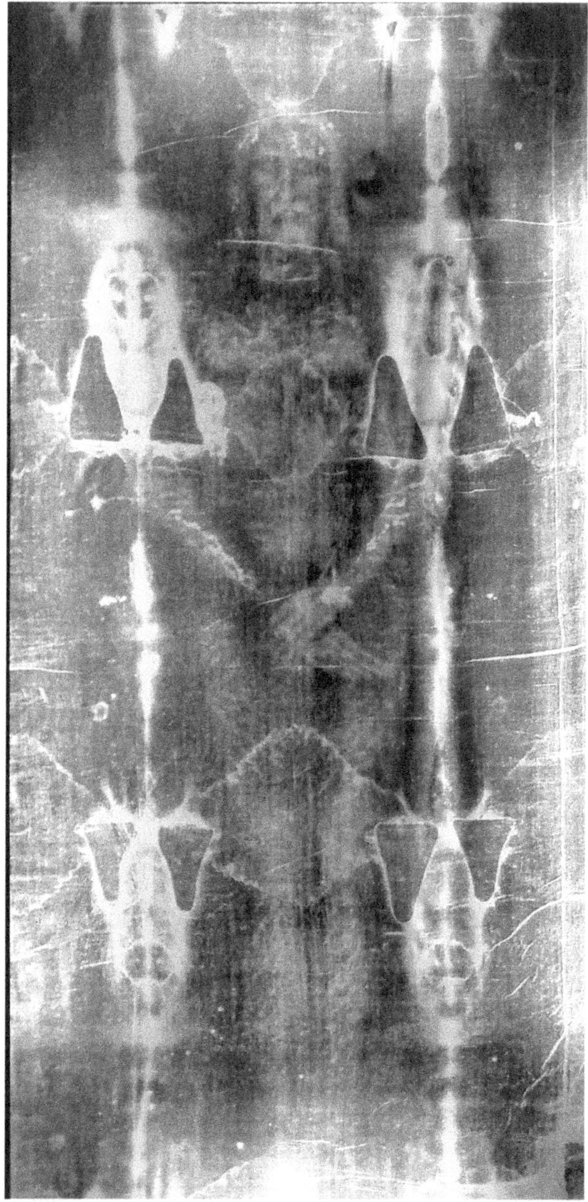

Figure 3.1 The negative image of the Shroud of Turin. Is this the image of Yēšūa the Māshīaḥ, known as the Great Healer? (Photographed at Saint-Sulpice, Paris).

believer in this Yēšūa. In fact, being an educated man, he embarked on a remarkable missionary journey and began to write prolifically about his new take on Judaism. His theology and familiarity with the life and teachings of Yēšūa were remarkable. Single-handedly he created the framework for a new religion—not one of Judaism, but a continuation of it. He knew the promised Māshīah had arrived. His kingdom was not of earth but was one of a spiritual nature. What was more, Paul found that, on occasion, he could heal as Yēšūa had. Wandering among the Jewish communities along the Mediterranean, he ministered to the infirmed and spread the words of the Māshīah. In an astounding anecdote, he, like his Māshīah, even raised a man from death who had fallen floors to his peril. In this particular circumstance, a crowd had gathered and agreed that the poor victim was soundly deceased. No, Paul said, life was still in him. With prayer to his Yēšūa, he brought the dead man to his feet, clearly alive once again. Those who witnessed this were dumbfounded and wondered about Paul's Yēšūa in whose name he had resurrected this victim. It was a convincing performance. Yēšūa must be the Māshīah, the son of David, as Paul declared.[25]

He was a dynamic preacher. A muscular man in his prime, Paul had energy and fortitude and was filled with a special ardor for this man he had never met—this Yēšūa. His words flowed forcefully but were laced with empathy, hope, and salvation. Those who listened began to believe in Paul's sermons. His theology, philosophy, and even psychology were sensible, understandable, and appealing. And this Yēšūa provided a glimpse into a dazzling world of the supernatural, the interchange of visible and invisible, and the possibility of life after death. The way Paul told it, Yēšūa had literally transported the heavens to earth. Paul's writings and many letters were in Greek, the language of scholars. He would refer to Yēšūa the Māshīah by his Greek name Ιησούς (Jesus) Χρήστος (Christos), Jesus the Christ. The followers Paul and other disciples were gathering would soon be known as people of Χρήστος, Χριστιανοί (Christianoi), "Christians." Yēšūa the Māshīah would become known around the Mediterranean world, not just the world of Judaism but the world of the non-Jewish: pagans, Romans, Syrians, Egyptians. Theirs was a Greek world, and Yēšūa the Māshīah would be better known as Jesus the Christ.

By his paranormal abilities, the bewildering Nazarene provoked a reconsideration of the natural and supernatural spheres of existence—the visible and invisible. Those who knew the Talmud remembered the words of the prophet Ezekiel, who wrote, "Thus saith the Lord God: Behold, I will open your graves, and cause you to come up out of your graves, O My people; and I will bring you into the land of Israel."[26] They wondered if the rumors that this puzzling Yēšūa had done so himself and had raised others were true and not some nonsense as their teachers claimed. What better way to endure the scourges of daily life than to know life continued after death. The learned Sadducees did not think the soul was immortal. Many rabbinic Jews felt reward or punishment for behavior would come from Yahweh in this life. But Yēšūa preached of an eternal life of body and soul, and pleasure or pain would be doled out by Yahweh in an afterlife based on righteous living on earth.

His invocation of the Jewish God Yahweh for demonstrations of bodily healing as a function of spiritual reconciliation added a novel dimension to traditional Jewish thinking. But more importantly, he altered the laws of Moses in favor of a new consideration of obedience. The covenant with Yahweh now entailed two basic principles: love of God and love of neighbor. No longer were any of mankind outside the realm of compassion or healing. No longer were afflictions the result of spiritual transgressions and therefore abhorrent to righteous people. Afflictions were not the work of Yahweh; they were the work of natural ideologies perhaps set in place by Yahweh as Creator but not necessarily delivered by Him. Belief and trust in a living, benevolent, and empathetic Yahweh, by virtue of his human form, Jesus would provide, if not physical mending, then surely spiritual reunion. As opposed to traditional Jewish beliefs and even Roman mythology, the promise by the God-Man Jesus of everlasting life made any infirmities of earth superfluous. Death, the decay of flesh, was not a finality. It was merely a physical barrier to be crossed.

The miracles of Jesus and his disciples—so notable in the first decades after his departure—would fade in frequency and even significance. Instead began the major focus of Christians: care of neighbor. Efforts by notable members promoted curiosity, skepticism, and even ridicule. How unusual for these people to occupy their time with society's dregs. Yet communities throughout the Mediterranean would profit immensely from their generosity, passivity, and compassion. By their kindness and actions, they became known as healers.

A few were so enthralled by the message of the Christ that they devoted their lives entirely to solitude and prayerful communication with their Jesus. They took to desolate spots—usually the blankness of deserts—and formed communities. Their houses would be ζήσει μόνος, ("zaysei monos": live alone) where they "lived alone." Those who passed by would call their hamlets "monasteries." These "monastics" coveted their education, though, and continued scholarly tasks as part of their lifestyle, hoarding precious documents of learning from the ravages of constant civil unrest and persecutions.

Some were even familiar with the healing arts. Now, they could incorporate their newfound spirituality as part of the healing method. At first, they cared for each other, but soon, pilgrims heard of their wisdom and compassion and traveled to seek their healing care. All who came were accepted. "[T]ake care to make the bed of the sick and not to be short of bread, and also, if possible, to find a pillow or a head-cushion, so that those who are weak may rest," the fourth-century CE aesthetic Pachomius told his fellow monastics.[27] These men of Jesus the Christ provided simple measures to ease suffering, salves and nostrums learned from men of the East and even from those *ιατροι*, those priest-healers of Asclepius. They provided an atmosphere of health—calming rest, food, drink, and prayer. Their way of living promoted tranquility. Their prayers promoted hope. Were many physically healed? Some, perhaps, were. Some afflictions likely responded to their prescriptions. Many were likely not. But spiritually, their subjects found conviction in a continued life after death—their Christ had done so and promised them a resurrection, too. With that consolation they could resign themselves to their fate, comfortable that their Jesus would come for them in the end. Asclepiads had done the same; their god comforted in dreams. But Christians offered this for free and did not demand sacrifices or elaborate rituals.

There was one such monastic, Hospicius, who, people told, had exceptional powers to cure. A witness told that Hospicius, coming upon a pitiful one, deaf, dumb, and wracked by fever, took hold of his hair and drew his head into a window. And taking oil that had been blessed, Hospicius took hold of his tongue with his left hand, poured the oil in his mouth and on the top of his head, saying: "In the name of my lord Jesus Christ let your ears be opened and let that power which once drove a wicked demon from a deaf and dumb man open your lips." Having said this, he asked him his name, and the mute, rid of the fever, answered in a clear voice. He had been cured by Jesus the Christ the monk declared, and by Paul and all the disciples of Jesus. When the cured man proclaimed the wondrous deed of Hospicius, the holy man replied. "Be silent, beloved brother, it is not I who do this, but he who created the universe out of nothing, who took on man for our sake, and gave sight to the blind, hearing to the deaf, speech to the dumb; who bestowed on lepers the skin they had before, on the dead life, and on all the infirm abundant healing." His fame spread. Among the local populace, there was no denying these remarkable accomplishments by those who professed allegiance to this Jesus the Christ.[28]

Non-believers were perplexed at this behavior. Why meddle in the distasteful and those of lesser worth? Why not strive for riches, privilege, and honor on earth? There may be nothing afterward. Romans in particular belittled Christians, hunted them, burned them, hanged them, tore them limb from limb, but they would not renounce. The Emperor Nero used them as human torches to light the nighttime streets after he blamed Rome's fires on them and had others, the lucky ones, torn apart by wild dogs for amusement.

Christians ignored their taunts, suspicions, and rejection. They quietly awaited their fate and suffered silently. So much so, the historian Tacitus wrote, that public sentiment swayed to their plight.[29] In the meantime, Christians ministered by healing as their Jesus had done. At their touch some lame walked, some lepers healed, some fevers vanished. But they reveled in healing by the spirit first. All would heal by this. Believe, they said, in the God-Man Jesus the Christ. He is *Ο Μεγάλος Ιατρός*, the Great Healer. He had taught them how to truly heal. Comfort the mind and the body will soon be comforted, he had said. So, they healed in His name. Hoping for intercession, Christians labored over the ill, pleading for them to turn to God.

To the Macedonians of Thessalonica, and the Greeks of Corinth and Ephesus the mercy messages of Jesus this Anointed One were strange, indeed. What was this charity toward the poor and needy, toward orphans and widows? Citizens of Rome shunned almsgiving or even pity toward the beggars of the street. Let them rot, Greeks and Romans might have thought before. Such was the will of their gods who blessed power, not poverty. Even the god Asclepius demanded payment and plentiful sacrifices only the wealthy could afford. Temples of the god were filled with those adorned in fine linens and the gold of jewelry, not in the rags of vagabonds. Perfumes permeated the air, not the stench of sweat. Only them would the god visit in dreams and wipe away illness. Only the Asclepian Hippocrates emphasized compassion. Do not be too unkind, he urged, and love man—*φιλανθρωπία* (philanthropia). But all men? Always? The honored physician Hippocrates had not said.[30]

Traditional Greek healers, steeped in the ways of Asclepius and Hippocrates, wondered: who were these people who healed as the god Asclepius would? Where were their temples, their sanctuaries, their medicines, their sacrifices to their god? Christians offered none of these. Christians offered shelter, warmth, food, water, and a life beyond life. Christians took nothing from the poor, the ill—no money, no possessions. Their healing was in the name of their God, Jesus the Christ, just as Asclepius would come in sleep to cure. Did they merely substitute the mysteries of their god-man Jesus for those of Asclepius? The miracles reported by these Christians were impressive, many felt. Perhaps this new God was even more powerful than

Asclepius. Learned men familiar with inner harmony—a central precept of the great Hippocrates—began to fill the Christian ranks and delivered a dual message: one of bodily healing body and one of spiritual contentment.

One disciple, Ignatius of Antioch, spoke of Jesus' healing power. He wrote *"εις ιατρός ἐστιν, σαρκικός τε και πνευματικός, γεννητος και αγέννητος, εν ανθρώπω θεός, ἐν θανάτω ζωή αληθινή, και εκ Μαρίας και εκ θεού, πρώτον παθητος και τότε απαθής, Ιησούς Χριστός και κύριος ημών.* ("There is one Healer, who is both flesh and spirit, born and yet not born, who is God in man, true life in death, both of Mary and of God, first passible and then impassible, Jesus Christ our Lord.")[31] Christians took in all comers, as *Ιησούς Χρήστος*, Jesus the Christ would have: the sick and suffering, the decrepit, the deformed, the wasted. They bathed their sores, bandaged their wounds, held their heads to retch, stroked their brows as they died. Christians offered shelter, warmth, food, water, and hope in life forever. Christians took nothing from the poor, the ill—no money, no possessions. They only gave. Christians offered unity with Jesus the Christ, the visible Elāhā, the visible Yahweh, the visible God.

But Romans were leery. Not a century after the death of Jesus, Justin of Samarian, of Roman citizenry and proficient in the creeds of the Stoics, Peripatetics, and Pythagoreans, knew well of Plato's philosophy. Perhaps, as Plato inferred, there was a supreme creator, Justin surmised. Proof of this became his obsession. By chance he met a wise old man, who, in casual conversation, directed Justin to read from the Jewish prophets and their predictions of an anointed one, a son of David. Scouring the Jewish scriptures and hearing rumors about this man Jesus whom people were calling the Christ, the promised son of David, he became convinced of their story. He himself accepted their religion. In his mind, Jesus was the God of Plato, the Supreme Being. What he admired most were the miracles of cures in Jesus' name. Healing was a focus of Christianity, he found. When the Roman Emperor Titus Antoninus Pius intended to persecute and eradicate the Christian cult because of reported dangerous actions to the emperor himself, Justin appealed as a Roman citizen. In explaining Christians and their Jesus, he alluded to Asclepius as healer just as Jesus the Christ was a healer of men. "When we say that He cured the lame, the paralytics, and those blind from birth, and raised the dead to life, we seem to attribute to Him actions similar to those said to have been performed by Asclepius," he wrote. Then he explained:

When, indeed, we assert that the Word, our Teacher Jesus Christ, who is the first-begotten of God the Father, was not born as the result of sexual relations, and that He was crucified, died, arose from the dead, and ascended into Heaven, we propose nothing new or different from that which you say about the so-called sons of Jupiter.[32]

Christians considered Jesus the Great Healer who restored body and soul. Still, these zealots did not strive for earthly power, he said. Little did the emperor hear. Rusticus, the prefect of Rome, rejected his challenge of Christian impropriety. Moreover, Rusticus ordered Justin and six followers to sacrifice to the Roman gods. Justin refused, willing to suffer for his God. "The holy martyrs glorifying God betook themselves to the customary place, where they were beheaded and consummated their martyrdom."[33]

Others, too, rose in protest, arguing that perhaps Christianity provided new dimensions in healing. One was a physician in the city of Alexandria named Cyrus. He was a respected ιατρός, well educated in the art, but he was drawn to the message of Christianity—care of all mankind. He outfitted a space for his practice, called an ἐργαστύριον, "ergastrion," meaning in the vernacular, a "work-shop"—what would be called today a clinic. In it he applied physical as well as spiritual methods of healing. In accord with Christian practices, he treated the sick without charge. By that reputation alone, patients flocked to him and were reportedly cured by his touch and his healing words. Those not with outward afflictions but who still suffered spiritually came as well: the depressed, anxious, and sorrowful. Just like the incurable leprous, Cyrus seemed to help. His message was the monastic message of repentance first, healing later. "Whoever wishes to avoid being ill should refrain from sin, for sin is often the cause of bodily illness," Cyrus preached. A corrupt soul will corrupt the flesh, and the sores of iniquity will fester aloud until the spirit is quieted. His popularity earned him no honor, though. Cyrus died at the hands of the madman Emperor Diocletian in his hatred of Christians, beheaded as he sought to protect the lives of innocent faithful virgins.[34]

As ridiculed as Christians like Cyrus were, their value temporarily skyrocketed during times of epidemics. With the awful plague that descended on all the Mediterranean in the third century, sick and dying cluttered homes and streets, the stench of their contagion could not be ignored, and the moans of the ill filled the air. It was "a horror like that of hell."[35] Fevers raged, mouths fouled with ulcerations, and fetid evacuations filled the gutters. Romans and all collapsed with the sickness, and the numbers of dying soared. The energetic bishop of Carthage by the name of Cyprian gathered Christians to him and assigned them care of rich and poor alike, to nurse, comfort, and bless the dying. Like many clergy, he was versed in certain health matters. To those of his kind, care of the sick was a standard part of their vocation. One contemporary wrote of the actions of Cyprian, who had no hesitation in roaming the streets looking for the destitute—a dangerous adventure in the days of Roman persecutions:

> On the people assembled together in one place he first of all urged the benefits of mercy, teaching by examples from divine lessons, how greatly the duties of benevolence avail to deserve well of God. Then afterwards he subjoined, that there was nothing wonderful in our cherishing our own people only with the needed attentions of love, but that he might become perfect who would do something more than the publican or the heathen, who, overcoming evil with good, and practicing a clemency which was like the divine clemency, loved even his enemies, who would pray for the salvation of those that persecute him, as the Lord admonishes and exhorts.[36]

For those benevolent deeds, as if Jesus the Christ himself had done them, Cyprian was banned from his city and his congregation. He also refused to submit to Roman gods and willingly walked to his execution spot where, in front of throngs of the curious, his head fell by the sword.

Cyrus and Cyprian, of course, were not alone. When the plague hit Alexandria, rulers of the city turned on Christians much like Nero did with the fires of Rome. One of their physicians, Origen Adamantius, was also an admirer of Christianity. He spoke often of Jesus the healer. In fact, he practiced the standard Christian blend of spiritual and physical healing. Under Jesus the Supreme Physician even wretched flesh would smooth, Origen believed, and the vile spirit would cleanse:

> Enter into this medical clinic, his Church. See, lying there, a multitude of feeble ones. The woman comes who was made "unclean" from birth. "A leper" comes who was segregated "outside the camp" for the uncleanness of his leprosy. They seek a cure from the physician: how they may be healthy, how they may be cleansed. Because this Jesus, who is a doctor, is himself the Word of God, he prepares medications for his sick ones, not from potions of herbs but from the sacraments of words.[37]

Origen healed like Cyprian—he took in all who sought his care. His nostrums appealed to body and mind. Soothing medications for fevers, sores, dysentery, and plague. Prayer and hope for worry. Origen, too, would not renounce his God. He could not escape the plague's resultant pogrom. Origen and fellow Christians were imprisoned and tortured. It was Christian sorcery, Romans felt. Origen would languish two years in the dungeon. Upon his release, so broken was his body that he lived less than a year.

Many other Christian heads would fall as well until their healing message was acknowledged by Roman rule. But their mission continued. However, their adherence to principles, their compassion, and their firm conviction of righteousness swayed public opinion from anger to pity to sympathy to admiration and finally, imitation.

But here rested the basis of Christian healing, that there was an unmistakable connection between sickness and sin. As for Jesus the Christ, he was not so dissimilar from other shamanic healers of his day. His ability to heal largely stemmed from hope and the purpose he instilled in his followers and the sense of community it fostered. And at the root of his philosophy attention to the spirit was a sine qua non of rectifying bodily distress.[38] With regard to healing practices, then, early church fathers, many of whom were very much involved in care of the sick, considered the healer—the physician—as one who "succors the ill, enduring unpleasant tasks in caring for the unhealthy, often [involving] necessarily painful means for effecting a cure." Yet they were first and foremost "physicians of the soul," the *medici animarum*, who adhered to the precepts of Christus, the Great Physician.[39]

CHAPTER FOUR

Galen the Inquisitor

In popular Greek culture, Asclepius the Healer reigned over all others. The magic of his eerie visitations calmed not a few troubled hearts. The standard healer, the *ιατρος*, could not do without him. But Greek physicians were also pragmatists; in many cases, they called upon their gods as a narcotizing intermediary. For palpable benefit they resorted to more urbane methods of therapy. Their armamentarium included a wide variety of botanicals and potions designed to take away or build up Hippocratic concepts of unbalanced humors or address disagreeable environmental elements. Suffering must abate, they reasoned, or else why the *τέχνη*—the art itself. And with pragmatism came a curiosity of the human body: its composition—the pulsing, gurgling, and ticking of inner workings—that fostered knowledge of their subjects. Perhaps the human body in all its complexities could be manipulated, adjusted, rearranged. Just maybe, harmony and health could somehow be restored by the very natures that disrupted them. Gods placated the intangible spirits within, man would placate the tangibles.

In the dangerous but exotic world of first-century Roman imperialism, an imaginative Greek healer emerged who would rearrange thinking about the human machine. He was known simply as Galen. Less spiritual than Yēšūa and his Christian cult, he was more earthy—perhaps bound more to mechanism than mysticism. Philosophically Greek, he exposed matters beneath the skin as so many fanciful articulations fueled by lubricating humors of bile and blood that worked at the whims of gods and nature and spirit. The will of man arose from it all. His were the projections of a rudimentary science and a manufactured but naïve logic.

Yet he would be perhaps the most influential figure in medicine for over a millennium. His were the first whispers of today's evidence-based practices.

While acknowledging the humoral theories of his predecessor, Hippocrates, he was not completely satisfied. He went further and mapped the interiors of the body, providing a network of reference for his interpretation of physical ailments and methods of healing. Galen's logic was flawed, his anatomic familiarity imperfect, part animalistic and part gladiatorial—he disassembled animals and reassembled gladiators—but at times, surprisingly accurate as he meticulously explored the open wounds of his human subjects. In his inquisitiveness he gave substance to theory and, until legitimate human dissection was permitted—necropsy was frowned upon in his day—he offered a foundation for medical thought that would last centuries. And imposed on his fledgling science of the flesh was a philosophical essence—call it "breath of life" or "spirit"—he insisted was also coursing through tissues and keeping mankind in harmony.

Galen was born Aelius Galenus in 129 CE in the Asia Minor town of Pergamon.[1] His father, Aelius Nicon, was a wealthy architect and prominent member of Pergamon's cultured world. With a wide interest in philosophy, literature, and agriculture, Aelius felt at ease among the community of scholars. He was a frequent visitor to the Asclepieion of Pergamon. Aelius began to gather the best medical teachers for the young Galen, who by the age of sixteen had already acquired the medical knowledge of practicing physicians. To further his studies, Galen moved on to the renowned center of learning at Smyrna, fifty miles distant, but then across the Aegean to Corinth and finally to Alexandria, Egypt. Alexandria at the time was at the forefront of medical science, particularly in anatomy, as they allowed human cadaveric dissection. Centuries before, Herophilus and Erasistratus demonstrated the marvelous intricacies of the body, particularly the brain and nervous system, assigning many structural names familiar today. Rumor had it, in fact, that the two did not confine their efforts to the deceased; they also performed vivisection on criminals supplied by the king. While still breathing, it was said, their bodies were cut open to observe internal organs splendidly perfused and functioning. It was likely here that the young Galen learned human anatomy from authorities in the field and which would shape his grounding as an anatomist.[2]

He must have been superbly trained. While he was a brilliant thinker, Galen was an arrogant man, firmly principled, convinced of his righteousness. He later wrote of himself:

> Is there someone who can not only shape in words, but demonstrate in deeds the limit of wealth that nature sets . . . if there is such a one . . . He heals a patient whose illness calls for the Hippocratic art, yet he does not think it right

to say with him always, but he treats the poor inhabitants of Cranon and of Thasos and the other towns . . . to wander over the whole of Greece since he must also write something concerning the nature of places.[3]

His rhetoric was intimidating. Galen argued persuasively about his ideas, to the point that his theories carried the approval of countless academicians and formed the working principles for all of physic. Even acknowledging his agnosticism, the sect of Christians subscribed to Galen's teachings as almost inviolate. Over time, so enamored did they become with him that challenge to his doctrines would be considered almost heretical and served to retard the progress of science until well into the second millennium.

Galen was a complex man: part pragmatist and part philosopher. He deeply pondered the unanswerable assumptions that allowed for life itself. What role did abstract notions of mind, cognition, and spirit have in the mysterious vitality of health? It was as much a question of philosophy as therapeutics. Others had grappled with those same issues before him. Any number of philosophers dabbled in the dynamism that instilled animation in the inanimate. Was it the mind? The spirit? Was it of nature or the supernatural?

He read Plato who had pondered the essence of man's vitality—those invisible qualities that gave animation. In his reasoning, Plato discussed diverse influences: ψυχὴ, the soul; αηρ, life-giving "air"; and, importantly, πνευμα ("pneuma"), the breath of living into flesh—the spirit as some would name it.[4] Galen acknowledged Plato's spiritual concepts. But he also subscribed to Hippocrates' moving force of φύσα ("phusa") that was the cause of all life—and the cause of sickness. This φύσα, Hippocrates felt, was the air that surrounded living things—perhaps the physicality of earthly existence—entering bodies and becoming *pneuma*. He blamed the omnipresent φύσα as a mischievous agent. "So breaths [he used the word φῦσαι] were seen to be the most egregious agents during all diseases," he wrote. His φῦσαι—his "nature's airs"—could even change the soul (ψῦχή).[5] These ethereal substances would become the root of φυσικη επιστημη (phusike episteme), the knowledge of natural things—physic.

Man was not a simple creature, Hippocrates had argued, to which Galen agreed. He was a mixture of elements and temperaments, a swirl of ψῦχή, *pneuma*, and visible humors. Hippocrates argued that if man were one single element, he would not suffer—but man does suffer, Galen argued. And if man were a single element there would be one cure for illness "but, in fact, there are many types of cures."[6] Galen carried this further. As man is a mixture of elements, then health and illness are consequences of good or bad mixtures:

[i]n health, there is an exact proper proportion in amount and force and the mixture throughout the whole, so, in the same way he proposed the opposite of this for illness, referring on the one hand to something lesser or greater with respect to the amount of substance or with respect to force, and on the other hand, to it being mixed with things in a poorly balanced mixture.[7]

He subscribed to Hippocrates' χυμός, "chumos"—the juices or humors that percolated through man: blood, phlegm, black bile, and yellow bile. His philosophy would eventually appeal to the rising influence of the Christian Church as it assumed the mantle of corporal as well as spiritual physician. Platonic in its philosophical leanings, Christianity favored the entirety of Galen's philosophy as it pertained to the spiritual natures of humanness. The possibility of a creating God and the likelihood of an immortal "soul" fueled a favoritism to Galen's corporal explanations as well. It fit with the bent of Christian healing as modeled by the *Christus* Himself—that, first, spiritual reconciliation be cemented, then physical pain relieved.[8]

But Galen was also pragmatic. He would learn much of τέχνη—the art—not in the academic halls of philosophers or dissecting rooms of academicians but in the bloody arenas of mortal combat. While Plato's ψῡχή enchanted him, the σώματα (somata), the body, consumed him. He could not ignore the graphic and bloodied machinery that would be laid before him. He became the gladiators' healer.

In the Roman Empire gladiatorial combat was public sport, much as American football is today. Crowds would gather in coliseums across the empire in raucous celebration to view these contests, a controlled microcosm of the brutal world in which they lived. As pitiless as the sport could be, extreme efforts were used to maintain the health and longevity of the combatants. They were prized fighters. Shortly after his return from Alexandria, Galen was awarded the distinction of doctor to the gladiators in 157 CE by no less than the high priest (*pontifex maximus*) of Asia Minor, who was the grand organizer and financier of this "sport." Gladiators were prized athletes, and taking care of them was considered of prime importance—both in training and combat. He learned a great deal of medicine tending to these valued combatants—diet, exercise, minor sports injuries. Adhering to the δίαιτᾰ—"way of life"—of Greek thinking, regimens of diet, exercise, sleep, and rest were essential to promoting health.[9] Wounded gladiators were treated intently, as the *lanista*, the owner, and the game's organizer had an investment in their health and durability. Most wounds, if not immediately lethal, were probably survivable, particularly injuries to arms or legs—more so if a competent healer attended. Galen was a student of anatomy and, unafraid to probe those vicious wounds, excelled in his powers to heal gladiatorial injuries. By his report he experienced only two deaths compared to sixty of his predecessors. In fact, at one point, Galen boasted that "not a single one of mine [gladiators] had perished either from a wound or otherwise." His talents were not ignored by successive "pontiffs" in charge of the gladiatorial contests, who, one after the other, entrusted him with the "duty of healing." While there appeared to be an "industry" of proper management of wounds by local physicians, "*medici*," he had done much more empirical work in the treatment of such wounds.[10]

For someone so talented as he, it was no surprise that Galen yearned to be in Rome, the center of all influence and learning. He did so at age thirty-two. There, he busied himself with lecturing and writing in addition to the practice of medicine. At the time, attitudes toward physicians in the city were mixed. Certainly, the types of Hellenistic philosopher-healers like Galen were highly prized for their theoretical expertise, but most were reluctant to treat commoners, preferring the intrigue of aristocratic imperialism. Then there were the street urchins. Many were former Greek slaves—some now freed or simply renegades—who practiced a form of rough and impersonal therapies, usually of a surgical nature, for the immediate irritants of everyday life. Others were household "healers," again, slaves given as prizes to the affluent—servants who may or may not have any knowledge of workable prescriptions. The city seemed overrun with these charlatans, privateers, opportunists, and frank quacks. Galen, however, found the busy metropolis and its degenerate form of medicine perfect for dissemination of his reasoned attitudes toward anatomy, humoral physic, and pension for influential teaching.[11]

From Rome he traveled broadly to Greece, Palestine, and Asia Minor, always inquiring, gathering drugs, encountering challenging medical cases, and enriching his fund of knowledge. After returning to Rome in 169 CE he served emperors Marcus Aurelius, Commodus, and Septimius Severus as their personal physician. So capably did he perform that Marcus Aurelius declared him "first among doctors and unique among philosophers." An academic wizard, he never ceased to be the clinician, welcoming all strata of patients: peasants, wives, children, and slaves of the rich, even random people he met in the streets. As a consequence, it was this time period when Galen was most prolific, drawing on his experiences from the past forty years of practice. He engaged in any number of lectures, debates, and even public animal dissections. He reportedly conducted displays on living pigs on the structure and function of respiration and vocalization, paralyzing intercostal muscles with ligatures, then, upon release, startled the crowd with a once again squealing animal.[12] In this, he departed from the theoretical to the theatrical, and used direct observation of anatomy to rationalize function, particularly that of the nervous system. He had become a new brand of doctor—an experimentalist. He did not wonder; he demonstrated.[13]

> Those who neglect practice in the Art . . . how can they treat dislocations, whether simple or compound, or fractures and sphacelus of bones; how can they even open abscesses, or excise gangrenes, or remove a missile or splinter properly . . . I expect beginners to practice all such methods first because I see their necessity, and second because if the time needed to learn them is but short, as they think, then the shame of ignorance is so much the greater.[14]

But then what about Hippocrates' fabled vital humors? How did they interact with the core of animation, the ψυχή? For Galen the humors were a puzzle. He could never clearly demonstrate their origin or interior significance, even by his detailed dissections of animals or in his sometimes-filleted gladiators. Yet they could be graphically seen in human excretions or expulsions—vomit, blood, bile, phlegm, urine, or feces. Such manifestations must signal internal disorder. Yes, Hippocrates had said, the body of man had in itself blood, phlegm, yellow bile, and black bile; that these made up the nature of his body, and through these he felt pain or enjoyed health.[15] In that, Galen agreed. The body was indeed a perplexing container of percolating liquids, coursing among softened substances of crimson sacks and squirming tubes, reaching to every corner of flesh with revitalizing fibers. Too much or too little? It only made sense that replenishing deficiencies and curtailing excesses should help in restoring equilibrium, a state Hippocrates called harmony.[16]

Galen tried to tie together his curiosity about anatomy and Hippocrates' theories of humors. His anatomic concepts were intriguing but faulty. In part based not on the human anatomy he had studied in Alexandria but on his animal dissections, he, for example, featured the liver, with its "five fingers" (lobes), clasping the nearby stomach to provide warmth for digestion of food. In his mind, it was this liver that was the source of sanguification—the production of blood from ingested food. The magnificent liver, he taught, transferred its nature to nutriments that, when mixed, flowed as purified blood.[17] Onto a speculative anatomy with which he had familiarized himself he put Hippocrates' concepts of humor and harmony. Which generates what, he pondered. His ruminations produced a three-book text he called *On the Natural Faculties*. Here he combined his theories on phlegm, bile, and blood with threats of nature's fire, earth, wind, and water. How did the mechanics of man readjust for those forces from without that upset delicate balances of internal harmony? And what, in the end, was the perception of illness and health? Was it not in part elusively spiritual? A feeling of well-being suffused the spirit. Likewise, a feeling of malaise did the same. Disease arose from the body, illness from the spirit. He wrote:

> Surely, whenever there is no impediment in any of the activities of all their bodily parts, people say that they are healthy, and think they have no need of doctors. But whenever they become aware that some one of their natural functions is beginning to perform either badly or not at all, they consider themselves to be sick.[18]

How then did Galen heal?

He was a free spirit—if not an arrogant one—unencumbered by the ranging doctrines of religious or theological advocates. In him there was no shortage of conceit. He felt himself a courageous individual, a maverick, often confrontational, even querulous with his contemporaries. Without doubt, he was ambitious and outspoken. His rhetoric, at times, seemed insufferable. He based it not on the metaphysical but on nature—the physical. Natural laws compelled actions accordingly. "Health is that which is in accord with nature. Disease is that which is contrary to nature," he wrote.[19] There were four different bodily occurrences that signified disease: impaired activity; the deposition that brought it about; its causes; and the symptoms that necessarily followed. In terms of causes, human temperaments—the individual manifestations of ψυχή—could be responsible. Then, he wondered, how best to countermand contrariness? In a rather vague way, with regard to therapeutics, he postulated that "the entire science consists in observation and recollection of what has been seen to go with what, what to proceed what, and what to come after what."[20] His therapeutics took into account bodily reactions, elemental forces, the suspected humoral disharmony, and individual temperament. He agreed with Hippocrates in that there were three aspects of medical treatment: the physician, the disease, and the patient. Galen wrote:

> If the patient agrees with the physician and does what he tells him, he helps him fight the disease. If he disagrees with the physician and does what the disease compels him [to do], he thwarts the physician in two ways: first, he leaves him, who is a single [person], alone, whereas they were at first, together with him, two; and second, he makes his opponent, who had been single and isolated, two by aiding it, and two are inevitably stronger than one.[21]

So here, he proposed, was the true art of healing. Inquire, he urged. Know your subject. The goal of inquiry was to discover cures for every disease. How was that to be done? Know the disease, what kind of disorder it was by nature; delve into the particulars of each patient for that will guide specific therapy. All humans were different just as all animals were different. Galen stressed a universal understanding of disease that applied to specific victims. Therapy would be guided accordingly. Therefore, the physician must know his patient and their peculiarities to design therapeutics. He, like Hippocrates, sincerely believed in the integrity of the healer. He wrote that such a practitioner of the art must already "possess all the parts of philosophy: the logical, the scientific, and the ethical. He must condemn riches and lives temperately." He firmly felt that "all the rash and unjust things that men do, they do because they are seduced by covetousness, or bewitched by pleasure."

> I do not think it needs further proof that philosophy is necessary for doctors if they are to use the Art correctly, when practitioners who are no physicians, but poisoners, are daily before our eyes: lovers of money who abuse the Art for ends that are opposed to its nature.[22]

And what of the metaphysical? As any studious observer might, he witnessed the ebb and flow of life—whether *pneuma* or *ψῡχή*. He had seen vitality dwindle at the end of a gladiatorial sword and wondered what immaterial substance fled at those moments of last breath, and where did it go. Was it as finite as the paling flesh before him or some vapor that yet hung in the air and possessed still all those temperaments of Plato? Did a hovering god snatch them away? In nature Galen saw a supernatural influence and pointed out that man looked to nature as if "he was worshiping a certain divine deity." But proper explanation of the science of medicine required acknowledgment to a "great good God," useful to the whole human race also to dispel the "false and portentous words, inextricable labyrinths of sentences." Galen also wrote that proper physicians should know themselves, both in body and mind, and acknowledge that certain deities arranged both in mutual symphony that becomes part of each man. He implied that nature and the supernatural were intimately linked.[23]

He knew of this strange religious sect called Christians. By then occasional public executions and exhibitions of these bizarre folk captured public attention. At the same time, as a healer, he was aware of their basic premise—that their god, Christ, healed, too. How did he perceive this new cult? They were peculiar in that they embraced the destitute and the sick. There was no avoidance of street urchins in all their smells, pustules, and putrid breath. He himself seemed to honor philanthropy, the willingness to treat everyone as Christians proclaimed to do. From *Remarks on the Book of Plato and the Republic*, he was obviously curious and, in a manner of speaking, per-plexed by their unorthodox behavior:

> From this we may infer that the people called Christians derive their faith from signs and miracles. Also, sometimes, they show such behavior as is adopted by philosophers; for fearlessness of death and the hereafter is something we wit-ness in them every day.[24]

How they healed he did not comment on but, as long as they abided by his same Hellenistic principles, he likely took no issue. What stood out was the benevolence and compassion they bestowed on each other and those of lesser ranks. He stubbornly subscribed to their benevolence in the care of the less fortunate—a tendency usually discouraged in Greek or Roman society.

Yet Galen's singular achievement would be his willingness to inquire, to investigate, to experiment. He brought to light a hidden anatomy imperative for human healing to progress. His keenness about structure and function, together with an imaginative mind, provided the seeds for future conjectures of health and disease. It is likely that Galen's gladiatorial experiences formed the basis for his anatomic curiosity. Certainly, his gladiator work gave him a perspective of the arrangement of muscles, nerves, and tendons of the limbs. The organs of the belly and chest were mostly inferences gathered from his work on animals—or maybe the occasional gutted human specimen. From anatomy, he then envisioned a physiology in part based on Hippocratic thinking and in part on his supposition of knowledgeable anatomy. He was certain that theory be based on logic and logic on evidence. Man's nature was a conglomeration of elements and tissues, intertwined as a complex of moving functionality, he reasoned. Only then, he wrote, can healers under-stand "the nature of the body, and the distinction between diseases, and the indications for remedies."[25]

But what suspicion about the patient's behavior did he feel was so critical to healing? It might stem from that indefinable essence of man—however philosophically defined—which, Galen contended, promoted temperaments favorable or unfavorable for the cure. But of matters of body or spirit, Galen focused mostly on the body. His interest was a novel physiology and novel anatomy. Like many healers of his day, a life-giving essence could not be denied, so he was compelled to contemplate, yet he began to orient healing more to the body while still acknowledging the spirit. And whatever hap-pened to this spirit after death—he could not tell—during life it facilitated or impaired the patient's ability to heal. Plato's ψῡχή was intangible but real. Without the patient's cooperation the physician could do nothing. All the faculties of trust and hope must be fully directed at attempts to heal—both for the healer and the ill.

As for the healer himself, mastery of the art was paramount. Learn. Investigate. Think. Practice. And physician, know your patient. Know their *ψῡχή*: their hopes, fears, passions, strengths, and weaknesses. These, Galen felt, were as important to healing as the intricate networks of nerves, arteries, veins, and tissues. To Galen, too, as with Hippocrates before him, healing was a sacred calling, one of excellence and art; one of guidance and compassion; one of devotion and immersion.[26]

CHAPTER FIVE

The Medievalists

Early medievalists who with their hands and crude instruments honed, sawed, sewed, set, and sliced the human body were an ignoble lot. They were the undertakers of the living, as much apart from the renowned physician as carriage makers from kings. It was hard to imagine that this unruly band would, with time, become the darlings of medical practitioners.

There was little argument in the world of the Middle Ages that restoration of bodily health was instrumental in mending a worried mind. The passage of a febrile crisis, resolution of vomiting and diarrhea and return of appetite, usually signaled departure of whatever evil had passed through. And with it a renewed sense of well-being—indescribable but as certain as the awful disease-driven dread that preceded it. Could physicians do anything to speed the process? Likely not. Illness was still a malfunction of bodily humors and therapy still aimed to rid or replenish those mystical fluids in imbalance. Rituals of humoral manipulation by purging, sweating, and bloodletting did little to abolish misery and frequently added to it.

These "internal" ailments were in contradistinction to the very visible external afflictions many fell victim to as well: boils, hemorrhoids, fissures, fistulas, tumors, fractures, and wounds. For these, one did not blame Hippocrates' and Galen's humors or ravaging epidemics—many were the consequences of daily life. Instead, the afflicted and damaged needed fixing and sought the services of laborers—of whatever sophistication—who could cut away or mend, much as a broken wagon wheel needed repair. Little did it matter whether humors aligned. Yes, diet and lifestyle still played a role, but the nostrums of educated physicians made trivial difference. Liberating pus, setting fractures, extracting bladder stones, or lancing bulging hemorrhoids did. Even then, such mundane practices were thought distinct from natural philosophy—nature's capriciousness on human physiognomy. And those practitioners adept at such barbarism were no more skilled (or academically valued) than the barbers who trimmed beards or the bone-setter or the tooth-puller. Such violations of the flesh were little more than blood sport, little more than the hacking and carving of war-injured in the carnage of Dark Age battlefields. Defilement of human tissue was horrid work, spurned by the Holy Church, and best left to tradesmen whose bloodied hands were not so different from the calloused fingers of carpenters and stone masons. Yes, repair of combat-mutilated was one thing. Necessary. As brutal as the wounds themselves. But cutting on virgin skin was quite another. It was hazardous incursion on the sacred nature of the soul—likely as not, sometimes, to snatch death from life as health from sickness.

It was nothing new. Hippocrates and his followers forbad refined *ιατροί*—those recognized as healers—from doing it. Health of the body was philosophical, not mechanistic. Physicians should, instead, dwell on the nature of things and the causes of all physical phenomena. The great Galen himself did not shy from surgery but held that faculties of the soul depend upon the mixture of the elements of the body, be they hot or cold or moist or dry.[1]

Those who defied tradition and cut, at their core, were journeymen. Usually, burly tradesmen did the work, capable of restraining a howling subject. They had few qualms about plunging into flesh or wrenching dangling limbs into place. So ruthless was their craft it was no wonder Hippocrates dismissed it. The most egregious task was to extract bladder stones—a procedure the Hippocratic school felt lethal. Healer beware. "Neither will I let them suffer from the stone [bladder stones], but will assign this task to those so trained," his Hippocratic Oath read.[2]

What kind of men could stomach this sort of brutality? They were what the Greeks would call *χειρουργόι* ("chirurgoi"): from the Greek words *χείρ* (hand) and *έργον* (work)—"hand work." They were craftsmen by their hands, not so different from woodworkers, blacksmiths, and potters. *Χειρουργόι* had nothing to do with medicine, at least not at first. These were little more than common hawkers. Yes, there was a *τεχνη*, a learned skill (at first, hardly the "science" of Hippocrates), but so was carpentry or blacksmithing. With time, such skills of the *χειρουργον* were limited to treating ailments and injuries—but not always.[3] In Umbrian Italy, for example, there were *salumieri* (sausage-makers) who were so adept with the knife in slicing pork that they were sometimes called upon to carve up living humans. In all their humble ranks, income from such work was modest, but probably adequate—although a bit of chicanery and deception might have helped. For the more scrupulous, they were well-intentioned but surely uneducated and unable to read or write. Some might even have been considered dullards, poorly equipped for much of anything but working with knives and tools. A few were quite gifted, though. So adept were the more gifted that the Greek polymath Aristotle considered talented χειρουργόι as almost artisans, refined craftsmen. His term was the sensual δημιουργοι ("daemiurgoi")—"creators" or "sculptors."[4]

For the better intentioned, how did they learn? Like many trades, most relied on a master and apprentice relationship. Dissection of anatomic specimens—dead warriors, slaves, or apes—was key, but not always possible. In lieu of that, many joined the military with abundant opportunities to chop, cut, cauterize, and splint on the battlefield. Surgical instruments, the tools of the trade, became quite familiar, and left few battle surgeons inexperienced using them. Most of their casualties were so grievously injured that any help—novice or otherwise—could not hurt and sometimes was miraculously successful.[5] Celsus characterized surgeons as providing "that which cures by the hand." He considered them of fluent fingers, clear eyes, and steely temperament:

> Now a surgeon should be youthful or at any rate nearer youth than age; with a strong and steady hand which never trembles, and ready to use the left hand as well as the right; with vision sharp and clear, and spirit undaunted; filled with pity . . . yet is not moved by his cries, to go too fast, or cut less than is necessary; but he does everything just as if the cries of pain cause him no emotion.[6]

Galen might have agreed. Surgeons were specialists in healing.[7] Such reasonable qualities did little for surgeons' image, though. Learned physicians of the day demeaned them. Tolerated but shunned. Necessary but brutes. Skillful but disgusting. For centuries, they remained on the fringe of medicine, so uneducated and illiterate that their talents rarely made it into writing. It was a craft of the streets, hardly one to embrace the wider principles of humors and commotions that guided health or illness. The link to divine intercession and soulful consideration was almost ludicrous. Flesh, blood, urine, and pus were surgeons' only guiding principles—or so licensed healers thought.

A scholarly profession, then? At first, hardly. Only sporadically would the written word appear—Celsus and Galen were notable exceptions. Not until the twelfth century was there any compendium of the art. Many apprentices could not read anyway. Italians were among the first to record much of anything. Perhaps they had greater freedom in exploring the interstices of the human body. Anatomical dissection was neither forbidden nor even discouraged. At the great school in Salerno, dissection had begun about that time, and King Frederick II of the Kingdom of Naples mandated in 1241 that anyone wanting to practice surgery must have mastered anatomy *on human bodies*.[8] The deceased lent their lifeless forms to professors who opened them up and exposed the glistening machinery within. Perhaps then was the first inkling that the human assembly could be fixed as methodically as wagon wheels, clogged sewers, or cathedral archways. Perhaps surgery, like natural philosophy, could be elevated to *sciencia*, "knowledge." To separate surgical *scientia* from the base operations of barbarous street urchins would be a formidable task. Most practitioners of the craft were hardly worthy of intellectual or moral acknowledgment, so spoke the Italian surgeon Bruno da Longoburgo (c. 1200–1286):

> Scarcely anyone who is illiterate can understand this art, but at the present time . . . those who exercise this art are for the most part ignorant and stupid peasants; and on account of their stupidity the worst possible diseases are generated in people by which indeed the patients are killed since the surgeons operate neither wisely nor according to certain reasoning.[9]

Yet the few surgical men of letters began writing about their vocation. Textbooks appeared. The *Practica Chirurgiae* (Practice of Surgery) of Ruggiero Frugardi (c. 1140–1195) was likely one of the first. Frugardi was from Salerno, Italy, an entry port for Greek and Arab merchants.[10] Others followed. The Italian Theodoric Borgognoni (1205–1298) copied the lessons of his teacher Hugo de Lucca, who taught at the school in Bologna, and published it as *Chirurgia* ("Surgery"). Theodoric himself was highly educated, schooled as a Dominican friar and appointed Bishop of Cervia in northern Italy. He was a student of surgical "hand work," even promoting cleanliness as a vital element in successful procedures. In his estimation, surgery "is the ultimate resource of medicine."[11]

In Italy, then, far from the crude manual workings of antiquity, surgeons became healers of the highest caliber. In fact, some romanticized them as the equals of Apollo the Healer. Like Celsus' description, surgeons were portrayed as the ultimate in masculinity. "[The surgeon] should be of a well-proportioned and temperate complexion," one Italian surgeon wrote. His hands must be "well shaped, [with] long small fingers, and his body not quaking [steady hands]." He must be versed in all the parts of logic, scripture, and philosophy. He should not be gluttonous, nor envious, nor niggardly. He must be kind, considerate, and understanding of his patients. His knowledge must excel. He must know all the parts of healing and know well all the human elements. He must be a paradigm of breeding, refinement, and education.[12]

Scholarly men such as Taddeo Alderotti (c. 1206–1295) were proficient in surgery as well as physic. Alderotti was one of the first to hold lectures in medicine at the University of Bologna, debating works of Hippocrates and Galen. One of Alderotti's pupils, Dino del Garbo (c. 1280–1327) published the first commentary on Persian physician, Ibn Sīnā (980–1037), called by the West Avicenna. Avicenna's influential text was *al-Qānūn fī al-Ṭibb*, or *The Canon of Medicine*. All healing, Avicenna professed, was tied to divine influence and the healer was, by inference, the instrument of God. "We render thanks to Allah, for the very excellence of His creation, and the abundance of His benefits," Avicenna opened his text. And as for medicine itself:

> [When] we say that practice proceeds from theory, we do not mean that there is one division of medicine by which we know, and another, distinct therefrom by which we act. We mean that these aspects belong together—one deals with the basic principles of knowledge; the other with the mode of operation of these principles.[13]

Avicenna believed surgery and physic to be a spectrum of healing, one blending into the other. Like Avicenna's spiritual connection, del Garbo argued that surgery reached far beyond a manual activity—his so-called *operatio manualis* (manual operating)—and was true *scientia*, or knowledge. Like physic, surgery was based on *res naturales*—natural things—primarily anatomy, and could be used to correct *res non naturalis*, "unnatural happenings." Del Garbo's mentor, Alderotti followed Hippocratic thinking in that disease was subject to certain laws of nature, and the body did not passively accept exterior insults but adjusted to counteract. Recovery, then, was also a work of nature, the healing power an effort to restore harmony. The physician's role was not superfluous. He observed and moderated factors of influence as proposed by the Greek δίαιτα "diata," a way of living. There were factors that could moderate—*res non naturalis*: air, food and drink, exercise and rest, sleep and wakefulness, secretion and excretion, and mental affectations. Sometimes alteration by manual means—discharges, repairs, or restorations with bare hands—would be necessary. But this required judgment. To practice surgery meant in del Garbo's mind not only the techniques of dexterity but also the discernment of what could be treated by hand work and what required more subtle adjustments of *res non naturalis*. As artisans of the flesh, surgeons lifted healing from the realm of the theoretical to that of the pragmatic. Cures were no longer necessarily a matter of faith but of human intervention.[14]

⌒

Still, for surgeons, if nothing else, religion stood in the way.

In medieval Europe, even on the Italian Peninsula, the Catholic Church had an iron grip on medical practices. Roman Catholic Christianity permeated all facets of society, and strict adherence to doctrines of faith was brandished as fundamental to eternal salvation. No less was Catholic dogma on healing. Natural and supernatural were inexorably tied, and divine permission to interfere was closely aligned to adherence to canon. Physicians were at the mercy of Mother Church. Canon 22 of the Fourth Lateran Council of 1215 pronounced it so: "we declare in the present decree and strictly command that when physicians of the body are called to the bedside of the sick, before all else they admonish them to call for the physician of souls."[15]

Yet secular studies began to challenge Church-sanctioned teachings. One such champion was Henri de Mondeville (1260–1320). He came from that rebellious Norman countryside which spawned restless figures like Rollo the Viking and Duke William the Conqueror. Any more precise location of his birthplace is largely speculative; perhaps the small hamlet of Mandeville, three miles from Caen or maybe the village of Emondville. Described as a handsome man of slender build but with sharp, distinctly masculine features, he first traveled to Montpellier and then to Paris to study medicine. He may have spent time with the masterful Theodoric Borgognoni in Italy. Borgognoni must have been a fascinating teacher, bringing to life his extensive text *Chirurgia* before his eyes. Returning to Paris, de Mondeville soon attracted the attention of Jean Pitard (1228–1315), a Parisian surgeon of renown whose academic position was beyond repute and had earned him the admiration of the French Court. Pitard took a liking to the young de Mondeville, perhaps one like himself, and groomed the young man in ways of nobility. It might have been de Mondeville's tireless energy and his unique passion for the art that drew Pitard in, but in any event, de Mondeville found an invaluable mentor in the aging surgeon.

The Norman Pitard was considered by some to be the "genius" of French surgery. He had studied anatomy in Bologna.[16] He probably fled back to Paris afterward, driven from Italy by wars and civil strife. By the age of thirty, Pitard had earned the confidence of royalty and dignitaries. Unencumbered by the theories of scholars, Pitard practiced a sensible art, as much from experience as from assumption. He became an intimate of the French kings, particularly the saintly Louis IX, whom Pitard accompanied to the Holy Land. Shortly, Pitard brought the gifted de Mondeville into his fold, and together, the two were described as "the most competent in the art of surgery of those [surgeons] who remained in France."[17]

As for de Mondeville, few had reached his level of prestige. By 1301 he, like his mentor Pitard, had been named surgeon to King Philip IV, grandson of Louis IX. He insisted that surgery was a divine calling. "The Savior exercised some work with his hand, similar to the office of surgeon, when he took his own saliva and applied it to a blind man's eyes and restored sight to him. By this deed he elevated surgery above all others [professions]."[18]

Yet in the early fourteenth century the practice of surgery was in shameful condition in France. And not without reason. Surgeons could be crass and poorly educated. Charlatans and butchers of their ilk roamed the streets preying on the impoverished and destitute. The Faculty of the University of Pairs, that paradigm of education, were aghast at the brutality of it all, and had tried to set down principles of practice for those doing surgery years before, but lacked royal awareness. It had worked elsewhere, they knew. Similar restrictions were in place on the Italian peninsula for the Faculty of Medicine at Salerno.[19]

Perhaps it had been the fault of the Church. From the second century on, monastics had assumed the role of healers of the body—and many of them did "hand work" as well. But the Church had long decried the letting of blood. In his encyclical *Ecclesia abhorret a sanguine* ("The Church abhors blood"), Pope Alexander III declared at the Council of Tours in 1163: "Blood has always frightened the Church." Furthermore, he explained, "this fear is natural, blood carries with it a horror which seizes us in spite of ourselves; whether instinct or childhood weakness, it is only by redoubled efforts within ourselves that we can overcome this repugnance which we feel at the sight of blood." Put bluntly was Alexander's feeling that "prejudice has regarded them [surgeons] as cruel men." They could practice their craft, Alexander finally allowed, but only if it were done far from the walls of academia (where ecclesiastic support was firm).[20]

Furthermore, Canon 18 of the Fourth Lateran Council of 1215 specifically prohibited any cleric from practicing "that part of surgery involving burning or cutting."[21] The Church clearly felt that surgery was insulting to the living body (or dead one, for that matter) and those who practiced this heathen craft were dishonorable. In Christian-crazed Europe, papal support for the healing profession was essential. Canon law must be observed. Faculty dare not waver too far from firm dogma and doctrine. Heretics were actively pursued. But in the shadows lurked those who ignored Mother Church. Far too many people were plagued by common ailments of the flesh: abscesses, hemorrhoids, stones, wounds, and difficult pregnancies. Far too many suffered and sought help. For them Church doctrine held no meaning. Relief was needed. So, they approached those willing to comply; who, with knife in hand, carried out chores formerly done by clerics. Skills varied of course. Some were near miraculous in their dexterity. Some were outright butchers.[22]

Reform was needed.

King Philip IV of France was not afraid of the Church. Philip had little patience with the distant papal authority, quarreling even with papal mandates. He intended to free his court from Rome's influence, jerking back any semblance of liege to Church authority. Called the "Iron King," Philip turned to consolidating domestic control. He was determined on several fronts to rein in corruption. As for healthcare, he tired of the itinerant practices of barely competent medical practitioners. In response, he decided to enforce previous declarations of licensure put forth by the Faculty of the University of Paris in 1271. In 1311 Philip issued a regal edict condemning "murderers, highwaymen, counterfeiters, [and] other vagabonds and libertines, tricksters, alchemists, usurers."[23] He knew well, from Pitard and de Mondeville, that Parisian streets were littered with largely ignorant and ill-equipped practitioners. Few were legitimate members of academia, those of the Fraternity of Saints Cosmos and Damian. His ill subjects, relying on the Crown for safety, had fallen victim to the wiles of these charlatans. Philip then decreed that anyone practicing surgery be first examined by "Master Sworn Surgeons."[24]

Violations carried penalties even to loss of life. But certification would prove difficult. Many so-called surgeons hovered in the shadows. Some cut hair, trimmed beards, and lanced boils. Others set bones and splinted sprains. Still others drew blood and pulled teeth. Some were midwives tending to birthings. More were frank quacks, milking the needy of precious coins, and commoners still sought them out.[25]

De Mondeville set out to change all that. He held both a diploma from medical school and an apprenticeship in surgery; he was a *médecins-chirurgien* (physician and surgeon). His knowledge incorporated not only theory of the ιατροι, the traditional healers, but also practical skills, probably one of the first true surgical scientists. It was time for a new medicine, he reasoned. Surgery and physic—hand and mind—must mesh. Healing demanded both. He would write it all down, a textbook of this new surgery:

> In this way the intelligent pupils who will want to learn surgery, will have joy and contentment, mainly those who are literate and know at least the general principles of medicine, and understand the terms of the art; because it is especially for them that a work of this kind is written

His book would be named simply *Chirurgia*—"Surgery." Before God and King, de Mondeville began, the healer had a sacred obligation to aid the infirmed but equally important—and in this required education—to properly interpret their illnesses. His descriptions of surgical technique which filled his pages were done explicitly to explain anatomy, the nature of ailments, and to "dwell at greater length on the explanation of all that is easy or difficult and useful in practice." Like Hippocrates, de Mondeville acknowledged the three elements of healing: the patient, the disease, and the doctor. Beware, he cautioned surgeons, to consider all factors in curing disease. The surgeon played only one part. The patients commanded a larger role. Always central in any effort to treat, de Mondeville emphasized, was the patient.[26]

It was an expansive treatise—a constitutional dissertation for a new surgery. His depictions of anatomy, while primitive, reflected Galen's interpretations of structure and function.[27] He discussed extensively the treatment of wounds, extraction of weapons, and arrest of bleeding. He detailed the most agreeable incisions to use for ulcers, venomous bites, and tumors. His roadmap was what he called the *Zodiaque humain*—the human Zodiac—depicting the twelve regions of the body and the astrological signs which governed them to determine the correct times for surgery or medication or bloodletting. He spoke of the cautery and its uses, of abscesses (apostemes) and their vile contents of blood, bile, and phlegm. His chapters roamed from female disorders to scabies to leprosy to lice and nits to burns, measles, smallpox, cockroaches, warts, and assorted growths. His pictured inventory of surgical instruments rivaled that of the Andalusian surgical genius known as Albucasis two hundred years before: cannulas, cauteries, scissors, syringes, speculums, scalpels, trephines, and tenaculums, drawn and described in minute detail for the curious reader.[28]

As revolutionary as it was, de Mondeville's book went unfinished. He could not conquer his own health. Cough, an annoying shortness of breath, and weakness plagued him. The Greeks had called it $\varphi\theta\acute{\iota}\sigma\iota\varsigma$—"phthisis"—a wasting condition most often, as it turned out, due to pulmonary consumption—tuberculosis. As so many of its victims experienced, his energy diminished. Toward the end of his writing, he could no longer endure. To his readers he explained, "I am not destined to live a long time, unless, by a special grace, God prolongs my existence. I am asthmatic, exhausted, and consumptive." He seemed to know his end was near. He had seen it in his patients. He was dying.[29]

More and more he took to his bed, writing now a distant desire. At the end he was totally infirmed, barely able to raise his head, his sputum the bright red of expectorated blood. And finally, without fanfare or spiritual revelation, he quietly died in 1320. His great book died, too. *Chirurgia* was not even uncovered until historian Julius Pagel from Berlin located the text in 1889, far too late to influence those around him or break with the overbearing resistance of Catholic Christianity to scientific progress.

⁓

A near contemporary, Guy de Chauliac (c. 1300–1368), would finish what de Mondeville started. De Chauliac was from the Auvergne, that hilly, central region of France cut through by the Loire and Allier River valleys. In ancient times, there resided the powerful Gallic *Aruernoi*, the Arverni, whose ferocious warlord, Vercingetorix, had battled Julius Caesar and his legions almost to a standstill. The Arverni tribe continued as a formidable vassal of the Île-de-France into medieval times. Likely a descendant of that fierce clan, Guy de Chauliac was from a small and insignificant hamlet called Claulhac (or Chauliac), containing just 140 residents. Guy's family were likely of peasant stock and simple farmers. Yet at an early age, de Chauliac earned the favor of the powerful Auvergne Lords and Dukes of Mercoeur, some of the first nobility of the French kingdom and rulers of the vast Mercoeur estate of the Auvergne.

Perhaps it was de Chauliac's agreeableness and intellect or perhaps it was something more mysterious.

Some said that an aura of the supernatural hovered like a mystical spirit over the young man. As the legend was told, the teenage de Chauliac had been summoned to the home of a wealthy merchant. It seems his niece had fallen from a horse on a hunting trip and fractured her leg. Fractures of that sort were dangerous injuries, likely to become infected or cause invalidism. The family, as was the rural practice, consulted a sorcerer (some might say, "witch") who informed them that "she will be cured by a peasant," and pointed in the general direction of Chauliac. Guy, as a suitable peasant boy, was called to the young girl's manor. His mere presence apparently had a miraculous effect, and, in two days, the leg was healed. Word quickly spread of his phenomenal talents. Of course, it was assumed Guy had invoked the Virgin Mary. Surely, this boy will be a healer, they might have said, he draws down the divine to intercede where man cannot.[30]

Despite his charisma, Guy de Chauliac was an uneducated, illiterate peasant boy. Ordinarily not fit for formal education, his association with the Mercoeur family probably earned him schooling by Church clergy. Only then did he qualify for medical studies at the University of Montpellier.

The Montpellier school of medicine, located near the Mediterranean coast of France, was founded as early as 1137 and was one of the most progressive of Europe. Its administrators encouraged a wide range of teachers from around the Mediterranean region to instruct. In fact, by edict in 1181 Lord William VIII of Montpellier wrote, "I will, command, praise, and grant in perpetuity that every [qualified] man, from whatever his origin and without interruption, [can] instruct in *physic* at Montpellier." As a result, talented physicians flocked to the place attracted by the academic liberalism of Montpellier.[31] Consequently, with such a renowned faculty, students of medicine eagerly sought admittance. De Chauliac reveled in the academics of physic there but had little exposure to surgery. Like many European schools, the Faculty of Medicine did not teach it. Yet, unlike some medical faculty, surgical interests were not discouraged at Montpellier. Some faculty, like Raymond de Molières, Master of Medicine, had no disdain for surgery and might have even encouraged de Chauliac to pursue it.[32] More probably, though, de Chauliac piqued his interest from surgeons in town. From Montpellier, de Chauliac, like other men who favored surgery, traveled to Italy. In Bologna he studied under the great anatomists, teachers such as Nicola Bertuccio and Alberto de' Zancari.

The availability of human cadaver work was peculiar to Bologna, and Bertuccio was an avid dissector. However, his teachings bordered on Church heresy. The Papal Bull of Boniface VIII, *De Sepolturis*, issued in 1299, strictly forbade tampering with corpses.[33] Perhaps academia turned a blind eye to the brilliant Bertuccio. Both he and fellow anatomist Alberto de' Zancari clandestinely continued their practical teaching even to the point of exhumation of the dead. In Bologna court records of 1319, it was claimed that four of de' Zancari's students exhumed a corpse hanged that very day (fresh cadavers were prized). The body was allegedly taken to the house of de' Zancari where he and his pupils set upon it with "razors and knives" as part of their "medical art." It was this man who opened the eyes of young de Chauliac to the surgical possibilities of healing practices.

From Bologna, de Chauliac settled in Paris. He arrived just after the deaths of Pitard and Henri de Mondeville. By that time, he was a man in his prime, perhaps mid-twenties. Portraits of him from the fifteenth century show an unshaven de Chauliac attending to a patient with a dislocated elbow. His demeanor is befitting an academician, cloaked in the long robe of the learned. He expresses a kindly face with benevolent features in that cartoonish quality of medieval art. Is it a true likeness? Scores of years later, it is doubtful. Who, by that time, could remember his appearance? Still, the setting is sincere. Surrounded by his students, de Chauliac in this portrayal is at once healer and teacher, showing them maneuvers for relocating the painful and twisted arm. From images of the sixteenth century, he is pictured as a man in academic regalia with a pleasing face, a subtle smile, and attentive eyes. He was a scholar, a master of medicine. As for his surgical skills, some of his fellow physicians labeled him as a barber, one of those itinerants who pulled teeth and let blood. De Chauliac was far from that. He understood medicine, was well-versed in anatomy, and used surgical tools only for sound therapeutic purposes. As one who had mastered medicine—much of it at the side of Bologna's Alberto de' Zancari—he functioned as a "*clerc*"—a term most likely meaning a graduate student (or trainee in residence)—and then was awarded Master in Medicine, the highest title conferred in France in the fourteenth century. He may also have taken Holy Orders, as he later referred to himself as "Household Physician and Chaplain of our lord, the Pope."[34]

Toward the end of his life, de Chauliac—like the much admired de Mondeville—wrote his famous compendium *Chirurgia Magna* in 1363. For de Chauliac there was little doubt how healing occurred: his God imparts knowledge (*sciencia*) of the medical arts and permits those knowledgeable (*sciens*) to effect divine cures. There can be no healing outside of it. Those who denounced God and turned to idols were no more than witches and sorcerers and fell under the broad condemnation of *maleficium* ("evil-doer"). Practitioners of the medical arts must be in God's graces and abide by authority of God's earthly representatives—the Holy Church.[35]

De Chauliac, too, knew the medieval world of academia was a world of letters. Only the literate—meaning only the educated—could read, so a true profession existed only in the Latinized pages of books. The street craft of surgeon-barbers had no need of this, but if surgical healing—healing with the hands—were ever to attain noteworthy status, they must be rationalized and standardized in precision-like writing. Not to discount "hands-on" training, but the transmission of science—at its essence, knowledge—from one generation to another demanded it. Almost certainly, de Chauliac knew nothing of de Mondeville's text—he never mentioned it. As far as he was concerned his majestic *Chirurgia Magna* was the first of its kind in France.

To be respected, de Chauliac considered, surgeons must have culture, manners, even patrician bearing. They should understand the outmoded but still popular natural philosophy of Hippocrates and Galen and how surgery applied to it. They should be dexterous technicians: good eyesight, slender fingers, and steady hands. Their judgment must be impeccable, bold yet considered, fearful of perilous things. Above all, they should be gentle and kind.[36]

And, like all healers, they must acknowledge the divine.

As for the true profession of surgery, it was very much a knowledge of healing, de Chauliac wrote: in theory like physic, in practice like artistry. It was "teaching the manner and quality of treating, principally by consolidating, cutting, and performing other manual operations, for the expressed purpose of healing people as far as possible," he explained. With apothecary and *diaeta*—the Greek "manner of living," probably the basis for all of physic—surgery was another arm of treatment.[37] Surgeons, however, had an added duty: the perfection of manual creativity. The surgeon's tools, extensions of his fingers, were the channels for his artistry. The *scalpendo*, the scalpel, was like the chisel and shaping tool of the sculptor, working the restoration of flesh.[38]

To de Chauliac an understanding of science—in its broadest sense—was essential. Without it, physicians were figuratively blind. Those *res naturales* of the Italian del Garbo such as anatomy and botany gave insight to healing efforts. Anatomic structures harbored essences of life: breath, spirit, humors, and virtuous airs. "For a surgeon ignorant of anatomy is like a blind man woodcarving," he insisted.[39] "For the Creator has given each bodily member a specific virtue, that it is not designed in vain or to remain idle," he wrote. Treat it as such, he admonished. God is in all things. Know when to invade and know when to retreat. If cure is not possible, retreat.

Chirurgia Magna was the foremost authoritative text on surgery for almost two hundred years. As for de Chauliac himself, he did not stay in Paris. It was most likely he settled in Lyon with other members of his family. The onset of the Black Death in Europe, though, found de Chauliac in Avignon at the service of Pope Clement VI. With the pestilence, patients succumbed quickly, he noticed. Some, stricken by continuous fever, died in the throes of coughing and gasping of air. Their sputum soon turned crimson, and death quickly followed. Then there were those consumed with fever who broke out in *bubos*, abscess-like excrescences under the arms and in the groin. Too quickly they also dwindled and died within days. As were many, de Chauliac was puzzled by the virulence of the plague, blaming it on supernatural influences, in this case, the astrologic alignment of Saturn, Jupiter, and Mars. This planetary position, he surmised, brought on terrible changes, the coming of prophets and great pestilences. It aimed to destroy human nature—as if God willed it. Despite his focus on earthly remedies and earthly diseases, he could not ignore the impact of the divine, still, on the arrangement of the natural. In his thinking, it would always be that way.[40]

Guy de Chauliac remained in Avignon, even after the death of Clement VI. His connection with the Church, for all its imperfections, remained solid. He was a man of God and welcomed divine influence into his healing practices. To that end, he never failed to invoke the supernatural in healing affairs of the natural. It is not known the precise date of his death, probably around 1370. His great book, though, would long outlive him. The dawn of scientific investigation—evidence and knowledge—was breaking. His anatomy and his surgical techniques provided a foundation for surgery, not as a barbaric spectacle, but as a legitimate component of the healing art, the manual arm of compassion.

CHAPTER SIX

Angelical Conjunctions

Repent. Let God heal your sins and then heal your body.

Whirlwinds of sickness still hounded both the Old and New Worlds as the Age of Reason—that epoch of intellectual curiosity of the seventeenth and eighteenth centuries—unfolded. Without respite, the complexities of health and the uncertainty of healing puzzled all. Accordingly, disease remained tightly linked to moral behavior and was generally viewed by those of faith as some signal of displeasure from God. Could healing be done without attention to the soul, then? Many felt not, and physicians of any repute continued to prescribe nostrums that would empty a troubled body of evils perpetuated by a troubled soul. The result was a blending of the natural and supernatural, one of medical scholarship might want to be adept at both, and preachers of formal education veered into the realm of physic as an instinctive tendency of their calling.

From the earliest days of Christianity, healers promoted an angelical conjunction as the proper working of spirit on flesh. No better place than the monasteries of the Church. These cloistered places relied on a mingling of Godly petitions and medicinal concoctions to alleviate illness. Few blamed diseases on natural causes alone. Perhaps, they reasoned, ailments had causes outside of heavenly realms, that disorders of mankind were corruptions, brought about solely by disturbances of *diaita*, the manner of living: diet, environment, health. Most reasonings invoked the supernatural. Divine trials and tribulations provoked internal disharmony. Beware, sinner, that God will punish your wicked ways.

Of course, medieval illness had been mostly speculation; fevers and epidemics puzzling, likely of divine origin. Hippocratic humoral theories still held sway. Yet by the seventeenth century, natural laws began to fall under the scrutiny of observation, deduction, and logical interpretation. It was to become the Age of Reason. The new philosophy of the French scholastic, René Descartes (1596–1650), focused on observation and analysis. Sensory encounter was the source of all knowledge. Descartes' Cartesian approach did not deny God, it simply operated outside of God. Now, slowly, religion and the newfound science of knowledge began to diverge; religion no longer an a priori necessity for understanding daily happenings.

Science was probing, experimenting, and observing. Knowledge of the invisible mounted that did not pertain to the spiritual world, as if workings still to be exposed were at play:

> That there are such Things in Nature, i.e. immaterial Beings, Substances naked of any Matter, or Corporeal Parts, invisible to the Eye, undiscernible to the Touch, without Flesh and Bones, as ordinary Creatures have; Beings hidden from our outward Senses, either filling or traversing the World, unseen, unobserved for the most part, by our weak Intellectuals; is so certain a Truth.[1]

For medicine, Andreas Vesalius and William Harvey dismantled Galenic thinking and showed that man could be anatomized as minutely as stars and planets. Humors did not necessarily determine health. The same physical laws governing astronomy and mathematics might be applied now to man. The human machinery should be analyzed as a mechanical spinoff of anatomy, they reasoned. Extend static anatomy to dynamic function. Hearts and arteries and lungs might have the same properties as pumps and pipes and bellows. As for the ghostly spirit, science tried to separate the two—one independent of the other. But sicknesses were still a conundrum. The hand of God must be in play, many thought. In this regard, few could completely divorce science from faith.[2]

As for cures? Rare, in truth, but when they happened, cures were occasions of wonder, as much blamed on God's mercy as not. Not through any prescriptions of man did seemingly miraculous happen but through divine intercession. All healing came from God, so claimed the English clergyman William Turner in 1697:

> From Miracles: Prithee, Reader, answer me, whether or no, those Wonders in Nature, which we call Miracles, be nothing else but a meer Lye and Forgery? If not; then how comes the World to be so generally imposed on? How comes not only the Christian, but Jewish Religion to be confirmed and ratified in so fixed a posture as they have been amongst Men? Or what makes our Scriptures and Annals, and Books of History, so big with them? If yea; then, I hope, they

speak a Divinity, and a supernatural Power concerned in the performance of them.[3]

~

But in the New World of colonial America, science lacked penetration. Religion and the Christian God were paramount and could explain all, and Hippocratic humors reigned. Disease remained a form of retribution or reward by the heavenly bodies and mostly a spiritual, rather than corporal concern. For the English Puritan sect, their sole purpose of colonization was "to carry the Gospel into those Parts of the World, and Raise a Bulwark against the Kingdom of Antichrist, which the Jesuits labour to Rear up in all Parts of the World."[4]

It was a sickly country, though. Existence in the New World was fraught with plagues, distempers, and dysenteries. "The Calamities that have carried off the Inhabitants of our several Towns have not been all of one sort . . . Pestilential *Sicknesses* have made fearful Havock in divers Places," the Puritan minister Cotton Mather later wrote.[5] Puritans demanded exacting accountability for human sinfulness, that the corruption of mortal bearings could be found everywhere. And nothing was more apparent than the wrath of a vengeful God shown by suffering. Clergy hounded their flocks to mend evil ways, that, with epidemics, God was punishing all for the sinning of a few. Would that the humble servants of the Lord in these colonies could relieve suffering by unctions and remedies of all sorts. But, alas, they could not. Disease ran its course unaltered and seemingly by divine whims. Only prayer and righteous behavior might stem the tide of calamities of health. And congregations and ministers prayed fervently that God reverse his punishment and hardships to favor healing.

Indeed, health was a matter of repentance.

Still, wellness faltered everywhere, and sickness took men, women, and children even at the pinnacle of wellness. Why such perturbations? The hand of God was to blame, the sinfulness of man the reason. Oxford scholar Robert Burton wrote *Anatomy of Melancholy*, a dissertation on disease in general but the mental agitations of melancholy in particular, published in 1621 and already in New England in the library of Puritan pastor Increase Mather by 1660. Burton alluded to sicknesses as the humbler of mortal pride:

Sickness, diseases, trouble many, but without cause. It may be 'tis for the good of their souls . . . the flesh rebels against the spirit; that which hurts the one, must needs help the other. Sickness is the mother of modesty, putteth us in minde of our mortality; and, when we are in the full career of worldly pomp and jollity, she pulleth us by the ear, and maketh us know ourselves.[6]

Avoid fear and sorrow, Burton encouraged. Instead suffuse the mind with mirth, constancy, good hope. Remove vain terror and all bad thoughts. The body's troubles, he claimed, stemmed from the soul. So, to rectify the flesh, satisfy the mind. If the mind remains bothered, the body will never heal. Use prayer and "physick" together, he admonished, if medicine be allowed to work at all.

Colonial clergy flailed on their congregations to search their souls for sinfulness. Repent, was their message. Penance, fasting, prayer. Puritan preacher Michael Wigglesworth (1631–1705) saw by 1662

> Our healthful days are at an end/ And sicknesses come on/ From yeer to yeer, because our hearts/ Away from God are gone/ New-England, where for many yeers/ You scarcely heard a cough,/ And where Physicians had no work,/ Now finds them work enough . . . We turn not from our sins./ We stopp our ear against reproof,/ And hearken not to God:/ God stops his ear against our prayer,/ And takes not off his rod.[7]

Wigglesworth himself was stricken with enormous guilt for his own perceived transgressions. Fearful of divine retribution, he struggled, as many did, apologetically for forgiveness. It was almost impossible to offer enough supplication to amend his sins. His God was one of anger and punishment, for as much as he would do, the evils of sin would rise again within the sordidness of his body:

> [I]n a word my heart and words and actions go wholly out of frame, and voyd of any thing of god, that I see my sin is above measure sinfull; I loath my self, and could even take vengeance of my self for these abominations.[8]

Wigglesworth was a sullen, selfish busybody, a parody of the New England Puritan.[9] Yet so typical were such feelings of inadequacy that it provided a ready explanation for the anxieties of New England life. Little could be done to stave off the menacing threat of sickness. Ministers had a particularly valuable role. Generally, among the most educated of colonial citizenry, they knew that healing was a matter of the spiritual, aided by various concoctions only the learned could decipher.[10] Even then, so-called humoral medicine reigned—the humors in excess or deficiency. Purgatives, emetics, bleedings, blisterings. All meant to counteract the perceived imbalance of natural humors. While ministers exhibited a modicum of restraint, others, less scrupulous, proclaimed themselves as healers—"doctor" was the term used—and could wreak havoc on their sufferers. "The doctors have no licenses, and by means of this very license (or lack of restraint) they are the worse," one prominent diarist wrote.[11]

And then there were the "piss prophets." Seventeenth-century physician-satirist Thomas Brian published an essay denouncing the great fascination some doctors had with urine. His pamphlet, titled, "Wherein are newly discovered the old fallacies, deceit, and juggling of the Piss-pot, Science, used by all those (whether Quacks, and Empirics, or other methodical Physicians) who pretend knowledge on Diseases, by the Urine, in giving judgment of the same," claimed the common man was so trusting and in awe of physicians and their ability to discern diseases as to be hard pressed to relinquish those misconceptions put forth by doctors pretending to knowledge that they would nary dare to admit the folly of their beliefs.

It was largely hogwash, Brian wrote. "There is no certain judgment of any disease by the Urine," Brian maintained, and those who profess to the contrary are charlatans holding flasks of urine as some prophetic accolade of their astuteness and skill in interpreting those excreted humors. Woe to him who ignores the more worrisome symptoms of disease such as fever, malaise, and cachexia and relies on the yellow waters of error. Why the choice of ill-educated physicians? Brian attributes the bad judgment to picking an "insufficient man" or, even with proper knowledge, one who is "no fit Physician for thee."[12]

Understandably, few trusted in physic. Rather, seek the Savior as the Redeemer, common wisdom said. The first allegiance of the sick was to God, not physic, so preached English theologian William Perkins. Forget the doctor, turn to prayer:

> And that is in the very first place of al before any other helpe be sought for. Where the Divine endes, there the Physician must begin: and it is a very preposterous course that the Divine should ther begin where the Physician makes an ende. For till help be had for the soule, and sinne which is the root of sicknes be cured, physicke [physic] for the body is nothing.[13]

For the soul is far more valuable than the corrupt body, Perkins believed. And man, by his very nature, was susceptible to evil. God's wrath was understandable as justifiable punishment for breaking His covenant. The body will decay but the soul is everlasting, in heaven or in hell. Repent. Only then consider medicine:

> First of all, he that is to take physicke, must not onely prepare his body, as physicians doe prescribe; but he must also prepare his soule by humbling himselfe under the hand of god in his sicknesse for his sinnes and make earnest praier to God for the pardon of them before any medicine come in his body.[14]

Cure or death, man is not to question the will of God, Perkins went on. "We must not judge of the estate of any man before God by outward things, whether they be blessings or judgments, whether they fal in life or death."[15] The children of God most dear to him, Perkins claimed, attained corresponding heights of everlasting happiness through their torments of last hours and days. God's plan is mysterious, and maybe contrary to hope, but such is the matter of faith.

As for doctoring, Perkins declared that prescriptions be morally justified and in line with soulful restoration. Healing would not be possible without cleansing of the immortal spirit in reparation for sins:

> And to conclude this point touching physicke, I will here set downe two especiall duties of the physician himselfe. The first is, that in the want and defect of such as are to put sicke men in minde of their sinnes, it is a duty specially concerning him, he being a member of Christ, to advertise his parties that they must truely humble themselues, and pray fervently to God for the pardon of all their sinnes.[16]

Of body and soul, few ministers brought both together like the Puritan pastor Cotton Mather (1663–1728). He was a man of immense religiosity but exquisite sensitivity. In a time of intense faith as shelter for the unpredictable quirks of nature, Mather keenly understood the susceptibility of man to precarious fluxes of health—and was terrified of it. By his bargaining with God, pleading sinfulness and deep contrition, he hoped to ward off the inevitable: his Savior's condemnation. Mather's hope of an afterlife saturated his thoughts and helped console his troubled and fearful mind—if only he were found worthy. His wordy writings, inquisitive as they were, vented his worries of earthly suffering. And, too, ministering to the ill—both of flesh and spirit—provided a distraction by comforting the miserable.

Mather knew his flock needed both spiritual and corporal attention. The worthy minister, Mather explained, was one dedicated to the divine, but also to worldly suffering. "He that for his lively ministry was justly reckoned among 'the angels of the churches,' might for his medical acquaintance, experiences, and performances, be truly called a Raphael [Hebrew *Rĕphā'ēl*, 'God has healed']," Mather wrote. He argued that ever since the days of the evangelist Luke, medical skills were practiced by those dedicated to the study of divinity. The Art of Healing was first given to those set apart for the care of souls. And now, in the dispersed communities of raw New England, this "angelical conjunction"—the union of the divine and the corporal—was necessary to cater to "the poor to whom the gospel is preached," and delivered by preachers moved not only by the Word of God but also the ravages of disease.[17]

Yet Mather was a worrier, obsessed by fears of his own suffering and death. "But, now Illness and Vapour, with an aguish Indisposition, growes upon mee, at such a rate, that indeed I live in exceeding Misery: and I can see nothing but a speedy Death approaching," he wrote in his diary.[18] Perhaps it had begun in childhood, an anxiety that left him hopelessly stuttering. Even then, a devout Calvinist, he thought his garbled speech a punishment from God. So fearful of heavenly retribution, he was never without the premonition of approaching death. By age thirty he felt stalked by the grim reaper. "O save mee! O heal mee! O work for mee, work in mee, the good Pleasure of thy Goodness . . . there is a desperate Wickedness, from which I am yet uncleansed."[19] He would pray daily and fast. In the evenings he would lay prostate in the dust of his home in supplication and beg for his God's mercy. This did not rid him of his private Devil. So mindful was Mather that he constantly fasted and prayed in order to put off temptations—"Distempers of the Heart," he would call them.[20] His entire life would be one spent in spiritual flagellations as proper penance for his wicked soul.

Nevertheless, with all his personal drama, the sicknesses of others endeared him most. These wretched folks drove him to libraries laden with medical texts where he would seclude among the stacks—even before the age of fourteen. Without formal medical education, Mather acquired a sense of "physick" through his readings from his father's private collections and at Harvard College. He was reclusive and studious, more at home alone than with neighborhood friends. His stuttering probably anchored him there, afraid of ridicule. At the same time, he turned inward, accepting harsh self-criticism and dwelling on his innate sense of unworthiness. Entering Harvard at age twelve he studied arithmetic, geometry, logic, ethics, politics, astronomy, Hebrew, and Greek. His father's intent was that the young man join the ministry, as many graduates of Harvard did. But stammering made him hardly fit for the pulpit. Only with extreme concentration would he overcome it. Later, in sympathy, he would wonder as to the cause. Of stutterers, were they inherently anxious, irritable, and impatient? In self-deprecation he would write of the problem: "[c]holeric of Disposition; and *Sooner Angry* than they should be." The remedy? Pray. "[W]hat a release from the Extremity of your *Infirmity* may be obtained, by your ardent and constant Prayers, to a SAVIOUR, who by one Touch of His Almighty Hand can *open a Door of Utterance* for you."[21] His own stammering was an embarrassment. Maybe for that reason he lost himself in medical texts. Perhaps, even, understanding life could help him reconcile his fear of death. "I composed Systems both of Logick and Physick, in Catechisms of my own, which have been used by many others." His fascination with medicine became almost a hypochondriacal obsession:

> I fell under the Power of Melancholy to such a Degree that I exceedingly wonder it had no worse Effects upon me, and studying *Physick at the time*, I was unhappily led away with Fancies, that I was myself troubled, with almost every Distemper that I read of.[22]

It might be that an impressionable (and, no doubt, neurotic) teenaged Mather was struck by the somberness of the smallpox epidemic of 1678 as he watched an almost endless parade of hearses transporting deceased to burial grounds:

> Never was it such a time in Boston. Boston burying-places never filled so fast. It is easy to tell the time wherein we did not use to have the bells tolling for burials or a sabbath day morning by sunrise; to have 7 buried on a sabbath day night after [church] Meeting. To have coffins crossing each other as they have been carried in the street; - To have, I know not how many corpses following each other close at their heels.[23]

As for his stuttering, he asked for the mercy of Jesus to rid him of his affliction. Then, when he was at Harvard College, an old schoolmaster visited him and offered salvation—in the manner of deliberate, thoughtful oratory. "By this *Deliberation* you will be accustomed anon to Speak so much without the *Indecent Hesitations*, that you'll always be in the way of it," the old man counseled. Following that advice, the stammering relented, and, as Mather later told, "the young Man [Cotton Mather, of course] soon became a Preacher in Great Congregations."[24]

His curiosity of physic stayed with him. He had no experience in bedside practices and had no formal education in medical matters. Mostly, he relegated that function to physicians. But he understood suffering. In those days death and misery were ever present. For one so convinced that sickness and death were the consequences of sin, awareness of medicine could offer some hope of physical, if not spiritual, salvation. As for his Puritan religion, there was a general support for the sciences, since the natural and supernatural were viewed as a harmonious relationship. He had dutifully abided by his father's insistence on learning and had read lengthy discussions from Boston's Philosophical Society. Besides, charity to others promoted "goodness." Mather believed that each individual was responsible for the dissemination of good deeds and care for the community. As for the downtrodden, the ill, the impoverished, he advised: "'Tis possible, 'tis probable, you may do well to *Visit* them; and when you *Visit* them, *Comfort* them. Carry them some *Good Word*, which may raise a *Gladness*, in an *Heart Stouping* [sic] *with Heaviness*."[25]

While he gladly accepted his primary role as that of Puritan minister, he never gave up his interest in medicine. The relief of misery appealed to his carnal as well as his spiritual nature. Sin was the ultimate cause of sickness. As a clergyman, he saw himself as a practitioner of health. Curing a troubled and sinful soul was paramount to curing an ailing body. Physic, in Mathers' opinion, was a mere supplement to religion. In fact, all of nature was a manifestation of God's goodness and supreme power. "When we contemplate the obvious wonders, and beauties of the world, and survey the operations of prolific nature, we are forced to acknowledge, that the Divine power is manifest in every part," he wrote in 1720.[26] Indeed, he was privy to such miraculous events. In September 1683, at age twenty, he had prayed over his dear friend, Avery, who was drawing near death with an unconquerable illness. As Mather prayed, his friend "felt as it were a Load, or Cloud, beginning to roll off his Spirits; and from that Instant, unto his own Admiration, hee began to recover."[27]

Like orthodox Puritans, he believed in witchcraft and demonic possession. For three successive days he beseeched his God to rid a young woman he thought hopelessly entrapped by devils. "Unto my Amazement, when I had kept my *third Day* for her, shee was finally and forever delivered from the hands of *evil Angels*."[28] The mischievous doings of Satan were ever-present threats. In March 1693 his wife delivered a son who died a few days later of an imperforate anus. Distraught by the death, Mather quickly blamed the convenient scapegoat, witchcraft.

> [B]ecause my wife, a few weeks before her Deliverance, was affrighted with a horrible *Spectre*, in our Porch, which Fright caused her Bowels to turn within her; and the *Spectres* which both before and after, tormented a young Woman in our Neighbourhood, brag'd of their giving my Wife that Fright, in hopes, they said, of doing Mischief unto her Infant.[29]

Mather clung to the belief that his God was a God of miracles, and, as with his friend Avery, fervent praying over the sick produced unexpected healings. One poor woman of the neighborhood, ill for years with an ailment no number of physicians could treat, and now near death, lay before Mather and a group of Christians who prayed and read the Bible. She surprisingly recovered as proof, in his mind, of "the wondrous Works of God."[30] He visited the infirmed often. Of distempers and tumors, he had only prayer and fasting to offer the sick, which he did in abundance, his arrays of medicines seldom employed. Whether recovered or not, it was the will of his God. Only the divine could provide reasoning for life's sufferings, he believed. "[T]he many Scores of sick Families in my Neighborhood, and yett it being my desire to visit them as far as tis possible," he wrote. If not the body, then perhaps the soul he could comfort.[31]

Even his own ailments perplexed him, aches and pains he could not explain. He wrote in his diary December 9, 1711, frustrated at the failure of worthy remedies to work:

> All Methods and Medicines for my Cure, fail me. I have used Unguents, and Plaisters, and Cataplasms, and Epispaspicks, and Sinapisms, and Cathartticks, and what not! But all to no purpose. My Physicians are of no value. My Pains this Morning are more violent than they use to be. I ly down like a Stag in a Nett with a very despairing Discouragement.

He pleaded to his God. "I acknowledged the Power of my Enthroned Saviour, over the World, and over Diseases; and His Empire over the mighty Angels." He begged forgiveness and for help, and his God and his Angels finally came to the rescue. "My Pains immediately went off," he then found. The Lord had cured him.[32]

But far worse was to come for his struggling congregations. In May 1721, "The grievous Calamity of the *Small-Pox* has now entered the Town."[33] Mather likened the epidemic to one of his destroying Angels standing over Boston. In typical Puritan fashion, he blamed wickedness for the contagion.

> The monstrous and crying Wickedness of this Town (a Town at this time strangely possessed with the Devil) and the vile Abuse which I do myself particularly suffer from it, for nothing but my instructing our base Physicians, how to save many precious Lives.[34]

"This miserable Town, is a dismal Picture and Emblem of *Hell*; *Fire with Darkness* filling of it, and a *lying Spirit* reigning there," he went on.[35] Prayers for the sick consumed more and more of his time. His fasting increased and private supplication became more obsessive. He implored his flock to make right with the Lord and be prepared for any eventuality the contagion might have readied for them. In a more practical vein, he urged doctors to use the new method of inoculation as a preventative measure.

Smallpox was a bane of New England existence. It had been part of Puritan life, almost from their first steps onto the New World. Very likely, smallpox had decimated the local population of Native American Narragansetts even before Puritans arrived. In fact, horrible epidemics followed the earliest settlers, felling thousands more Native Americans, and almost annihilating their tribes. In Boston, within a year of its founding in 1630, smallpox struck. Epidemics in the city followed in 1636, 1638, 1640, and six more times before 1700. From the pulpit, of course, fire and brimstone rained down on congregations, spiritual behavior the obvious culprit: "The still outstretched hand of God's powerful wrath over this poor country, smiting down our pillars, plucking up our stakes and taking from us the breath of our nostrils is a matter so doleful, solemnly awful and tremendous."

It was a wicked infirmity. Such virulence could only be divine in origin. The spreading plague panicked any household of the day, as children and adults were vulnerable. Contagion! Windows were shuttered, doors barred. Quoting from Lamentations (5:16–17), preachers admonished "Woe unto us that we have sinned!"[36] Among those was smallpox, such a disease feared by both indigenous and immigrant peoples. The Massachusetts physician Zabdiel Boylston gave a vivid description of the horrors of the unchecked disease:

> Some of the bad Symptoms attending . . . Purple Spots, the bloody and parchment Pox, Hemorrhages of Blood at the Mouth, Nose, Fundament, and Privities; Ravings and Deliriums, Convulsions, and other Fits; violent inflammations and Swellings in the Eyes and Throat; so that they cannot see, or scarcely breathe, or swallow any things, to keep them from starving. Some looking as black as the Stock, others as white as a Sheet; in some the Pock runs into Blisters, and the Skin stripping-off leaves the Flesh raw, like Creatures flea'd. Some have a burning, others a smarting Pain, as if in the Fire, or scalded with boiling Water.[37]

Mather knew well of the consequences of smallpox epidemics. Of his observation on Native epidemics, not one in ten survived, he wrote.[38] To him it was but another manifestation of the displeasure of God on his community. "There is a *Great Plague* which we call, the SMALL POX, wherein *the Misery of Man is great upon him*," Cotton Mather wrote of the disease. Mather railed at mankind for the folly of sin that gave rise to this horrid distemper, "Wilt thou not from the View and Sense of this *New Evil Devised* against thee, Humble thyself *under the mighty Hand of God?*"[39] His chief advise for the treating physician was to "steer and rule the Passions, and keep up the

Hopes of the Patient." Of course, the various concoctions of the day were to be tried, including emetics to cast out the "Morbid Matter" in vomit. Diarrhea, if present, was to be encouraged to pass down the "Peccant Matter." Narcotics, either laudanum or diacodium, were indispensable, and bloodletting on occasion, Mather felt, life-saving. Most of all, though, the victim should turn to God. "Thou wouldest without Delay, Sett apart Some Time to go through a *Process of Repentance* and *Lay hold on Eternal Life*." Prepare for death, Mather advised. Turn to God and ask mercy and forgiveness. Reject your wretched soul.[40]

Despite acknowledging the divine, albeit capricious will of his Lord, Mather could never reconcile suffering and death with a merciful God. Thirteen of his fifteen children and two of his three wives died before him. That it be God's will was ever on his mind, yet he seemed perplexed at the seeming injustice of such tragedy befalling those of sound moral character, faithful, and righteous. Was it a God who delivered hardships to strengthen the soul or a God meting out punishment for some unrecognized transgression? Still, it was imperative to hold a strong faith. Little else could explain the hardships of this life. Physicians were powerless. Only a divine plan, invisible though it was, could provide an answer. Despite his misgivings, Mather stolidly provided comfort and unyielding faith in his God's mysterious plans:

> My Kinsman at Roxbury, lies a dying; full of Distress and Darkness about his future State. With much Importunity and Impatience, he calls for me to be fetch'd over to him. I have the Satisfaction to strengthen him in his Agonies, and advise him, and comfort him; and leave him with a sensible Satisfaction, and a good Hope thro' Grace arrived unto him.[41]

He died the next day, blissfully, Mather indicated (but that might have been hopeful conjecture).

In 1724, four years before his death, Mather wrote *The Angel of Bethesda* that would be the only compilation of medical knowledge found in the English-American colonies. In his words it was an "essay upon the common maladies of mankind," incorporating a "rich collection of plain but potent and approved remedies." Yet throughout his text, he still could not separate disease from punishment, flesh from God, natural from supernatural:

> If we enquire after the Origin of DISEASES, we shall not Enquire wisely after this Matter, if we do not find we SIN against the Holy and Blessed ONE, to be the Root of Bitterness, from whence they have all arisen.
>
> The *God of our Health* is never praised with the Acknowledgments that are due unto Him. Nor indeed has he Skilful *Physician* always the *Esteem* and *Reward*

that he deserves. He that appears like an Angel while the Cure is yet expected, appears in quite another Shape after it is accomplished.. . . But, syrs, tis the *Health of the SOUL*, that is most of all to be wish'd for. [42]

His grasp of human anatomy and physiology was remarkable for one lacking formal education in medicine. "The body of man, being most obvious to our view, is that with which we will begin; a machine of a most astonishing workmanship and contrivance. My God, I will praise thee, for I am strangely and wonderfully made," he wrote, almost mirroring the views of a distant renowned Dutch physician, Herman Boerhaave.[43] His fascination with the human form was palpable. "In the body of man the lodgment of the parts is as admirable as the parts themselves."[44] His anatomy was exacting—nerves, arteries, viscera, brain, eyes, ears. He detailed anatomic structures and provisions for warding off evils, namely secretions of glands. Lastly, he recognized the soul. "[T]he stupendous faculties of the soul! the wisdom, with which a soul may perform wonderful things. It is the wisdom that God puts into the heart of a Solomon."[45]

Yet practicing medicine was far more than the studious pursuit of knowledge. To Mather physic was a complex and dynamic process, as much spiritual effort as scientific. Physicians had onerous responsibilities to the community. He wrote of this commitment in his work, *Bonifacious*—how Christians should look not to the heavens but to earth for opportunities to distribute God's love for mankind. Particularly, for physicians:

> Sirs; You will never count your selves to be such *Adeptists* [skilled alchemists] as to be at *a Stand* [complacent] in your Studies, and make no further Progress in your Enquiries, into *Maladies*, & after *Medicines* . . . [instead] you will be Diligent, and Studious, and Inquisitive; and still *Read* much, and *Think* more, and *Pray* most of all; and be Solicitous, to *Find out*, and *Give out*, Something very considerable for the *Good of Mankind*.[46]

And for his congregations, trust not solely in physicians, he admonished. "T'wil be a very foolish and faulty thing, to fall into the Distemper of him Concerning whom it is left upon Record: *In his Disease he Sought not unto the Lord, but unto the Physicians. . . .* But place the Dependence on God alone to Direct and prosper them." Rather, for the glorious cure of disease "My Help Cometh from the LORD who made Heaven and Earth." The physician was ordained by God to perform miraculous wonders but his strength and skill came not from schooling but from the heavens above. And disease arose not from the flesh itself but from the tarnished, corrupted soul. But too often, in his opinion, did physicians become bogged down in the more earthy aspects of human existence. He, too, rankled at the preoccupation with urine some physicians manifested. Those ignominious "piss prophets." Such goings on, he felt, were "meer [*sic*] Fallacy and Imposture." The victims were unsuspecting patients who placed their trust in such apparent nonsense.[47]

Cotton Mather was the personification of angelical conjunction. It was his term and his practice. For one more committed to spiritual health, he knew the vital components of bodily healing, that the soul become one with a divine nature and, in union, accept the whims of an imperfect earth. His was not a unique perspective. Interplay of the physical and metaphysical wove its way through many cultures and seemed inseparable from the natural laws that governed both.

~

CHAPTER SEVEN

Heȟáka Sápa, Lakȟóta Healer

It is nature that surrounds us. Nature also brings the manifestation of supernatural might—thundering skies, rolling seas, trembling ground. Such terrors that even the psychologist Sigmund Freud admitted were "forces majestic, cruel, and inexorable," which led mankind to appease their authority through a religious construct of the invisible. Might these energies also fall within the purview of sickness and health—perhaps whimsical, perhaps purposeful? Might they be the metaphysical that defies scientific explanation? Those who lived closer to the earth understood this and appealed to the spirits that not only possessed them but also coexisted in their surroundings.[1]

Nineteenth-century ethnologist, "Indian Man" James Mooney, spent time among the Native Americans of the Plains and was taken by their spiritual lifestyle. He wrote, at one point about their response to disease and illness:

> The faith of the patient has much to do with his recovery, for the Indian has the same implicit confidence in the shaman that a child has in a more intelligent physician. The ceremonies and prayers are well calculated to inspire this feeling, and the effect thus produced upon the mind of the sick man undoubtedly reacts favorably upon his physical organization.[2]

For Native Americans nature was their constant companion. Spirits hovered everywhere and were as much a part of their surroundings as flesh and blood.

Healing in the world of the Lakȟóta (Lakota), a Native people of the northern plains, was a spiritualization of physical infirmities. Common-folk remedies proved useful much of the time, but those more serious afflictions demanded the presence of a healer, a holy man, or what is sometimes called a "medicine man." This person would ritualistically invoke the powers of the invisible world. By their ceremonies—prayers, songs, and gestures—the victim might feel a presence of healing. Whether real or imagined did not matter; if tranquility was the result, cure was a success.

Lakota healing is best explained through the eyes of one such man, the remarkable *Heȟáka Sápa*, known to white men as Black Elk. Years after his role as shaman to the Lakota, Black Elk told his elaborate story to ethnographer John G. Neihardt in the 1930s. Neihardt fashioned a novelistic retelling, but Black Elk's transcript was later published verbatim by fellow anthropologist Raymond DeMallie.

Black Elk was a *wakȟáŋ wičháša*, a holy man. To him was given a divine mission, that of communicating with the Lakota spirit world. In that sense, he was a healer, one who was called when standard folk remedies failed. He was the interpreter of illness, the maker of magical herbs, and the conductor of rituals designed to invoke spiritual intercession. As a man, he was utterly Lakota. He presented the slim but subtle muscular build of the Plains Indian, high cheekbones, aquiline nose, the epicanthic eyes of a distant Asian heritage, bronze skin, and a neutral gaze of one interpreting all before expressing any. His look was intimidating, the stony gaze of a scrutinizing Lakota. Within Black Elk was embedded the stolid bearing of Lakota ethos.

His account is a story of rich Lakota culture. It is a story told in great detail, sometimes disjointed, sometimes repetitious, but a story of healing and inner peace as Lakota interpreted it. As holy man and healer, he cared for the ills of his people. His healing rituals were elaborate, methodical. Each event, each word, each movement was a priestly function that plaited a fabric of Lakota life and beliefs. Like the ancient Greeks, theirs was a culture of mysticism and magic. And, like the Greeks, it served to placate an existence sometimes fraught with fear and danger. But Black Elk's story is also one of tragedy: the attempted annihilation of the Lakota people and the forced replacement of one culture—one healing—by another.

By tradition, priestly Lakota shamans, the *wakȟáŋ wičháša*, were anointed after a long process of development, instruction, and visionary phenomena that usually began in early childhood. In Lakota thinking, holy men were chosen by the spirits, not by man. Such was the story of Black Elk. To understand him and his people is to know his background.

That foremost, Black Elk was a brave Lakota, there was no doubt. He was a member of the Oglala band. The Oglala were one of the seven tribes of Lakota, members of the *Očhéthi Šakówiŋ*, the Seven Council Fires. Although not for sure, he thinks he was born sometime around 1863 on the Powder River, somewhere within the present-day Wyoming borders, in "The Winter When the Four Crows Were Killed" (December). Black Elk's mother was named White Cow Sees. His father was a *wapiyé*, a healer—one who makes new. His father was a cousin to Crazy Horse's father (making Black Elk a second cousin). The iconic Crazy Horse, *Šúŋka-Witkó*, was the bravest of all Lakota. He was a formidable chieftain, cunning warrior, and fearless combatant.

Black Elk also knew troubled times. He endured the "Indian Wars" of the late 1800s. In fact, according to his telling, it was "The Moon of Making Fat" (June–June 25, 1876, the exact date) that Custer was "rubbed out." That morning the sun was thick with heat, he remembered. For the Lakota, the season of roaming and hunting was at hand. Tipis ranged as far as the eye could see. But on that day, his people would not hunt buffalo, they would hunt white men. He heard that "blue-coat" soldiers were coming. He was not yet a teenager, but the memories were vivid. Black Elk saw many Lakota warriors paint their bodies, grab spears and arrows and guns, and mount their ponies. They wore no clothes, a sign, he knew, of impending combat. *Hokahey* he heard them yell—"Let's go!"—and felt the ground tremble with the reverberation of horses' hooves. Then he saw them. White men—*wašíču*—were galloping across the Greasy Grass (Little Big Horn River), hollering and shooting. These *wašíču*—these fat-takers and big-talkers— were crazy people. Now they were chasing Lakota as they had chased the sacred buffalo and wanted to kill them all. What for, who knew. Oglala women and children were running for the hills to save themselves. Then gunshots, shouting, screaming, and splashing. Lakota warriors were converging on them. The *wašíču* soldiers tumbled from their mounts into the stream. Black Elk's father gave him a six-shooter to take to his brother over at the Hunkpapa camp. He took the gun, flipped onto a buckskin mare, and sped to the Greasy Grass himself, excited to be a young warrior, too, although he was not yet thirteen. Maybe he could count coup like a man. He came upon a blue-coat soldier in the water, thrashing about. "Boy, get off and scalp him," a painted Lakota shouted to him. Black Elk took his knife out and tried, but the *wašíču*'s hair was short and he pulled away, grinding his teeth as Black Elk sawed. Frustrated, Black Elk stopped, pulled out his revolver and calmly shot the soldier between the eyes. Back on his pony, he rode to his brother, gave him the pistol, and galloped on to find *wašíču* to scalp. There were plenty. He took his hairy hides back to his mother who yelped with pride.

The maturing Black Elk had been a quiet child. Obedient. Observant. He saw and heard but rarely spoke. Events and people made deep impressions on him, and he stored away those experiences and lessons. He would say his mind was a gift that saw beyond the ordinary. It was almost expected, in Lakota culture, that those destined to become *wapiyé* would have such visions. Experiences in the spirit world were essential for healers to understand their connection with nature and their favor with Lakota spirits. At age four, he says, he heard voices singing. By age five he had his own pony. One day, when he was riding in the woods, he saw a thunderstorm coming and heard a voice in it. Then he saw two men with lances appearing from the cloud. They were singing a sacred song. A kingbird fluttered by and told him to listen. He heard the men sing: "Behold him, a sacred voice is calling you. All over the sky a sacred voice is calling you." He had no idea what they were telling him. The ghostly disappeared, but Black Elk would hear those voices from time to time. Afraid he might be called crazy, he kept their messages to himself.

Then when he was nine, he fell ill. So sick was he that his arms and legs swelled and he could barely stand up. His worried mother and father put him in their tipi and laid him down. He must have lapsed into delirium because his dream-like visions began. The same two men he saw at age five were coming toward him again.[3] As he later told it, his revelations were very complex, confusing, and startling. He remembered vividly, though, his meeting with spirit-figures who seemed to summon him for a holy mission.

The first two men who appeared beckoned him to follow them into the clouds. "Your grandfather is calling you," they said. He rose and did so, climbing aboard a cloud with them as he saw his mother and father looking on. He felt sad to leave them but knew he must obey his dream.[4] And then his vision sharpened. He met twelve white horses who spoke to him and led him away to his grandfathers. He was taken to a place on a cloud under a rainbow gate and there he met his six grandfathers (*Tȟuŋkášila Šákpe*). They represented the six directions: east, west, north, south, above, and below. The grandfathers spoke to him one by one and gave him courage that he would be a great warrior, but more importantly, that he would be very powerful in medicines and kill all sicknesses of the earth. Giving him a peace pipe, one said, "Behold this, for with this whatever is sick on this earth, you shall make well."[5] The fifth grandfather was the Great Spirit, *Wakȟáŋ Tȟáŋka*, and changed into a spotted eagle, *waŋblí glešká*, that would fly to the sacred four corners and then touch the earth. The spotted eagle flies the highest of all creatures, he was told, closest to *Wakȟáŋ Tȟáŋka*. His feathers were rays of the sun. To wear such feathers as a head bonnet was to assume the character of *waŋblí glešká* and to be nearer to *Wakȟáŋ Tȟáŋka*. Black Elk was then given a bow and arrow to destroy and a cup of water to heal. In particular, water was the great power, he was told. From water all herbs grew, and herbs were designed to cure. All then faced the four directions and Black Elk saw the whole earth, from Pikes Peak to the Missouri River. At one point he passed a tipi and all got up to honor him. "That's the way you shall save men," the southern grandfather said. From that point forward, Black Elk was to be a sacred man, a *wakȟáŋ wičháša*, a holy one.

In this dreamy state he would be instructed by the spirit-grandfathers on how to live his life, traveling the good Red Road. The Red Road was the path called by the Lakota as the walk of an honorable life, to achieve good things. "Give your sacred herb to your people; also give them your sacred wind so they will face the wind with courage," he heard his grandfathers say. He saw the future and saw that he would cure them. He said that the spirits of the universe had taken him "all over the world and showed me all the powers." Then he left his grandfathers and returned to earth and his tipi.[6]

He had been sick twelve days, his parents told him. Now he felt well, but his vision did not leave. He remembered the wonderful places he had been and seen and wanted to tell everyone about it but could not. It was not time. He knew no one would believe him. But others knew something had changed. A friend of the family took one look at Black Elk and "could see a power like a light all through his body."[7] Was such a young boy to be a *wapiyé* like his father? No one would understand the strange vision and the talk of the grandfathers. No one would trust yet the powers given to him to heal.

After his vision, Black Elk witnessed a healing ritual himself. Oglala had fought federal troops under General George Crook, called by the Lakota "Three Stars," near the Rosebud Creek in Montana Territory (June 17, 1876). As it was recorded, Crazy Horse found Crook and his soldiers camping on the Rosebud. Lakota and Cheyenne warriors surprised the contingent and, in Lakota lore, killed many *wašíčus*.[8] But in that battle, a wounded warrior named Rattling Hawk had been shot through the hips. It seemed impossible that he could recover. A *wapiyé*, Hairy Chin, was preparing a healing ceremony. He asked Black Elk to participate. Did Hairy Chin already sense Black Elk's healing gift? He could not tell. According to ceremony, his sons painted themselves red, and Hairy Chin painted Black Elk yellow. Each put on bear skins. They went into the tipi with Rattling Hawk, and Hairy Chin began singing, "At the doorway the sacred herbs are rejoicing." He gave the wounded man a red stick—a holy stick. At Hairy Chin's instruction two women first gave Black Elk and then Rattling Hawk a cup of water and herbs. The cup of water was the healing water, Black Elk knew. As Black Elk and others began to growl like bears, Rattling Hawk stood up and the two women helped him out of the tipi to face south. "The man [Rattling Hawk] was not strong enough to fight the next day, but he got well," Black Elk remembered. In Black Elk's mind this all made sense, it was the way of the grandfathers—like his vision had told. Black Elk knew that the *wapiyé*

Hairy Chin saw his power and that, someday, he would have to perform the healing ceremony himself.[9]

When he was seventeen, Black Elk had another premonition. There was no mistaking the message now. He heard a voice saying, "Your grandfathers told you to do these things. It is time for you to do them."[10] Now his parents accepted his role, and that he must prepare for it. His installment was elaborate. A Lakota *wakȟáŋ wičháša* must fulfill certain requirements before considered worthy of healing. First, he had to appease the Thunder-Beings, those sky spirits that brought thunder and lightning as manifestations of their power. Then he purified himself in the sweat lodge. The only "shrine" in the Oglala religion was the sweat lodge, ordinarily when not in use, a rather flimsy, profane, and drab looking structure—but reflected Oglala austerity and simplicity. Their true "cathedral" was the entire universe. The purification ceremony in the sweat lodge (*inípi*) used all the powers of the universe: water, fire, earth, and air. The water mixing with the hot stones caused steam which was interpreted as purifying the occupants' bodies. The occupants sweated and appealed to *Wakȟáŋ Tȟáŋka*:

> O Grandfather and Father *Wakȟáŋ Tȟáŋka*, maker of all that is, who always has been, behold me! And you, Grandmother and Mother Earth, you are *wakȟáŋ* and have holy ears, hear me! We have come from You, we are part of You, and we know that our bodies will return to You at that time when our spirits travel upon the great path. By fixing this center in the earth, I remember You to whom my body will return, but above all I think of *Wakȟáŋ Tȟáŋka*, with whom our spirits become as one. By purifying myself in this way, I wish to make myself worthy of You, O *Wakȟáŋ Tȟáŋka*, that my people may live![11]

Finally, as an emerging *wakȟáŋ wičháša* he had to complete the horse dance. This was another ritualized ceremony involving a number of horses (four each for the four directions), sixteen riders, and maidens. The horses were of specified color; the sixteen riders were naked, each painted a different shade: black, white, red, and yellow—highlighted by streaks of lightning; and the maidens, too, had specific roles. They wore red garments and painted their faces red. They were to bring Black Elk the *čhaŋnúŋpa* (peace-pipe) with an eagle feather, a cup of water, herbs, and bow and arrow. Black Elk himself was smeared red and on his mare was painted a spotted eagle. Six old men representing the six grandfathers were there, too. Each group of four horsemen took their steeds and faced north, east, west, and south, singing songs honoring the direction they faced. Then, seemingly on cue, dark clouds rolled in from the horizon and, according to Black Elk, thunder—the boom of the Thunder-Beings—shook the gathering. Yet neither lightning nor hail nor rain fell near. The Thunder-Beings were appeased and approved of Black Elk. He then prayed to the grandfathers acknowledging their gift of wind and herb and, holding up the sacred stick and sacred hoop, said, "I have presented your sacred stick to my nation and the sacred hoop. Grandfather, you have power to guide this sacred stick that I have presented to the people Guide the people that they may bloom on your sacred stick." Here, again, Black Elk remembered floating outside his body. He felt he had left the earth and hovered above it. Then he had the sense that "my people were cured all over for their sicknesses." The next morning, he awoke feeling more powerful, as if something inside had awakened and filled him with energy. Now he felt, he could bring up the healing wind for all in ill health.[12]

It was time for Black Elk's first cure.

During "The Moon of Making Fat," in his nineteenth year he would be called. They were living near Wounded Knee in "square houses" issued by the federal government. "It was a bad way to live," Black Elk said. "There can be no power in a square." The circle of the tipi gave strength and harmony. Square lodgings gave neither.[13] As he let it be known, he was a *waphíya wičháša*. A man named Cuts to Pieces came to him about his son who was very sick and likely to die. He thought Black Elk had special powers and could cure. Black Elk hesitantly agreed. He had not done healing before but had seen others do it and would follow their example. He trusted he now had the power to practice as a "medicine man" and to cure the sick of his people. With proper etiquette he hoped to call down authority from "the outer world."[14] He prepared himself. Dressed in headdress adorned with sacred herbs and with hallowed ornaments around his neck, he painted his body with lightning streaks and carried a square drum to represent the sound of thunder.[15] Cuts to Pieces brought him the *čhaŋmúŋpa*, the pipe with eagle feathers, which Black Elk lit and offered it to the four corners, the Great Spirit, and mother earth. He entered the tipi in ritual fashion and saw the boy. He was about four years old and nothing but skin and bones. He sat and gathered a drum, his herb, an eagle bone whistle, a cup with water, and his pipe. He began by calling, "[M]y Grandfather, the Great Spirit, you are the only one and to no other can anyone send voices. They have said you have made everything. The four quarters crossing each other you have made, and you have set a power where the sun goes down . . . you have given me power." Black Elk continued his prayer that the water he brought would be healing. Through its power all would live. Then he prayed that the herb he found would have power, too. "All beings that are not able will thus walk through your herb you have given me." He went on. "You have given me a sacred wind [from the west]." He then said, "with this wind I will breathe

the power on the weak that they may see a happy day." He walked to the little boy with his cup of water and saw him smiling and knew that he had the power and the boy would be cured. He would always think that, if the sick one smiled as he brought the water, he knew he could cure. He then drank some of the water and stamped his feet. He put his mouth on the boy's stomach and "drew the north wind through him," as if he were cleansing the sickness from him. Then the women tending him helped the boy to his feet and walked him from the south to the four corners. The boy recovered and lived almost thirty years.[16]

From now on, Black Elk, a *wakȟáŋ wičháša*, was a holy man on a sacred assignment, a task granted by *Wakȟáŋ Tȟáŋka* to aid in healings and to drive away evil influences. He was endowed to communicate with the grandfathers, the spirits of east, west, north, and south, the dwellers of the earth and sky, and all creatures who inhabit. They would come to him in times of distress and perplexity to interpret, assuage, and cure. Why could he do this? His mind received the mysterious visions and instructions allowing him the privilege. Even as the visions were confusing and tumultuous, he understood. To him the teachings of the grandfathers made sense, that each of their directives crystallized into meaning, and their way of life, the Good Red Road, was a way of honor and value.

Others of his people would see this in him. Somehow his favor with the spirit world showed—perhaps in his eyes, perhaps in his walk, perhaps in his speech. He was set apart from his brothers and sisters. And they would flock to him with their ills, when the simple measures of herbs and salves were to no avail, when nothing was left but to find one who could see beyond the visible and know the will of the spirits. He was their link between the earth and the sky. With this knowledge he could persuade, mollify, and entice goodness and deter evil. He could heal.

It was done through the *yuwipi* ceremony. *Yuwipi* was the major rite of the Lakota for healing. All Lakota recognized its restorative potential. To them it was strong medicine for the suffering. Black Elk performed it. He would heal with it. As a *wakȟáŋ wičháša*, a holy man, a medicine man, he was qualified. He alone could talk with the spirit world, and he alone could cure Indian diseases. *Yuwipi* was known as a most sacred ceremony, the calling of spirits for the purpose of healing, much as Black Elk had performed for Cuts to Pieces' son. In his upbringing and training, the *wakȟáŋ wičháša* learned the details of the *yuwipi* ceremony just as Black Elk had. There were prayers, songs, and material objects with which he must become familiar—his *čhaŋnúŋpa*, gourds, drums, ropes, and sage. These were personal items kept by the *wakȟáŋ wičháša* for *yuwipi* gatherings. They were usually destroyed after the *yuwípi* man's death. Above all, as Black Elk knew, the *yuwípi* man had to be morally unassailable, righteous, and giving. He was a priest of his people, a shaman who was trained to cure "Indian sickness," those illnesses affecting the Lakota before the arrival of the white man.

What were "Indian sicknesses"? Any number of maladies might have qualified. Headaches, fevers, vision problems, earaches, stomach issues, the wasting of consumption, chronic wounds from trauma, muscle and joint aches, paralysis, depression, even more ominous disorders like bloody stools, bloody urine, visible tumors, and seizures. Lakota were people of nature. They were among nature and dependent on nature. In times of stress, illness, or danger they watched for signs of the impending mood of nature spirits, whether favorable or ominous. Many of the tribes had plentiful agendas of botanicals—plants, roots, and herbs—to treat everyday discomforts: decoctions of cedar leaves for cholera, wild onions for inflammation, wild licorice for fevers, pursh (probably *Penthorum sedoides*) for consumption, hops for wounds.[17] It was only when those nostrums did not work that the victim was considered to be in the hands of spirits, either good or evil, and needed the attention of the "medicine man" who performed *wapiyapí*—healing rituals such as *yuwípi*.

But it was not like European "medicine." Lakota knew little of the theories of physic and of science they knew nothing. The Lakota world was not a world of measurement and experiment and analysis. Theirs was not a world of squares and angles and money and material. The Lakota world was a world of nature and seasons and symbiosis with plants, trees, and animals—it was a sacred circle. To embellish this was an array of mythology and spirits and supernatural intrigue—not so different from the Greeks of antiquity. They were content not to know more, to think that *Wakȟáŋ Tȟáŋka* was just that—a great unknown. So, to Lakota and other Native tribes, the term "medicine" simply meant "mysterious" much as *Wakȟáŋ Tȟáŋka* was the "great mysterious," the "great spirit." The Great Mysterious was in the heavens above the sky: the grandfathers. The space between earth and the heavens was their father. The earth was their grandmother. Whatever grew on the earth was their mother. They would rely on their holy men to interpret all else, but meddling with the spirits was not for most. Those *wapiyé* who appealed to *Wakȟáŋ Tȟáŋka* were able to use their special gifts to communicate and draw forth the spirits from sky and earth. Only they could cure disease inflicted by the spirit world.

On the other hand, white man's diseases were much more ominous, those of an infectious nature such as smallpox, measles, typhoid fever, syphilis, or influenza. If the *yuwípi* man thought the sufferer had a "white man's disease" he would send that person to the white man's clinic or hospital. If there was a good outcome, the *yuwípi* man would take credit. If a poor outcome, it would be the blame of the white physician. In that way, the *yuwípi* man, the *wakȟáŋ wičháša*, would retain respect.

The *yuwípi* healing ritual was a fascinating display of Lakota mysticism. Like many traditions, it was a very complicated ritual that had to be followed precisely. Even before a *yuwípi* began, the one to conduct the ritual, called the *wapiyé*, or the healing priest, would go through a purification ceremony in the sweat lodge to pray to *Wakȟáŋ Tȟáŋka* that he be deemed worthy to cure. Meanwhile the hut or tipi was prepared where the sick would lay—all in darkness. Once purified by sweating, the *wapiyé* entered the blackened tipi in a ritualistic fashion and prayed: "*Wakȟáŋ Tȟáŋka*, there is no one higher than you to whom I can speak. Somewhere between this earth and the clouds there are animals I will engage to help me. The animals are at the Four Winds. Some of them are here towards the earth. Some of them guard the earth. *Tȟuŋkášila*, help me. . . . We offer you this pipe so that we may gain knowledge."[18]

The *wapiyé* allowed himself to be bound and tied; this was the meaning of *yuwípi* (in Lakota: "to bind"). He was then placed face down on sage facing west. Then more singing and rattling began, petitioning to the four directions for help and calling on *Tȟuŋkášila* to visit them. Then there would be the boiling and feasting on dog meat as part of the ceremony.

At some point the *wapiyé would* announce that *Tȟuŋkášila* had heard the songs and they were happy. Now they would help the sick. There would be more singing and dancing. The actual curing happened in darkness where no one could witness. The sick one would feel the presence of powerful spirits. Others who were sick then also stood up to be cured. As they called out to the *wapiyé* their complaints, the *wapiyé* then prayed to the curing spirits to help those who were ill. Prescriptively, the patients then stood up and faced the wall. The sound of dancing rattles approached. Singing continued. Sometimes the sick said they could smell sweet grass—said to be the aroma of spirits. Sometimes they sensed a touch. Sometimes they simply felt wind pressing against their head. The sick then took a seat. Tobacco was offered up and rattling continued. It was total sensory immersion for the supplicant. Until the tipi darkened there was the sight of the costumed *wapiyé*, the smell of tobacco smoke—maybe even of "spirits"—the sound of rattles and the shuffling of feet, light touching, perhaps the whiff of breath, and the low percussion of distant drums. Surely, the subject thought, the spirits would listen now.

After a while, the rattling and singing ceased. Unbound now the *wapiyé* would tell the people that it was up to *Tȟuŋkášila*, that everyone should still pray. If there was no improvement of the sick, the ceremony would be repeated the following day. "*Wakȟáŋ Tȟáŋka* continue to hear this boy's prayers and answer them, and if you do he will offer up thanks to you in the years to come," the *wapiyé* prayed.[19] Then the shaman continued, "So hear all of our prayers, *Tȟuŋkášila*, and remember us. And *Tȟuŋkášila*, wherever there are common people who are sick and suffering or are in danger, protect them and help them regain their health."[20]

When Black Elk performed the *yuwípi* ceremonies, it was said his power was so strong that women's voices could be heard singing all around the room. His "medicine" was convincing. He often cured, they said, with his songs, prayers, and herbs. He was a most impressive *wapiyé*.

The Oglala *wakȟáŋ wičháša*, George Sword (Lakota name *Míla Wakȟáŋ*, "Mysterious Knife" or, according to the Lakota, "Sword"), explained how vital Lakota holy men could be to their tribal members:

> Disease is caused by the mysterious or mysterious-like. The evil mysteries may impart their potencies to the body and this will cause disease. Poisons and snakes and water creatures cause disease in this way. A magician can cause disease by his mysterious powers. A holy man can cause disease by his songs and ceremonies.[21]

Those *wakȟáŋ wičháša* favored by *Wakȟáŋ Tȟáŋka* with special privilege were so valued and respected that they seemed almost godlike—perhaps a Lakota version of Asclepius—in their communities.

> They are looked upon as a species of demi-gods. They assert their origin to be miraculous. At first, they are spiritual existences, encased in a seed of some description of a winged nature, like the thistle. Wafted by the breeze to the dwelling place of the gods, they are received to intimate communion. After being instructed in relation to the mysteries of the spirit world, they go forth to study the character of all tribes. After deciding upon a residence, they enter the body of someone about to become a mother, and are ushered by her into the world.[22]

Sword said the holy man was the most potent person in treating the sick. Only he could speak with the Great Mysterious, *Wakȟáŋ Tȟáŋka*. Sword added that the holy man's ceremonial bag was much like a white man's doctor bag. It was called *wóphiye*. In the bag there were various medicines: cedar weed for wounds, powdered turtle's heart for wounds, holy tobacco for wounds, cedar medicine to cleanse, soap weed for swellings, blue medicine for weakness, calamus root for delirium, sweet medicine for menses, yellow leaf medicine for swelling, and yucca powder for stomach aches. As Sword described it, the holy man prayed to his bag but he had to know the right song to sing. Still, it was what the bag contained that treated the sick. That which was in the bag was called a *wašičuŋ* (a medicine bundle). Sword then explained that "a holy man does not give medicine to the sick unless he is a medicine man. If he is a medicine man, he may give medicines and invoke his ceremonial bag (*wašičuŋ*) also, and the bag will compel the medicine to do as he wishes it."[23]

It was not pure fantasy. Seemingly miraculous cures were witnessed by visiting anthropologists. One described the supernatural abilities of a Dakota medicine man:

> Ten Dakota were very sick with a contagious disease. The White doctors could not cure them. They were removed from the other people, to be treated elsewhere, but the White man's efforts availed nothing. A medicine man announced that he could cure them. He cured every one of the 10. After doing this, he invited the White doctors into a room and sat down in the center by a stone which he had painted red. When he sang, the stone went in a circle about the room, in front of the White doctors. All of them talked about the feats this man could perform.[24]

Another Catholic missionary priest, Father Augustin Ravoux, witnessed such a ceremony for the sick in the 1840s. He had heard that the ability of the Dakota medicine man was astounding. When summoned, the conjurer would prepare for the ritual. He would come to the tent of the sick, stand over him, shake his gourd-seed rattle and utter horrible sounds all the while stamping his feet. Sometimes the conjurer would apply his mouth to the patient's body and, with much fanfare, pretend to draw the disease out of the subject. As a priest observed, "The sounds emitted by the operator were the most disagreeable that I ever heard, and his whole appearance the most revolting of anything to be seen among the Dakota." If the patient lived, the conjurer received all credit. If the patient died there were explanations without blaming the conjurer.[25]

And now, the heartbreak.

⁓

Black Elk had been recruited by Buffalo Bill Cody to participate in the traveling Wild West show. He even went to Europe and met Queen Victoria, who flattered his people much more than any *wašíču* ever had. She told the Native Americans who had gathered to meet her:

America is a good country and I have seen all kinds of people, but today I have seen the best-looking people—the Indians. . . . If I owned you Indians, you good-looking people, I would never take you around in a show like this. You have a Grandfather over there who takes care of you over there, but he shouldn't allow this.[26]

When Black Elk returned in 1889, he saw that his people were living in poverty. "They all looked pitiful," he remembered. There had been a great famine. The Lakota signed a treaty with the government but had not received the promised food. There were no buffalo to hunt. They lived in white man's square houses and did nothing. Black Elk said, "they had shut us up in pens."[27] With famine and inadequate food stores, Lakota were starving. In their desperation, Lakota and other Native Americans turned to the supernatural. Black Elk had heard of a man called the Messiah, who was a Paiute named Jack Wilson—Wovoka was his native name—who preached in an area of South Dakota called Wounded Knee. Like many Native Americans, Jack Wilson had a prophetic vision. According to his telling, he was to be the son of the Great Spirit and he had come to resurrect Lakota pride and self-sufficiency. They were to live apart from the white man and once again subsist independent of them. This would all come about with a ritualistic ceremony called the ghost dance, *wanáǧi wačhípi*. A ghost dance was another sacred ritual that united the living Lakota with the dead. "[T]here is another world coming," the ghost dance would reveal. A world is coming "just for Indians." This world would come and "crush out all the whites." Only those outfitted appropriately could live in this new world. It would come like a cloud.[28]

It was not a dance of rebellion. It was a dance of coexistence. "The great underlying principle of the Ghost dance doctrine [if truly the Lakota held to any written doctrine] is that the time will come when the whole Indian race, living and dead, will be reunited upon a regenerated earth, to live a life of aboriginal happiness forever free from death, disease, and misery." From this, each tribe would adapt such a hope to their own mythology.[29] There were obvious features of Christianity in all this, as Jack Wilson would interpret it.

Black Elk visited Wounded Knee, now a vast encampment of Lakota people and the site of a great ghost dance. He danced the ghost dance day after day. As he remembered, those were happy times. After all their misery, the Lakota now believed their life would improve. Many were almost delirious with happiness, experiencing visions themselves and thinking that they would be taken back to the old ways of living and that the spirits of earth, air, and stars would return to them again.

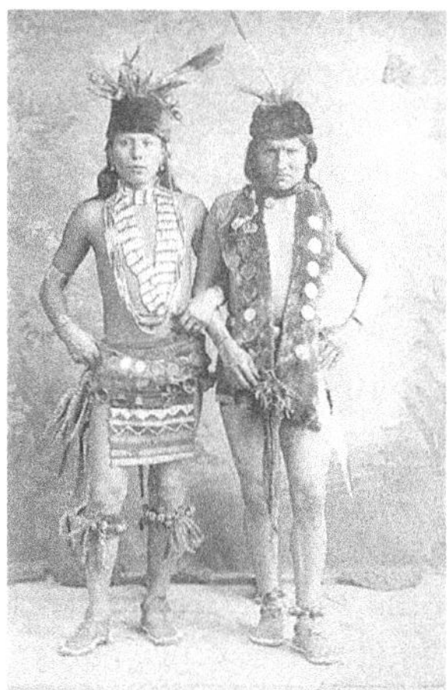

Figure 7.1   Black Elk (left) and Elk of the Oglala Lakota when performing in Buffalo Bill's Wild West Show 1887 Elliott Fry, London.

The ghost dance would be the end of the Lakota.

The white men had a different interpretation of the ghost dance. It was a radical and militant movement of Native Americans that very well might threaten treaties and the welfare of white settlers farming and ranching lands formerly occupied by tribes such as the Lakota.

Black Elk heard the cannon the morning of the Wounded Knee massacre, December 29, 1890. He prepared for war and put on his sacred shirt with a spotted eagle outstretched on the back. It was the hallowed blouse with pictures of his vision that would give him protection that day. He painted his face red and wore a single Eagle feather in his hair. He rode with some other men and urged them to take courage, their relatives are lying dead. He himself prayed to his grandfathers. "Today my people are in despair, so, six grandfathers, help me."[30] When he arrived, he saw the shooting and the white soldiers running around killing men, women, and children. He and his men would charge the soldiers and he could feel the bullets flying by but he held forward his sacred bow and the soldiers, he said, fled. At one point, he was shot near his waist and was ready to die. "It is a good day to die," he said and tried to charge again. An old man ran up to him and told him to hold back, that it was not his day to die, his people needed him. There would be a better day to die.[31]

After the shooting stopped. Black Elk wandered the battlefield. In some places there were heaps of bodies, young and old entangled in protective clumps. Some bodies had been torn apart from the mounted guns. When he saw this slaughter, he wished he had died, too. Among the dead were numbers of *wašíču*. Outnumbered Lakota warriors stood their ground and, even though death was certain, continued to fire until they dropped. They managed to kill twenty-five bluecoats and wounded dozens more. After the soldiers left snow fell and covered the bodies of women and children "who had never done any harm, and were only trying to run away."[32] Estimates varied, but as many as three hundred Lakota may have died that day.[33]

The Messiah was wrong. A new world was coming but not for the Lakota. Their world was finished. Their world lay before him there at Wounded Knee. Heaps of bodies covered in snow was their legacy. Black Elk said, "And I, to whom so great a vision was given in my youth—you see now a pitiful old man who has done nothing, for the nation's hoop is broken and shattered. There is no center any longer, and the sacred tree is dead."[34]

∼

In 1892 Black Elk married Kate War Bonnet. They settled on the Pine Ridge reservation. It was a time of wrenching change, though. The traditional activities of men—hunting buffalo—were no more. Farming was little more than women's work and despised by menfolk. Black Elk tried to show them new ways, and the Oglala bargained with the federal government on raising cattle and horses. Ranching allowed a roaming lifestyle for the men, and women did most of the planting. Black Elk helped his people do things that would please the federal government and prevent officials from diminishing their rations. He continued to be their *wakȟáŋ wičháša* and, he recalled, cured many sick.[35]

Even before the ghost dance and massacre at Wounded Knee, in 1884 the visionary Lakota leader Red Cloud had converted to Catholicism. Many Lakota had done so because of the work of the Jesuit missionary Pierre-Jean De Smet. Four years later, Jesuit missionaries arrived at Pine Ridge and set up the Holy Rosary Mission. Many Lakota chiefs said they wanted a "Blackrobe [Jesuit] school and no other." The Jesuits converted several "big chiefs" to Catholicism as well, men like Big Turkey, Two Strike, He Dog, and Big Head. Black Elk's wife soon turned to Catholicism, but Black Elk was not so enthralled. At least, not at first. A Jesuit priest, incensed by his *yuwípi* healing rituals, had barged in and destroyed his sacred objects, claiming pagan customs. His blatant disrespect understandably offended Black Elk. The boy recovered nevertheless, but the priest was killed soon after in falling off his horse, Black Elk told—undoubtedly feeling his spirit world had extracted retribution.[36]

But over the years, he was slowly drawn to Christianity, and perhaps felt the priests had more power than he in spiritual matters. Anyway, *wašíču s* had ended Lakota hopes at Wounded Knee. "A people's dream died there. It was a beautiful dream. . . . There is no center any longer," he later said.[37] Now he studied spirits of the white man. The theology of the Society of Jesus was similar to Lakota. The Jesuits believed God was in all things, like *Wakȟáŋ Tȟáŋka* was in all things. In the early 1900s he finally converted to Catholicism and, once and for all, put away his Lakota religious ceremonies and healing rituals. He now concentrated on the shepherding of his people toward the Christian faith and professed the charity that it held sacred. It allowed Black Elk to organize Lakota communities and preserve Lakota tradition, free of interference from the federal government. No doubt, he never dismissed the instructions of his ghostly grandfathers, to care for his people. It was his vision as a Lakota *wakȟáŋ wičháša* and remained his vision as a Catholic Christian:

> Those of us here on earth who are suffering should help one another and have pity. We belong to one family and we have only one faith. Therefore, those who are suffering, my relatives, we should look toward them and pray for them, because our Savior came on this earth and helped all poor people.[38]

When a man is alive, he has his *wóniya* (breath of life) and his *naǧí* (spirit). His *naǧí* is not part of himself. His *naǧí* cares for him and warns him of danger and helps him out of difficulties. When he dies his *naǧí* goes with his *wanáǧi* to the spirit world, far beyond the pines. His *wanáǧi* stays near for a while but soon it will go to the spirit world. Whether Lakota or Catholic, the breath of life and the spirit within are shared by all mankind.

CHAPTER EIGHT

Healing the Incurable

Damien of Moloka'i

The certainty of death is as lonely as death itself.

Then how does one heal the incurable? Too often, they are the biblical lepers of today. As if their fatal disease is somehow contagious: the smell of death a repellent to intimacy. They become the "unclean," tainted by the specter of corruption and decay. Like lepers of old, their features whither from a malicious internal pestilence, drawing and wasting a seeping vitality: eyes sunken, luster vanishing, strength receding. They become an outward ugliness to be shunned. One cannot heal the disease—to be labeled as "incurable" or "terminal" such remedies are far beyond comprehension. But the suffering mind anguishes beneath, not yet perished. Nor incurable. As if imprisoned in flesh that has betrayed them, their spirits reach through bars to touch, again, sanity. They yearn for comfort, for hope, for peace. It is that which can be tended. There lies the healing. Reach inside. Let their pain wash over you. It is not contagious, it is redeeming.

On January 6, 1866, the first native Hawaiians with advanced leprosy, twelve in all, were deposited at the mouth of the Waikolu Valley just east of the Kalaupapa Peninsula on the north shore of the Island of Moloka'i. They had been rounded up and screened at the Kahili Hospital in Honolulu, Hawai'i, boated for the ride to Moloka'i, and unceremoniously dumped. The looming *pali* blotted out the sun as if into darkness they had been relegated. It was still miles overland before they arrived at their new settlement. On foot they trudged, over roots and brush that tore into the ulcerated feet of the diseased. Perceived as an existential threat to the Kingdom of Hawai'i, this vanguard of the unclean had been consigned to exile by decree of the Hawaiian Board of Health. Led by the efforts of King Kamehameha V just one year prior to stem the tide of another "Western" disease sweeping over his subjects, his Board of Health had acted. Indeed, dwindling numbers of *kānaka maoli*—native Hawaiians—had captured the attention of Kamehameha and health officials as possibly turning into the serious threat smallpox had posed years before—when thousands were wiped out. "Whereas, the disease of Leprosy has spread to considerable extent among the people, and the spread thereof has excited well-grounded alarms," the Board of Health proclaimed. For a disease with no known cure there was only one option available. Segregate and isolate. More intent on removal than sustenance, the Board of Health vaguely made provisions for establishment of a hospital "where leprous patients *in the incipient stages* [italics mine] may be treated in order to attempt a cure." The Board also expected a "reasonable amount of labor" from the refugees and decreed that to finance the whole endeavor, lepers' property could be seized as payment for their confinement. The Board of Health was given authority to "reserve and set apart any land or portion of land . . . to secure the isolation and seclusion of such leprous persons as in the opinion of the Board of Health or its agents, may by being at large cause the spread of leprosy." Those suspected of leprosy were first screened in Honolulu, and if their fate was confirmed, forcibly removed from family and friends and sent in exile, likely for the rest of their lives. Only a wealthy few would be able to bring uninfected *kōkua*, or helpers, with them. In effect, lepers had been criminalized.[1]

Kalaupapa's vanguard lepers did not have "incipient" disease. They were sick, bedraggled, and riddled with illness.

Leprosy was an affliction of antiquity, as vile and revolting as any contagion in history. Its disfiguring progression, distorting and animalizing human features turn victims into grotesque caricatures. If not the sight itself, then their putrid discharges set them apart. For its grotesque manifestations, the sickness was the ultimate in suffering. And to what did the *kānaka maoli* attribute this affliction? Surely a disobedience to their gods held the answer:

Heaha la ka'u hala nui, e ke 'kua,
I ai kuia paha a'u, i ai aia,
I ai aia ia'u, e lakou nei.
O ka hala ia la e Kaneikawaieola . . .

E ola e, e ola hoi a'u la, ko pulapula

What is my great offense, O god!
O have eaten standing perhaps, or without

giving thanks
Or these my people have eaten wrongfully
Yes, that is the offense, O Kaneikawaieola . . .

O spare; O let me live, thy devotee[2]

For these twelve suffering lepers, some numbed from the neurologic effects of the disease, and many disfigured by signature distortions, tumors, and foul ulcerations, the sea voyage on board the schooner *Warwick* to their exile had been nothing short of miserable. In an advanced stage of leprosy, they had poor tolerance for a rough sea ride with high waves, sea sickness, and the sudden separation from loved ones. Their destination, the Kalaupapa Peninsula, was a flat finger of land extending into the ocean no higher than seventy feet above sea level and surrounded by the formidable 1,500 feet vertical *pali* sea cliffs, extending fourteen miles along the northern coast of Moloka'i that made escape for impaired lepers almost unthinkable. They landed a haggard group, shabbily clothed, hungry, sick, and confused. Without substantial provisions at first, the lepers were expected to plant crops, make their own clothing, and care for themselves, a tall task for these twelve whose missing limbs and gnarled hands made field labor and sewing all but impossible. Separated from loved ones and afflicted with a hopeless disease, they were broken in body and in spirit. At first the lepers remained at the mouth of the Waikolu Valley as it opened to the peninsula, but as more patients accumulated, they slowly wandered two miles northward to the settlement of Kalawao on the eastern side of the peninsula. Both places were relatively inhospitable as the shoreline was rocky, making passage difficult, and water access was treacherous due to unpredictable seas and rough, rocky coastline. At least at Kalawao the sun shone longer, the ground was flatter.

Such was Moloka'i, the land set apart—*Moloka'i Nui A Hina*: Great Moloka'i, Child of Hina:

Moloka'i of the Hawaiian Islands, like a human child, was born to a mother and father: Wākea, god of the sky, and Hina, goddess of the moon and weaver of the clouds consummated their affair that birthed Moloka'i. This traditional legend of origin establishes that the island of Moloka'i, like a child, is small and fragile—unlike a large continent.[3]

Moloka'i's 3,500-acre Kalaupapa Peninsula seemed divinely destined for incurables. The outcropping of land jutting from the massive, almost vertical sea cliffs was from afar as remote and desolate as it appeared up close.

Forbiddingly isolated, the Kalaupapa Peninsula was ideally constructed for quarantine and segregation. Even access by sea was foreboding, the unpredictable waters often precluded safe landing of even small whaling boats.

In the nineteenth century, the Hawaiian island of Moloka'i was the least populated of the eight sizeable land masses comprising the archipelago. In truth, the island hosted areas of fertile fields and lush valleys, but the shoreline was inhospitable. Only ingeniously designed fish ponds on the southern shore promoted an active aquaculture of consistently available marine life. Most people, as a result, lived on the southeastern shores opposite Mau'i in the distance. Those lands had gentle sloping ranges, fertile soil, and their characteristic fish ponds. However, in terms of population, Moloka'i would remain itself a land apart. The few rickety harbors could not compete with the robust landings of Mau'i or O'ahu. Lack of fresh water and adequate provisions added to discourage stopovers of the lucrative whaling trade or trans-Pacific commerce.

Prior to Western influence *kānaka maoli*, native Hawaiians, were spared many diseases and pestilence. Their health regimen was reasonable: diets high in fiber and starch, vitamins, and fastidious personal hygiene (frequent bathing and strict public sanitation). Physical exertion was commonplace in work or play. Health education was first and foremost the responsibility of every *'ohana* (family). Health was defined by proper balance of *mana* (personal energy) and *pono* (proper personal harmony or order). Illness happened with loss of *mana* due to lack of personal *pono*, including relation with spiritual forces. Public proper *pono* was directed by the *kahuna* in establishing *kapu* or sacred restricting behavior. *Kapu* emphasized self-discipline and responsibility for personal hygiene, illness prevention, and public sanitation. For any perceived illness, treatment consisted of restoration of proper orientation of *mana* and *pono*. The descendants of *Hawai'i Loa*, the legendary South Sea seafarer who stumbled onto the islands, had prospered by their virtual isolation.

Few serious disorders were seen. According to anthropologist Craighill Handy, physical ailments and even death were thought to be from psychic conditions rather than physical causes. Evil forces intent on man's destruction were either demons acting of their own accord or at the request of a god or malicious person's behest.[4] Mostly local infections, such as dental caries or troublesome carbuncles, plagued the population. The bulk of healthcare involved repair of traumatic wounds, childbirth, and consequences of aging. Personal reflection and self-correction were the first steps for any affliction, but if results did not happen, the ill one would seek an experienced *kahuna lapa'au*. By virtue of their selection and training, these priestly healers were not charlatans or miscreants. They were reputable practitioners and had received extensive education and training in their art. *Lā'au lapa'au* was the traditional way of healing, bringing together cultural and spiritual dimensions often ignored by Western medicine. The dispensers of *lā'au lapa'au*, the *kahuna lapa'au*, were highly valued by the *kānaka maoli* and readily sought for any stubborn illnesses. The *kahuna lapa'au* might employ a combination of psycho-spiritual methods (prayer, faith healing, sorcery, group therapy), physical measures such as manipulation, enemas, massage, and pharmaceuticals rich in ritual and symbolism. Sometimes, even surgery would be done for superficial afflictions such as carbuncles, fistulas, and the like.[5] Their temples of healing, vaguely reminiscent of Asclepian sanctuaries, were called *heiau hō'ola*, dedicated to one of the four great gods: Kāne, Kū, Lono, or Kanaloa. Only the *kahuna lapa'au*, with their proper training and dedication, could communicate with the spirit world and bring to bear their spiritual powers to heal. While not exorbitant, the *kahuna lapa'au* did not provide their services for free. Usually, some type of barter payment was made, such as a fattened hog or produce.

With the coming of the *haole*, the white man, the isolation of the Hawaiian Islands ceased, and spread of new, malevolent sicknesses rampaged.

Shortly after British explorer James Cook's initial visit to his "Sandwich Islands" in January 1778, Western disease made its appearance. The *kahuna lapa'au* were said to have first encountered venereal diseases brought to willing native girls by Cook's sailors. Females of the islands were far from shy sexually, and had no qualms in being bedded by hungry seafarers—particularly those of the peculiar white complexion whom they called *haole*. Surgeon John Law aboard the HMS *Resolution* on Cook's return visit in March 1779, remarked that "[w]e heard today also for certain as it was confirmed afterwards by many of the Natives that when we were here the last Time we gave them the venereal disease, they [*kahunas*] had a method of curing it but it was a long time first."[6]

At the time of Cook's landing the total population of the Hawaiian Islands was estimated at near one million natives. Infectious devastation followed. By 1893 this population would dwindle to around forty thousand. But that was not all. Progressive Western influence and arrival of proselytizing Christian missionaries with their disapproval of traditional *kanaka* ways, would gradually dismantle both *'ohana* (family) and *kapu*. In 1819, in despair, Hawaiian leaders formally abolished the sacred *kapu* laws. Pollution and unsanitary conditions began to rise. Epidemics of dysentery (squatting sickness), cholera, smallpox, typhoid fever, and tuberculosis in addition to syphilis and gonorrhea felled numbers of previously healthy *kānaka maoli*.

Their *kahuna lapaʻau* were powerless to stop it. Even the *kahuna Lonopūhā* who appealed to the god *Lonopūhā*, the traditional god of healing (more or less, the Hawaiian Asclepius), to guide their treatment, could not make sense of it. Hawaiians were becoming a weak and dying culture. Their stringent concerns for public health teetered, and all the preconditions for contagion surfaced: poor hygiene, inadequate diet, and the intimate social natures of the *kānaka maoli*.[7] Of the decline of *kapu* the Hawaiian scholar Samuel Kamakau wrote:

> [W]ith the coming of strangers, there came contagious diseases which destroyed the native sons of the land. No longer is the sound of the old man's cane heard on the long road, no longer do the aged crouch about the fireplace, no longer do those helpless with age stretch themselves on their beds, no longer do they remain withering in the house like the cane-blossom stalks plucked and dried for the dart-throwing game. . . . The smallpox came, and dead bodies lay stacked like kindling wood, read as singed hogs. Shame upon those who brought the disease and upon the foreign doctors who allowed their landing.[8]

And then the scourge of leprosy appeared.

It is difficult to say when leprosy first emerged in the Hawaiian Islands. Missionary Reverend Charles Stewart, landing at Honolulu in April 1823, had no problem recognizing it and wrote that some natives already manifested the

> [F]requent and hideous marks of a scourge, which more clearly than any other, proclaims the curse of a God of purity, and which, while it annually consigns hundreds of this people to the tomb, converts thousands while living into walking sepulchers . . . many are as unsightly as lepers.[9]

Whether these were truly leprous individuals was indeterminate, but they showed many of the stigmata of the disease. However, in the years to follow, anecdotal cases of leprosy were authenticated and recorded. Some blamed imported Chinese laborers brought to man the burgeoning plantation business and called the affliction *maʻi pake*, "the Chinese disease." Others thought the disease came from the Azores, Malaysia, or Africa. It is inescapable that leprosy was imported, and Western exploitation furnished the opportunity. By 1860 cases were so numerous and found throughout the island chain that matters were taken to the Board of Health in 1864.

Christian zealots blamed the Hawaiians themselves. The entirety of native life there was distasteful to Westerners. The *kahuna lapaʻau* and their gods were not welcomed by Christian missionaries and physicians, feeling Hawaiian culture was contrary to Christian beliefs and emerging scientific medicine. The *kānaka maoli* were savage, paganistic, and immoral. It was not a stretch to think that before long, victims of leprosy degenerated in the eyes of whites to dehumanized freaks. In fact, one evangelizing minister argued that the weakness facilitating physical decay of the Hawaiian "race" was due to "unchastity," drunkenness, *kahuna* sorcery, idolatry, and rampant epidemics.[10] The specter of an inferior race loomed over this interpretation at a time when American thinking favored a racial polycultural—and uneven—distribution of Christian-friendly monogenesis, loomed over this interpretation. Some societies, such fanatics reasoned, by virtue of their environment assimilated traits that, with time, became ingrained and almost immutable—an acquired form of polygenesis.[11] In Christian logic, *equal but unequal.* The terms "savages" and "pagans" peppered their rhetoric. The opinion was that *kānaka* had brought it all on themselves. They were lazy, dull, and sinners and idolaters to boot. Their flagrant immorality and uncleanliness sunk them to levels like the pitiful, leprous beggars of the Old Testament. God had stricken them in their wicked ways. Where Jesus the Healer was in all this reasoning cannot be known. He was clearly forgotten by most.

By all parameters, leprosy was a horrible disease. History had relegated it to the worst afflictions of mankind, disfiguring, demoralizing, and eventually fatal. The leprous "unclean" littered the alleyways of antiquity, the medieval world, and even early modern times. Whether a form of syphilis, as many moralizers believed, hereditary, or just an outward manifestation of inner moral corruption, those with the disease were set apart, the unaffected afraid proximity itself would lend to communication. It was a disease characterized by skin lesions at first flat but eventually coalescing developing into enlarging nodules termed tubercles. These tubercles often ulcerated and discharged their rotting contents. Lesions were found not only on the skin but also in mucous membranes such as the mouth and throat. Additionally, the disease attacked peripheral nerves, producing loss of sensation and trophic disturbances to the limb leading to necrosis and self-amputation. The leper in the full throes of the disease could be a hideous creature, unable to ambulate, filled with putrefaction and palsies, and missing amputated digits. The face took on leonine features from the disfiguring tubercles. Scalp and eyes lost hair. Death usually came from debilitation, wasting, and pneumonia.

Even ancient Jewish Law, of course, prohibited any contact with lepers, whose open, pus-filled sores were ready avenues for transmission. Spread among Hawaiians was likely due to the culture itself. Few *kānaka maoli* feared the disease and continued to touch, eat with, and be intimate with the infirmed. For Hawaiians, leprosy was not the unclean sickness of biblical times—that was the doing of Westerners. What they feared was separation.

Instead, they would call leprosy *ma'i ho'oka'awale'ohana* (the disease that separates families). Despite the efforts of the Norwegian investigator Armauer Hansen in identifying the microbial culprit of the disease, the second half of the nineteenth century still considered leprosy a fatal diagnosis. That segregation was peculiar to Hawai'i is not correct. Even the distinguished Canadian, Sir William Osler, in his great textbook of medicine, remarked that "cases should be isolated," as "there are no specific remedies for the disease."[12]

Its disfigurements debased humanness. Of the horrors of Moloka'i, visiting author May Quinlan wrote:

> They stand out like creatures from some under-world; so brutalized, so hideous, so awful, that they appear to have lost all semblance of human kind. In and out, they creep among the rocks, for some are weak and ill with disease. Others, whose limbs have dropped off from the rotting joints, crawl along the ground like the brute beasts.[13]

Few Westerners wanted any part of it. Let them rot in isolation. Their depravity brought their punishment. The Belgian missionary Joseph de Veuster was to be the exception. Joseph was born in the Flemish town of Tremeloo near Louvain in 1840. His upbringing was rural and agricultural. He grew physically to handle the numerous tasks of farming from animal husbandry to carpentry to planting. Yet his calling was religious. Despite his father's eagerness to keep him on the family farm, Joseph was determined to serve his God. "Do not stop me [from the priesthood] because to forbid your son to follow the will of God . . . would be an ingratitude that would bring down cruel punishment on you," he wrote his father.[14] Like his older brother Auguste—soon to be known as Pamphile—Joseph was admitted to the Congregation of the Sacred Hearts of Jesus and Mary and took the religious habit under his new name of Brother Damien. That he had a curiosity about medicine was evident from his choice of Damien, adopting the name from the brotherly physician duo, Cosmos and Damian, who healed miraculously in the third century. Perhaps he had hope that he and his brother could do the same. Damien adapted quickly to clerical life. At first deficient in the classical languages, he soon mastered the necessary courses by diligent overachievement. On October 7, 1860, he took his vows and began preparation for ordination. However, a serious case of typhus struck his brother Pamphile, who had been assigned to the new mission in Hawai'i, and Damien, eager to salvage a family opportunity to contribute to the mission field petitioned to take his place. It was granted. After 139 days in transit his ship, the *R.W. Wood*, dropped anchor off of Honolulu March 19, 1864. Damien was greeted by a tumultuous welcome. Hundreds of *kānaka maoli* lined the wharf and proudly displayed their rosaries while showering him with *alohas.* His adventure had begun.

In Honolulu he completed his requirements for priesthood and was ordained on Sunday, April 17, 1864. He lay prostrate on the hard stone floor, a symbol of death that will give rise to life. He heard Bishop Maigret intone those ancient words: "O Jesus, our great High Priest, hear our humble prayers on behalf of your priest, Father Damien . . . In his loneliness, comfort him; in his sorrows, strengthen him; in his frustrations, point out to him that it is through suffering that the soul is purified." In posterity the now consecrated Joseph de Veuster would be known simply as Father Damien

Yes, Damien's priestly work would be one of suffering.

His first assignments were on the big Island of Hawai'i covering expansive territory that made travel from one community to the other almost a continuous necessity. However, his determination and dedication provided a sound ministry to the Catholics under his care. He was particularly adept at refurbishing and constructing chapels that had fallen into disrepair across his enormous district. "Here I am a priest, dear parents," he wrote to Belgium, "here I am a missionary in a corrupt, heretical, idolatrous country."[15]

As if the remoteness of the neglected native population of the Big Island were not enough, the leper colony of Moloka'i caught his attention. The settlement was expanding at such a rate that proper spiritual—and certainly, bodily—care of the lepers was failing miserably. There was no minister (or doctor, for that matter) to tend to the needs of flesh and spirit for the residents. Protestant ministers were reticent to venture in for fear of exposing their families to risk of contagion. Catholic priests, being celibate, seemed perfect candidates. Damien, in his forceful style, volunteered. His bishop, the Reverend Louis Maigret, reluctantly agreed. Damien informed his brother of the decision. Prior to his departure, Damien also wrote his parents: "[l]eprosy is beginning to be very prevalent here. There are many men covered with it. It does not cause death at once, but it is very rarely cured. The disease is very dangerous, because it is highly contagious."[16]

Together with fifty lepers, Damien went ashore at Kalaupapa from the interisland steamer *Kilauea* on May 10, 1873, to join 800 other lepers of the colony. He was thirty-three years of age and would never leave. By his own efforts he had to construct a place for him to live, not at Kalaupapa but a few miles distant at the original settlement, Kalawao. It was now a dirty, ramshackle hamlet. The huts in which the lepers lived were unusually squalid and vile, containing numbers of lepers that only accentuated the filth of the place. Eventually, he and able-bodied lepers would refurbish Saint

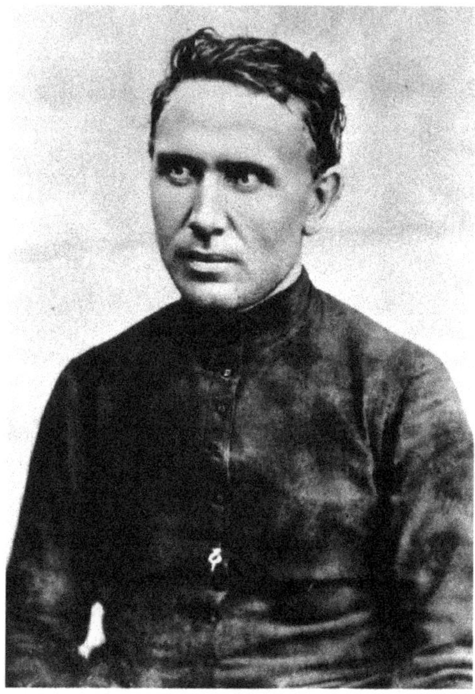

Figure 8.1 Father Damien (Joseph de Veuster) before he sailed to Moloka'i in 1873.
Henry L. Chase

Philomena chapel, build a hospital, suitable lepers' quarters, and an orphanage. But on that windswept day, he remembered his first impression:

> [T]he poor people were without any medicines, with the exception of a few physics and their own native medicines, from which, I judged, it had been the same from the inauguration of the Settlement. It was a common sight to see people going around with fearful ulcers, which for the want of a few rags, or a piece of lint and a little salve, were left exposed to dirt, flies, and vermin.[17]

Aside from the inherent dangers, Damien seemed a perfect choice. His record of church-building and ministry on the Big Island had impressed his superiors, and his working medical knowledge allowed some capacity for caring for the lepers. He was physically fit and energetic. "My dear Brother," Damien wrote on November 25, 1873, "God has deigned to choose your unworthy brother to assist the poor people attacked by that terrible malady so often mentioned in the Gospel, leprosy."[18] There was no doctor to minister to them. He sensed the general feeling was that the disease was incurable, so why bother. Without hesitation, he took to the task of physician, drawing on instructions he had received in Hilo from a local Protestant physician, Charles Wetmore, when he was on the island of Hawai'i. Wetmore had been a godsend to Hawai'i, offering medicine, treatments, and even some surgical procedures. He was more than willing to instruct the curious Damien on some of the more common remedies available, including opium and calomel for dysentery and quinine for the periodic fevers of malaria. On Kalaupapa Damien did not waste time. He daily visited the sick, changed their filthy, pus-soaked bandages, cleaned their wounds—sometimes filled with maggots—and applied clean dressings. There was no question in Damien's mind that, although leprosy had no known cure, premature deaths occurred because of secondary infections and malnutrition. All too often, he found, "anyone getting a fever, diarrhea or any other of the numerous ailments . . . was carried off for want of some simple medicine."[19]

He found conditions deplorable and the awful consequences of the disease challenging. Sanitation was nonexistent, the water supply was inconsistent, and foodstuffs were unpredictably delivered by boat. The seas around the Kalaupapa Peninsula were often just too hazardous to dock. So often, he harangued his superiors and the Board of Health to facilitate transport. His lepers were close to starving, he would argue, and malnutrition was another enemy of their health. He wrote to his brother Pamphile of his challenges:

> Their clothes were far from being clean and decent, on account of the scarcity of water, which had to be brought at that time from a great distance. . . . Many a time in fulfilling my priestly duty at their domiciles I have been compelled to run outside to breathe fresh air. To counteract the bad smell, I made myself accustomed to the use of tobacco, whereupon the smell of the pipe preserved me somewhat from carrying in my clothes the noxious odor of the lepers.[20]

Faced with the dismal conditions of Kalawao, Damien anguished over how to comfort the suffering. He launched into simple measures such as replacing their thatched shacks with sturdier housing and fixing better ventilation in their dwellings to circulate the putrid air from their wounds. Even the roofs leaked. He worked to shore them up so that with the frequent storms that swept the peninsula his lepers would not get soaked as they lay immobilized in bed, covered with scabs and open sores. As for the disease itself, Damien found it detestable. "The flesh is eaten away, and gives out a fetid odor," Damien wrote his brother, "even the breath of the leper becomes so foul that the air around is poisoned with it."[21] For terminal cases, those about to die, he tried to alleviate their pain (likely with opium), and pray with them since no cure was forthcoming. "We can only hope in a supernatural gift" for these pitiable people.

It was not just the physical effects of the disease, tragic as they were. Leprosy spawned an overall social deterioration. Lepers became as predators, the strong preying on the weak. Those too ill simply allowed it to happen, powerless to fight. Lawlessness reigned. Deprived of the scarce resources available—foodstuffs, clothing, and building repairs were squandered by the healthier—victims suffered a crippling apathy in addition to their infirmities. And deterioration of the spirit hastened deterioration of the body. One visiting physician to Damien's colony observed that

> The terrible disease which afflicts the Lepers seems to cause among them as great a change in their moral and mental organization as in their physical constitution: so far from aiding and assisting their weaker brethren, the strong took possession of everything, devoured and destroyed the large quantity of food on the lands, and altogether refused to replant anything. . . . In fact, most of those in whom the disease had progressed considerably showed the greatest thoughtlessness and heartlessness.[22]

Above all, most lepers of Moloka'i were left without family or friends. This in itself was cause for profound depression. They knew they were doomed to live and die there and never leave. There was a feeling of complete despair. How to help? Damien visited them and spent most of his time among them, particularly the hospitalized ones. "[H]e cared for their bodies as well as their souls; he would himself feed them, putting the food in their mouths when the terrible malady had deprived them of their hands, and bring little sweetmeats and delicacies."[23] By doing so, by touching them, talking to them, and sitting with them he did what must be done for the incurables: show them they were not alone. Damien might have wondered, as psychologists later discovered, that physical hardships—hunger, thirst, cold, fatigue, exhaustion—magnifies the mental impact of desolate, forlorn suffering. As if creature comforts can actually bolster the sagging framework of hope and provide glimpses of a not so despairing future. That a small amount of spiritual recompense could, in fact, radiate outward to illuminate a fading optimism. Perhaps Damien wished himself that by imparting some degree of physical relief to his fated lepers he could foster a sense of meaning, even in grim hours, as Holocaust survivor Viktor Frankl later wrote: "[w]e must never forget that we may also find meaning in life even when confronted with a hopeless situation, when facing a fate that cannot be changed."[24]

Even faced with their misery, Damien tried to oust their pagan tendencies. He found what he considered rampant immorality. The lepers were living "promiscuously without distinction of sex and many an unfortunate woman had to become a prostitute to obtain friends who would take care of her." He also objected to the *hula*. To him it was a heathen ritual "under the protection of the old deity *Laka*, who had his numerous altars and sacrifices."[25] *Laka* was goddess of forest growth and the *hula*. While dancing the *hula Laka* was to be the inspiration, causing the *hula* movements. The *hula* was considered objectionable because it told the story of Hawai'i based on any number of gods and goddesses in mythology—and often sensuously carried out by topless women. It seemed to unnecessarily conjure up their ancient mythology. Yet Damien found that the *kānaka* were less bound to their "pagan" ways than other non-lepers, even when he set about stopping the *hula*. He felt they had reached "the climax of despair, both of body and soul," a forgivable dalliance perhaps, and were more amenable to hearing his preaching.[26]

But the *kānaka* were lighthearted people in spite of their awful affliction. Gatherings in their hovels were frequent and sometimes boisterous, made all the more cheerful by drink and music. They would guzzle fermented sweet potatoes, sound the *uliuli* (a gourd-like musical instrument), and revelers would start the offensive *hula* dance. Not one for frivolous socializing, Damien had no time for their irreverent fêtes—particularly the wanton *hula*. "If Damien arrived, the hilarious feast would abruptly break up . . . party goers would hurry to dodge out the back door to escape his big stick, for he would not hesitate to lay it on good and hard on the poor hapless person who happened to come within reach of his cane," told admirer and leper, Ambrose Hutchison.[27]

In some sense, Damien, like many Westerners, had preconceived notions of the *kānaka maoli*. He thought of them as "children." Despite their physical prowess and initiative in building churches and residences and their devotion to singing at Mass and their general cheerfulness, he felt there was another side to their character. He often featured them as he would a "bad child": willfully disobedient, unteachable, and even "irredeemable." He was particularly offended by their blatant sexuality. As Cook's sailors had found, they were uninhibited in dress and sexual self-expression. Damien wrote at one point "corruption is so precocious among the young *kānaka*! The children have scarcely learned to talk before they know more than a young theologian still has to find out." He, of course, was poorly equipped to make such judgments. He was not an anthropologist, and his frame of reference was little better, a sheltered child himself enamored with his Western Catholicism. It was as Rudyard Kipling penned during those colonial times, "The White Man's Burden": to bind fellow humans to exile, "half devil and half child."[28]

Damien knew just the same that he was witnessing what no human should suffer alone. He wrote to his brother January 31, 1880:

> I have now been nearly seven years among the lepers. During that long period, I have had the opportunity of closely observing, and as it were touching with my hand, human misery under its most terrible aspects. Half the people are like living corpses, which the worms have already begun to devour, at first internally, afterwards externally, until the most loathsome wounds are formed, which very rarely heal.[29]

He apparently was burying an estimated two hundred people each year. Many of the graves he dug himself. The Catholic cemetery at Kalawao was close to his house. He wrote his brother that frequently at night he would go there. Amid the sea breezes and distant rhythmically rolling surf his mind would take him beyond. He called the dead his "spiritual children." He would stand and meditate over their graves about the "unending happiness which so many of them are already enjoying." He confessed to his brother that the cemetery and the hut of the dying were a "benefit of my own soul."[30]

He labored on their spirit, the faith of life after death, the end of their earthly agony. This may have been his true healing potential. For one so caring and dynamic, surely words of redemption would carry a heavy impact. "Ordinarily, they listen attentively to the word of Salvation, which I spread among them according to their disposition. . . . Here, I give words of sweetness and consolation, there, I mix in a little bitterness . . . I threaten the impenitent with terrible punishment."[31] He knew his lepers, every one, by name, and knew their temperaments and propensities. It was something one so committed must do. It was with that knowledge he could work on their mind and their spirit. He individually directed each to look inside, amend their flaws, and seek a closer union with the supernatural. For those too sick to reflect, he simply sat with them in silence.

Damien's patience and simple companionship seemed to help. Some months after Damien's arrival, a local newspaper, the *Ka Nuhou Hawaii*, printed a report by William Ragsdale, then superintendent of the raggedy Kalawao Leprosy Hospital. Of Father Damien, Ragsdale wrote:

> [Damien] is very dedicated in separating and planting the seeds of life among the members of his church, and he is also dedicated to searching for everything that makes the grieving lives of the patients comfortable in some places. He constantly goes among the patients who are seen to be experiencing troubles in their lives, giving hope to [the hopeless].[32]

Damien's reputation as the selfless leper-priest spread quickly. American author Charles William Stoddard, eager to meet this fabled Father Damien, told of his first visit with him and tour of the colony.

> From cottage to cottage, across lots, through garden spots ablaze with brilliant flowers . . . lepers were everywhere waiting to receive us; they crouched under the thick banana hedges, or in the smallest of verandas . . . [with] spirits comparatively gay . . . dwelling within the sound of the busy hammer that is shaping the coffins which are to enclose their remains!

His duties were never-ending, Stoddard observed, Mass in the morning at Saint Philomena, then continuous rounds of his lepers at home or in the makeshift hospital "to ease the anguish of the sick and dying." Religious services in Kalawao were highlights of the colony life. Yet Stoddard found that High Mass there was celebrated in more of a spirit of requiem than salvation. Invariably, the small chapel was packed, the unmistakable odor of leprosy hanging in the air. He saw all the participants were doomed; the living "well-nigh dead." But the chapel would be filled with sweet singing and smiling faces. Their devotion was remarkable, he saw. Life beyond the grave was their only salvation.[33]

What kind of man was this imperfect but saintly character who would forego personal safety and health for the sake of the miserable outcasts of a remote civilization? One of the lepers, Ambrose Kanewalii Hutchison, who arrived in 1879 and would spend over fifty years at the settlement, described Damien in quite mortal terms:

> There was nothing supernatural about Father Damien. He was a vigorous, forceful and impellent man with a big kindly heart in the prime of life and a jack of all trades, carpenter, mason, baker, farmer, medico and nurse, grave digger. . . . He was that type of man of action, bull headed, strong will high minded . . . of determined tenacity to attain results of his aspiration, but of kindly disposition toward all who came into contact with him. . . . Father Damien's relations with non-Catholic Christians were amiable and friendly.[34]

As for his personality, physician Arthur Albert St. Mouritz came as the resident doctor for the Kalaupapa community in 1883. He faced a weathered Damien by that time, the priest in the throes of leprosy himself. Considered an authority on leprosy, Mouritz at first did not appreciate Damien's supercilious attitude on treatment as a non-physician, although, by that time, Damien himself had ten years of experience. Nevertheless, he could not help but admire the man and characterized the leper priest as active, vigorous, and tireless. He had the calloused hands of a worker; fingers of a common laborer who toiled almost daily to maintain the physical shoring of the settlement. Mouritz went on to write that:

> His temperament was mixed . . . He was easily excited, easily peeved, super-sensitive, and difficult to get along with at times. Damien and I clashed and snapped repeatedly. His years of residence at the Settlement had made him an autocrat on all matters; he had very fixed views and brooked no interference with his will. His unyielding attitude on many affairs outside his proper sphere of work brought him in conflict with the Board of Health and the workers connected with the other religious sects at the Settlement.[35]

Yet Mouritz was constantly amazed at Damien's disregard for personal safety. He would touch, clean, and bandage the leprous lesions without hesitation, a behavior Mouritz strictly avoided, using a cane to lift clothes and examine ulcers. But Damien, with bare hands, gently teased the sticky dressings off open sores; wash, pick, and wipe away the gummy exudate that had accumulated; then unroll and wrap with new bandages. He would feel the rising tubercles, search their mouths, and even examine the moist under-pinnings of their genitals. Some lay in liquid excrement—dysentery was a constant accompaniment—that he would dutifully scrub away. Mouritz felt Damien's methods were pure suicide. His manner with the lepers was gentle and patient. More than one observer told of this. He seldom argued, one said. He was not impulsive, and remained calm—even for deviant behavior, like drunkenness, he rebuked but did not humiliate. One leprous woman, Kaili'ohe Kame'ekua, who eventually lived to be 115 years old, likened Damien to Jesus Himself. "Watching him [Damien] I learned about Jesus. They were both alone. No one took care of them. They had no 'Ohana [family]."[36]

Despite groundless accusations that he was flirting with non-leprous women sent to Kalawao to help with house cleaning and cooking,[37] Damien's care of the lepers never diminished. Day after day he would make his rounds. Each deserved personal attention, both physically and emotionally. It was so time-consuming that some days were spent doing little else. He would see them arrive, mark their deterioration, and watch them die. Never a thought of his own safety, he would dip with them from the same bowl of *poi*, smoke their pipes, and sit on their filthy mats. Of his brushes with the incurable leprosy, Charles Stoddard wrote,

> Father Damien's escape [from leprosy], after eleven years of intimacy with the worst known cases; after having nursed the sick and buried the dead—more

than 1,600 of them—can be looked upon as almost miraculous. He is working with them and for them night and day; his intimates are lepers; his house is hardly ever free of them.[38]

In fact, he was extremely curious about the disease and would often transcribe his parishioners' medical histories for the benefit of visiting physicians. He recorded ten in great detail, including "salmon-covered spots," "hands and feet insensitive," "eyes always open, flesh wasted away." By the time he submitted his account two of the ten were already dead. In that report he finished with the prophetic line, "perhaps I have the germ of leprosy in system, I am not sure."[39]

Indeed, he would not escape and there would be no miracles. On return from a visit to Honolulu in the early 1880s, Ambrose Hutchison was on the wharf unloading supplies when Damien stepped ashore. His left foot was bandaged. "Naturally I asked the Father how he hurt his foot? And came the prompt answer, I did it with hot water . . . I think I have the disease." Damien added. He had noticed pain in his left foot for some time, thinking maybe it was sciatic nerve trouble. But the numbness was another indicator. Examination by a visiting physicians detected the telltale cord lateral to the head of the fibula—an inflamed peroneal nerve, a hallmark of leprosy.[40]

Instead of his customary "you lepers" with which he often began his Sunday sermons, Damien would now begin "we lepers."

In 1885, Damien wrote Bishop Koeckmann in Honolulu: "I cannot come to Honolulu, for leprosy has attacked me. There are signs of it on my left cheek and ear, and my eyebrows are beginning to fall; I shall soon be quite disfigured." The news of the disease he kept from his ailing mother, but she discovered it anyway. The Belgian papers announced it and someone read the report to his mother. "Well," she commented, "we shall go to Heaven together." She died August 5, 1886.[41]

Not surprisingly, Damien's routine remained unaltered. One leper, sent to Kalawao in the last year of Damien's life, found "his charity towards people maybe made him imprudent regarding infection, but he couldn't act in any other way if he wanted to help them."[42] Yet Damien, like other lepers, suffered the torment of loneliness and, as one so religious, began to doubt his worthiness for heaven. He even managed a trip to Honolulu to go through the new treatment devised by the Japanese Gotō Masafumi and his son Masanao, who peddled their regimen of therapy across Japan and the Pacific with baths and ingestion of the foul-tasting Seiketsuren pill—more or less a self-declared "purifying" substance. Encouraging at first, the regimen soon failed. The baths sapped his strength, the numbness of his foot remained unaltered, and his facial lesions were progressing. Most distressing was his easy fatiguability. He had lost his joy in physical exertion. Damien resigned himself to his fate. Ironically, as he weakened the numbers of lepers on Kalaupapa decreased as well. There had been only forty-three admissions in all of 1886—an all-time low.

By 1887 he was still performing his backbreaking duties for the leper colony and, by sheer determination, had not slackened in the least on his busy schedule. "Though leprosy has a pretty strong hold on my body, and has already disfigured me somewhat, I continue to be robust and strong, and my terrible pains in the feet are gone . . . I continue to say Mass every day."[43] He continued to be the only priest on Moloka'i despite his diagnosis.

Despite the inexorable progression of his leprosy, Damien continued his vigorous physical labors, even helping to enlarge the chapel of Saint Philomena. Then, while saying Mass one day in October 1888, he collapsed and needed help to retire to his quarters, unable to proceed with the service. His appearance withered. That December, visiting nuns alarmingly remarked that "his face and lips [were] deathly gray, covered with purplish red inflamed tubercles. . . . His voice was gone. . . . He looked so cold. . . . And yet he was so happy and cheerful."[44]

On February 19, 1889, Damien wrote his brother, Pamphile: "I am happy and contented. . . . Kindly remember me to all the Fathers and Brothers of Louvain, to Gerard, Leonce, and all the family . . . I do not forget any of you." He then asked that "God fortify me and give me the grace of perseverance and a good death." This was his last letter.[45] Despite his weakness and fevers, Damien dragged himself to Saint Philomena's each day for prayer and meditation. When that finally became impossible, he would lay on his thin mat on the floor, not allowing it to be replaced with a comfortable mattress and clean sheets until he was too weak to object. On April 13, fellow priest Father Conrardy anointed him with the sacrament of Extreme Unction: "From the realm of death deliver my soul, O Lord. Once I was dead but now I live—forever and ever." Words that Damien must have uttered countless times to the dying lepers under his care.[46]

Consumed with pneumonia, Damien passed peacefully on April 15, 1889.

There was a spontaneous outpouring of adulation from Hawaiians for the man who had sacrificed his life in the care of the shunned incurables. Worldwide his reputation was already revered. He had become, even before his death, a living saint. He was truly a martyr, one who is a witness to God. Among the destitute he brought companionship; among the suffering, compassion. Among the forlorn he brought faith. One biography summed up Damien's solution to hopelessness:

He was therefore a slave in their bodily service, their nurse, their doctor, the builder, the carpenter, the farm laborer, the coffin-maker; the versatile and many-sided genius who evolved order out of chaos, cleanliness, self-respect and happiness out of abject misery, a well-ordered community in pretty villages with churches, hospitals, and orphan-houses, and all accomplished practically single-handed.[47]

Damien provided creature comforts, dignity, and respect. He saw to sturdy walls, sound roofs, clean floors, clean skin, and fresh clothing. He laughed with them, wept with them, mourned for them. He restored a sense of normalcy to lives never to be normal. This is how he healed the incurables. May Quinlan quoted a contemporary who said of Damien, "[m]en are so made that they have a hunger for human sympathy, a need for someone who can heal the bruised spirit, or where the injury is deep, bind up the broken heart."[48]

For the *kānaka* incurability was not death; despondency was. Loneliness was. Healing was not cure; comfort was. Family was. And for them companionship was the essence of living. Human connection defined not physical health, but spiritual tranquility, Damien saw.

~

CHAPTER NINE

Aequanimitas

William Osler

There was perhaps no more central figure in the integrated method of healing than physician Sir William Osler (1849–1919). He was a character of complexity. Highly intelligent, spirited, inquisitive, and yet, in all his scientific acumen, Osler remained acutely aware of the profound nature of man. At his core, in his practice of medicine, he fully comprehended the dramatic impact of disease on the psyche. In 1893 at the Johns Hopkins Hospital Historical Club meeting in Baltimore Osler quoted the Greek philosopher Plato, whom he greatly admired,

> there is no proportion or disproportion more productive of health and disease and virtue and vice, than that between soul and body. In the double nature of the living being if there is in this compound an impassioned soul more powerful than the body, "that soul, I say, convulses and fills with disorders the whole inner nature of man . . . we should not move the body without the soul or the soul without the body."[1]

Quoting Plato again in his famous farewell speech "Aequanimitas" in Philadelphia before his new posting in Baltimore, Osler emphasized that "the body cannot be cured without the soul." They are interdependent. They are in sympathy with each other.[2]

Osler was one who understood the convolutions of human nature and the impact of disease. "The processes of disease are so complex that it is excessively difficult to search out the laws which control them," he spoke at McGill University in 1895.[3] To be a physician—to be able to heal—one must be at the crossroads of the earthly and spiritual—what Cotton Mather had called the angelical conjunction of medicine and divinity. To his listeners he preached *caritas*, the art of caring. It is a sacred duty. He would assert that "the practice of medicine is an art, not a trade, a calling, not a business, a calling in which your heart will be exercised equally with your head." Furthermore, he warned that "often the best part of your work will have nothing to do with potions and powders, but with the exercise of an influence of the strong upon the weak, of the righteous upon the wicked, the wise upon the foolish." Patients are not burdened with the mere incongruities of their physical disorder but are torn by the anxieties of ignorance, doubt, and hopelessness. In the end, he would advocate for humanism, "of a humanity that will show in your daily life tenderness and consideration to the weak, infinite pity to the suffering and a broad charity to all."[4]

William Osler knew about healing. And his passion for teaching would impact countless students in their quest to be like him. To be as riveting and compassionate and wise as their master.

His story is one of a personal quest as well, for what he later termed *aequanimitas*, the calmness of mind that comes with a realistic appreciation of what can be done and what is not possible. This applied not only to an inner tranquility but also a projection of that same imperturbability to patients in their suffering, that the healer understood and, with an unnerving confidence, would guide them through their illness. It would not be an easy search and would bring him to a point where he himself found that elusive equanimity beyond his reach.

Osler was Canadian by birth. His father, Featherstone Lake Osler, had immigrated from England as a missionary evangelical to the backwoods of the dominant English settlements of Upper Canada. Featherstone was avidly Christian and preached with passion on the salvation of immortal souls. His son, "Willie" as he was known, was not so swayed as a youngster, participating in the usual antics and misbehaviors of typical adolescents. In fact, at age fifteen young Willie was tossed out of Dundee (Ontario) Grammar School for allegedly locking a gaggle of geese in a rival public school overnight and removing all the desks and chairs. Things were little better at his new grammar school, Barrie, where he quickly rose to lead "Barrie's bad boys," he and fellow boarders who could not stop their antics with their foes, the "day" students. Despite his bad boy image, he managed to graduate and enter Trinity College School on scholarship in Weston, Ontario, beginning in 1866. His reputation as a rabble-rouser continued there when he and fellow students were actually arraigned for assault. Even though he may have been the ringleader, charges against him were eventually dropped.[5] Pugilistic tendencies aside, his initial desire was to concentrate on the classics and divinity studies in anticipation of entering the ministry. He was a man of religious faith. The influence of loving parents was unmistakable and instilled deep spiritual beliefs by their words and behavior. In fact, his mother, Ellen, wrote to him of that issue in May 1866. She was delighted that one of her boys had an interest in ministry.

> It is a matter not to be decided hastily any more than is any other profession . . . above all search your heart for the motives inducing your decision, for remember that God always judges of us by our motives while man can only judge of our actions. If you ask God he will give you wisdom and guide you in the right path.[6]

Despite a sincere desire to focus on his Christian faith, Osler could not help being attracted to the more corporal mysteries of life. He finally made the switch to medicine and entered the Toronto School of Medicine in 1868. The art of healing intrigued him. It was a knowledge of the natural applied to the unknown. He imagined himself a descendant of the Hellenic cult of Asclepius, even. From the start, Osler proved to be an avid fan of history and viewed medical progress as a lineage of "apostolic succession."[7] Medicine, he later claimed, had evolved due to the wisdom and energy of Hippocrates, Galen, and others to emancipate the profession from priest-craft and shape it as the profession of cultivated gentlemen.[8]

In 1870, Osler, at the advice of mentors and friends, moved to nearby McGill University in Montreal, considered the pinnacle of medical care in Canada, if not all of North America. In his time there, Osler became something of a loner but an avid student of the life sciences: anatomy, pathology, medicine, and surgery. It was from there that he received his Doctor of Medicine and *Chirurgiae Magister* (Master of Surgery). But like many North Americans, any further training would have to be done in Europe. Osler chose the University of London. There, he concentrated on research in physiology and pathology and in 1874 continued on to the continent where he studied in Germany and Austria. After taking advantage of the best of Germanic specialists, Osler returned to America that spring of 1874, and took the position as lecturer in the Institutes of Medicine at McGill University. As one of his pupils observed:

> I saw him first as he entered the lecture-room to open his course. . . . Quick and active, yet deliberate in his walk and manner, with a serious and earnest expression, it was evident that he looked upon his lectures as serious, and at once imparted the same feeling to others. . . . When I look back upon that period it is evident that 1876-7 was the beginning of a period of *renaissance* for McGill, and Osler the moving spirit.[9]

He was a remarkable physician and educator. Osler easily conveyed his sense of compassion and consideration to his students, who quickly bonded with him. They saw in him a wise, gentle person who understood the essence of the physician. He seemed to grasp the inherent obligations of doctors to unite in suffering with their patients, to understand their pain and anxiety, and to address the spiritual misery many ill could not escape. This was important to him that he send the same message to his students, that they understand the gravity of their profession and the duties they assume as physicians—not only as diagnosticians but also as literal conferrers of charity.

Yet Osler had reservations about the German system of medical schooling. He was leery of unbridled experimentation if not done contextually in the attitude of compassion. The basic function of the university—of Academic Life—was to educate. It stemmed from the root of the word. In Greek Ἀκαδημία ("Academia") referred to the grove of trees in Athens under which Plato discoursed. In such an academic inclination, Osler cautioned unbridled science:

> It is very hard to adjust the two great functions of a University. . . . The work which shall advance the science . . . is the most attractive, and in German laboratories occupies the chief time of the director. . . . On the other hand, the teaching functions of an Institute [University] is apt to be neglected in the more seductive pursuit of the "bauble reputation."[10]

In Osler's estimation, teaching was not glorious or glamorous, but it was the very intellectual blood of life, the driving force for civilization—the passing of wisdom from one generation to another. Instruction in the art by those of proper bearing could afford a balance of healing: attention to ramifications of illness—withering of body *and* mind.

In 1884, Osler was offered a coveted position at the University of Pennsylvania in Philadelphia. It was a bold move by the trustees of the university, more inclined to consider only native Philadelphians. Yet men of such distinction as Silas Weir Mitchell and Samuel W. Gross lobbied hard for the man, so impressed had they been at meeting him. Trustees agreed and the offer went out. Osler could not resist. He freely admitted to his colleagues at McGill that it was a matter of ambition. He accepted the posting as chair of Clinical Medicine and moved from Montreal to Philadelphia. What prompted the change is largely unknown, and Osler had no clear explanation other than the opportunity to accept a leadership role in, perhaps, the most prestigious medical complex in the United States. He was handsomely supported by Philadelphians who had witnessed his glowing reputation in Montreal and felt, if an outsider was to be chosen, there was no better man than Osler.

Outwardly, he seemed a peculiar choice. Osler presented not as the crisp, aristocratic academician to which Penn students had grown accustomed. On the contrary, his behavior seemed disheveled. In his rush to the lecture hall, he was often seen to jump from his street care—not horse-drawn personal carriage—looking a bit rumpled, a tawny-skinned person with a drooping mustache, perhaps more akin to bartender than physician. He then would rush into the classroom, carrying a satchel with his lunch and with bunches of books and papers under his arm barely under control. He was not a natural orator, they found. His speech was halting and peppered with anecdotal examples of disease that he used to accentuate his points. It was not until his pupils saw him in his more familiar setting on ward rounds that they discovered the true brilliance of the man. The bedside was Osler's true pulpit. This was where his instructions were most impressive. His rapport with his patients was unique and fostered such an admiration that clusters of students gathered to see his bedside chats and examinations. He was a master of the hands-on method of teaching, commanding his residents to accompany him on his rounds, tutoring them in examining patients, and extracting from them the ability to link their findings with pathological processes. He would guide them on palpation, percussion, and auscultation, pointing out irregularities impossible to learn from books or lectures. He was so at ease with his patients, it was as if they were fast friends or even family. He would chat about their hobbies, their likes and dislikes, their joys and sorrows, and, in due course, about their illness. All the while he would puncture their stolid exterior and find a measure of their spirit. Thus, he would unite disease and illness. This style would become his trademark for years to come. Teaching would prove to be a sincere passion of his and would shape the expectations of his educational efforts.[11]

His reputation quickly grew. One former graduate remembered that Osler "was gracious to his elders, cordial to his contemporaries, encouraging to his juniors, and jovial almost to the point of frivolity with all." But the salient feature was that he knew his subject matter through and through and knew how to teach it well.[12] As one colleague said, Osler had the peculiar power of "inseminating their minds."[13] There is no teaching without the patient as a textbook, he famously said at one point. The best teaching, he added, was by the patient himself. "The whole art of medicine is in observation, as the old motto goes, but to educate the eye to see, the ear to hear and the finger to feel takes time, and to make a beginning, to start a man on the right path, is all that we can do."[14]

Through it all his Christian principles remained firmly entrenched. A physician remembered that during his student days, destitute as many students of medicine were, he encountered Osler on the streets of Washington, a man with whom he was only vaguely acquainted. Sheepishly, he asked Osler for twenty-five dollars to get home. Unhesitatingly, Osler gave him fifty. Twenty-five was not enough he said. In fact, Osler exuded humility and gentleness. A friend from university days remembered:

> Ever since I knew Osler—as quite a young man—he had always the same quiet serious manner, with unperturbed features and dark-complexioned almost expressionless face—so that strangers were entirely unprepared for the humor which would sally forth at the most unexpected times, without any relaxation of countenance or any change in tone of voice . . . indeed, people sometimes would take a remark which was entirely jocular *au grand serieux*, and wonder that it should have been made by so sedate and learned a person.[15]

It was in 1884, after moving to Philadelphia, that he developed a strong friendship with Samuel W. Gross, a surgeon at cross-town Jefferson Medical College. Gross, of course, had pushed for Osler to come to Philadelphia. Samuel's father, Samuel D. Gross, had just died the preceding May. Samuel D. Gross had been known for his hospitality and, in this vein, his son Samuel W. and daughter-in-law, the socialite Grace Linzee Revere Gross, followed suit. Grace, seventeen years her husband's junior, seemed the devoted spouse and had become involved in various social and philanthropic activities around Philadelphia. She herself was the great-granddaughter of Paul Revere of Boston and had been raised in all the patrician privileges such heritage provided. She was quite the flirtatious woman, an eye-turning beauty, charming and engaging and adding a spark to her more reticent husband. They invited the newcomer Osler over for an October Sunday dinner, which Osler quickly accepted. He knew no one in Philadelphia and had become stricken with a bit of Canadian homesickness. Besides, his spartan quarters had been overrun with mosquitoes in the uncharacteristically humid Philadelphia autumn. From then on, nearly every Sunday night, Osler had dinner with the Grosses at 1112 Walnut Street.[16]

And then Osler got wind of a new effort in the city of Baltimore. With a generous gift from the philanthropist Johns Hopkins, a hospital was to be built, centered around research and education. It was to furnish "advanced study in medicine and surgery" and recruit the finest of clinicians and academicians in the country.[17] John Shaw Billings had been named by the president of the new Johns Hopkins Hospital. The hospital was to represent state-of-the-art medicine and the pinnacle of American healthcare. Heavily endowed by the railroad tycoon Johns Hopkins, he instructed his board to "secure for the service of the hospital, surgeons and physicians of the highest character and of the greatest skill." Hopkins had specified that the hospital was to be for "the indigent sick of this city and its environs, without regard to sex, age, or color, who require surgical or medical treatment," in particular, the destitute and poor.[18] Billings had begun spending time with Osler in 1888 at medical meetings, and was seen so often with him that suspicion arose. He had won Osler over. Not long afterward, Billings offered Osler the position of Physician-in-Chief. "I have received a definite offer from the J. H. [Johns Hopkins] authorities & have determined to accept it. I shall leave you with deep regret. You have been like a good, kind brother. There need be no hurry about any official action, & I only write this so that you may be the first to know of it."[19]

Just before leaving Philadelphia tragedy struck. His dear friend Samuel W. Gross took ill with pneumonia. Despite the efforts of prominent Jefferson doctors and Osler, too, he died in a storm of fevers and delirium at age fifty-two.

On Wednesday morning May 1, 1889, Osler gave his farewell address to the University of Pennsylvania students—his celebrated 'Aequanimitas' address. In his oration, he acknowledged the death of his friend Samuel.

> We mourn to-day, also . . . the grievous loss which she has sustained in the death of one of her most distinguished teachers, a man who bore with honor an honored name, and who added luster to the profession of this city. Such men as Samuel W. Gross can ill be spared.[20]

He emphasized the quality of equanimity. "How difficult to attain, yet how necessary, in success as in failure," he added. Later, addressing the faculty, he admitted:

> While preaching to you a doctrine of equanimity, I am, myself, a castaway. . . . [T]o-day I sever my connection with this University. More than once, gentlemen, in a life rich in the priceless blessings of friends, I have been placed in positions in which no words could express the feelings of my heart, and so it is with me now. The keenest sentiments of gratitude well up from my innermost being at the thought of the kindliness and goodness, which have followed me at every step during the past five years.[21]

As for Samuel Gross' widow, Grace, intrigue was in the air. Ostensibly only dear friends, Osler's first public encounter with the widow Grace was during a trip in the autumn of 1889 to the Island of Grand Matan, where he met a boat bringing "two mysterious friends," "the Widow Gross . . . and Miss Woolley" who made the rest of the trip with Osler. What serendipity, one might think. Was it?[22] Then, in 1891 he offered a courting relationship but she refused, perhaps knowing he was preoccupied with writing his medical textbook. At length, she was visiting friends in Baltimore when Osler appeared with a big red book under his arm. He gave it to her with the words, "There, take the darn thing; now what are you going to do with the man?"[23] He finished his grand textbook, *Principles and Practice of Medicine* in 1892. There could be little doubt Grace, at that point, acquiesced. A secretive courtship began.

Osler visited his mother, Ellen, shortly after the publishing of his book, perhaps to tell of the news of his attachment to Grace. His mother was not surprised. As a mother might, Ellen long suspected an allure. She promptly wrote a friend:

He let Father and me into his secret when he was up, but we were not at liberty to make known the fact — these young things always think their love affairs are secrets to the outside world, whereas lookers-on often see plainly enough.[24]

On May 7, 1892, Osler took a train from Baltimore to Philadelphia and then straightaway to 1112 Walnut Street. Planned well in advance and hidden even from the household help, Grace had packed trunks delivered to the train station. They were eloping. And in all the clandestine intrigue that had surrounded their romance, they were finally married. How the whole affair had unfolded can only be a matter of speculation. Neither Grace nor Osler hinted at their mutual romantic appeal. The fact that they kept company was usually attributed to friendship only. Of course, that was not the entire truth.[25]

Within months of their secretive wedding, Grace became aware of her pregnancy. The baby was born at home with Johns Hopkins surgeon Howard Kelly in attendance on February 6, 1893, almost nine months exactly from their wedding day. Osler was delighted, feeling he had given Grace something her first husband did not—a live child. Grace had delivered a infant to her first husband, Samuel, in 1877. An easy birth, as Osler recounted. But his new son, Paul Revere Osler, did not thrive. Osler worried to a friend, "the young doctor looked very touchy; tho fine & strong he has developed a bad jaundice which has benumbed his nerve centres more than usual," Osler remembered that, although the birth was outwardly uncomplicated, the baby was "a little asphyxiated." The newborn struggled for several days but died a week later. "He seemed all right for five or six days and then developed a sudden coma," Osler wrote. His presumed explanation for the death was a meningeal hemorrhage at birth.[26]

By early 1895, Grace was pregnant again. That December, she gave birth to their son, Edward Revere. Osler announced the birth in his usual casual fashion: "Mrs. Osler had a small boy last week—both are doing splendidly. We are of course delighted, and he looks a strong and durable specimen."[27] A man reticent to share his private life, Osler no doubt was deeply moved by the event. Grace, less reserved than her husband, shared his private musings with her mother:

> You must please excuse the proud father if he leaves unsaid what you want to know, for he is really very much excited. . . . Before he left last night, he said he had kissed him [Edward] five times. He brings all his medical friends up to look at him.

Father and son were exceedingly close. William and he shared a number of activities, including their favorite, fly fishing. Academically, Edward excelled and would eventually gain entrance to Christ Church College at Oxford the spring of 1914. Osler suspected that Edward, whom he and Grace would informally call "Revere," would indeed be his protégé.[28]

After eight years of service, Sir John Burdon-Sanderson resigned as the Regius Professor of Medicine at Oxford University, England in 1904. It was a position of regal importance, founded by King Henry VIII in 1546. Such a prestigious position demanded the utmost consideration of one so sympathetic to the furtherance of medical science at Oxford—one, who the graduates insisted, to be held by a physician who is representative of Medicine in its widest sense—and preferably one of its alumni. Such a position was long in prestige but quite short in remuneration—£400 per year. Who would leave their lucrative careers for such a downturn in financial security? It is not certain who first suggested Osler's name. Sanderson, on hearing Osler's name submitted, immediately approved and forwarded it to the Prime Minister Arthur Balfour, as the position was a Crown appointment. Osler, burdened by increasing amounts of clinical responsibilities at Johns Hopkins—and with the enthusiastic approbation of his wife (afraid he would literally work himself into an early grave)— accepted.

> You will be surprised when I tell you that I have accepted the Chair of Medicine at Oxford; — to leave next Spring! 'Tis a serious step, but I have considered it well from all points. I am on the down grade, the pace of the last three winters has been such that I knew was riding for a fall Better to get out decently in time, & leave while there is still a little elasticity in the rubber.[29]

Osler, Grace, Revere, and their belongings sailed from New York on May 19, 1905, and arrived in Oxford Saturday evening May 27. And so began the next chapter in this illustrious life. He was the new Regius Professor of Medicine.

His house had open doors for his residents and students. Every facet of their existence concerned him. He and his wife Grace extended open invitations for residents to stop by, so much so that they were referred to as Osler's "Latchkeyers." His home was open for visits, tennis, swimming, and idle conversation. Saturday nights in particular were his weekly "evening talks." They were inviolate. Nothing was to interfere. Students sat around his dining room table with beer, books, and tobacco discussing all the nuances of medicine. Grace did not demure; she was the perfect hostess making sure all had adequate supplies of food, drink, and smoke.

Osler was always cognizant of the spirit. In fact, he was quite curious about things mystical. He would lose himself in contemplation, particularly when surrounded by the otherworldly portrayals of artists. On one cathedral visit, he remarked:

What manner of men were they who could, in those (to us) dark days, build such transcendent monuments? What was the secret of their art? By what

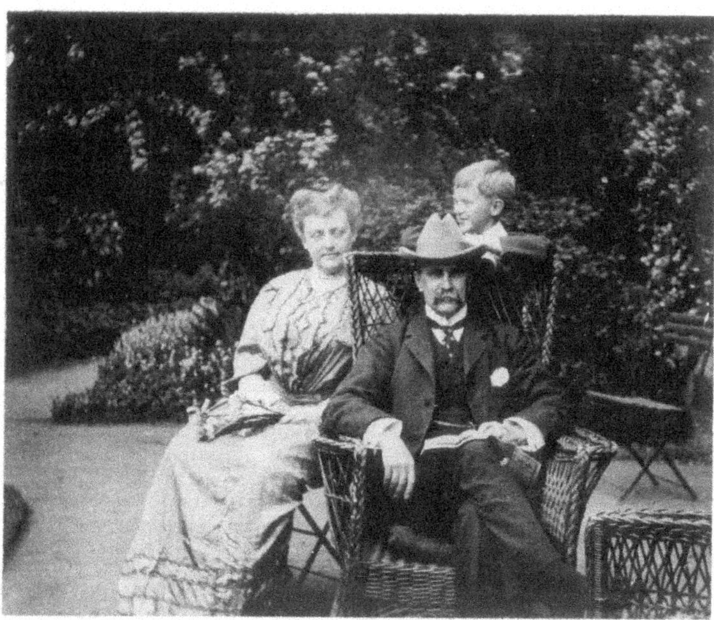

Figure 9.1   Sir William Osler, his wife Grace, and young son Revere. Colin Kerr Russel.

spirit were they moved? . . . Here was the answer. Moving in a world not realized, these men sought, however feebly, to express in glorious structures their conception of the beauty of holiness, and these works, our wonder, are but the outward and visible signs of the ideals, which animated them.[30]

In a paper read before the Philadelphia Neurological Society on November 28, 1892, on the classical Greek influence of medicine, Osler commented: "in the Golden Age of Greece, medicine had as today a triple relationship, with science, with gymnastics, and with theology." He went on to say that "[s]o much of the daily life of a civilized community relates to problems of health and disease that the great writers of every age of necessity throw an important sidelight not only on the opinions of the people on these questions, but often on the condition of special knowledge in various branches."[31]

Perhaps it was this tendency to entertain the metaphysical that led him to be soft with the cheerlessly ill and make every attempt to cushion discouraging news. "The careful physician has but one end in view—not to depress his patient in any way whatever." On one occasion a former student of his was mortally ill. As one nurse recalled, "Dr. Osler came, a gentle, tender presence, in a huge fur coat, and sat down by Dr. Swan [his former student]. . . . He talked to him like a sorrowing tender Mother for her little boy, and then he put his arm around him and said, 'Now Swan I want you to let this good woman here give you some morphia tonight so that you may relax and sleep, for that is what you need; and I want you to do this for me, your old Professor and friend.'" The man took the drug and slept magnificently that night. He felt better the next day but died soon afterward.[32] It was his observant nature that deciphered the spirit of the patient. "How much his eyes will see that would escape most of us." He would first fix his gaze into the patient's eyes, a penetrating gaze that saw through to the soul. Then he would examine every inch of the body, looking for additional clues. Infinite patience and "ever-tender charity" were his principles. He was quick to recognize that unique feature that concerned him the most when encountering patients. All other behavior, no matter how incongruous or irritating, he put from his mind. His focus was on the problem at hand. In that regard he was merciful and masterful. Aloof, intimidating behavior he strictly avoided. No long faces around his patients. That would only add to their worry and depression. To his students he imparted the immutable features of life—a heritage of sorrow and suffering as ancient as time and as constant as the heavens, unaltered by the most stupendous of scientific discoveries. Tragedy will always be with us, he counseled. Prepare. Patients need a kind presence.[33]

This was a major theme of his instruction. Amid the elation and despair of the profession, one must keep an even temperament, yet able to enlighten and comfort the most cantankerous of patients, he argued. In his Harvard lecture May 1904 on "Immortality of Man" he elaborated:

As perplexity of soul will be your lot and portion, accept the situation with a good grace. The hopes and fears which make us men are inseparable, and this wine-press of Doubt each one of you must tread alone. It is a trouble from which no man may deliver his brother or make agreement with another for him. Better that your spirit's bark be driven far from the shore — far from the trembling throng whose sails were never to the tempest given — than that you should tie it up to rot at some Lethean [Lethe, one of the rivers of Hades in Greek mythology signifying oblivion or forgetfulness] wharf.[34]

In 1911, as part of his coronation, King George V of England conferred a baronetcy—a hereditary knighthood—on Osler, the man his parents called "Willie," for his contributions to medicine. It was now to be Sir William. Grace Osler would henceforth be called *Lady* Osler. "They have been putting a baronetcy on me—much to the embarrassment of my democratic simplicity, but it does not seem to make any difference in my internal sensations," he humbly wrote to Marcia Noyes, his librarian friend from the Maryland State Medical Society. He jokingly made light of it with his American family, deprecatingly referring to himself as that irrepressible "bad boy" of his childhood and that he had fooled his compatriots with such honors. He signed the letter "Sir Billy."[35]

Osler's Oxford library was extensive, filled with texts on medicine since antiquity. One corner, though, was of special curiosity. He called it humorously as the section of "Death, Heaven and Hell." It contained books on spiritualism and its many manifestations—dreams, ghosts, witchcraft, immortality, resurrection, and the like. He was in high demand for travels, lectureships, and committee meetings. Osler had reached the pinnacle of his career; he was preeminent in the field of medicine. His social circles included visits from international dignitaries, including United States Army General John J. Pershing and Herbert Hoover. Grace reveled in the swirl of festive events, rubbing shoulders with the British Douglas Haig and the French commander Joseph Joffre.

And then tragedy struck.

His only child, Edward Revere Osler—called, informally, Revere—on whom Sir William and Grace doted, had grown to adulthood with that unblemished look of the privileged and the serene gaze of confidence and assurance that somehow his destiny would unfold in the most comfortable of terms. With fair complexion and strikingly blue eyes, he gave an air of good breeding and remarkable potential. Edward had the legacy of American patriots and British nobility. And now in 1917 the eager Revere Osler would look askance at the camera for his portraiture in the dress of the Canadian Royal Army Artillery.

Youthful enthusiasm for the glory of military service seized many young men, full of bravado but so ignorant of the tempests that lie ahead. No less was the ardor of Revere. At age nineteen Revere, as he was called, was struck with an abiding desire to serve. No doubt many of his countrymen had already joined, and any able body male of his age would be pressured—inwardly or outwardly—to do the same. Despite the pleas of mother and father, "[he] has made up his mind about the first steps to take," Grace wrote to her sister. The father was beside himself with it all and could not even talk any longer to his son about it. Grace knew that her husband was "breaking his heart over giving up his boy to this awful risk [military service]."[36] She had noticed a change in her husband ever since the war began—an uncharacteristic soberness at times, as if it were the prelude to enormous tragedy. Eventually, through his many contacts, one of whom was the commanding officer of the No. 3 Canadian General Hospital, Herbert Stanley Birkett, Osler got his son assigned a position of some relative safety.

Revere had not been content with the posting his father had arranged— that of a medical service officer with a Canadian hospital. Life behind the lines was flat, valueless. He considered his hospital mired in a "turbid mud hole, rank with unrest and discontent."[37] It was not the kind of duty a patriot like himself felt sufficient. Even transfer to a field ambulance unit was not enough. In March 1916, Revere shifted from the Canadian Medical Corps to the British Army as a forward artillery observer—a posting that invited danger, as he would be subjected to all the hazards of trench warfare. But he seemed satisfied despite the horrors of his position. "Not an inch of earth that has not been upturned is left, and in places the shell holes are twelve feet deep, and filled with putrid mud and occasionally with a corpse at the bottom," he wrote his father in November 1916. Regardless of his worries, Sir William complimented his son on the occasion of his twenty-first birthday, "[y]ou have been everything that a father could wish, a dear good laddie."[38] Revere learned well the depravity of war. "This has been a bad place for Germans. The poor fellows lie all around us, with very little on their bones but a few tattered rags of flesh and are being gradually cleared away by the rats."[39]

It was in those horrid conditions in an area known as Passchendaele on the Belgian front on August 29, 1917, that Revere's unit, Battery A, Royal

Field Artillery, was bridging shell holes, trying to haul forward their heavy, eighteen-pounder gun. With the suddenness that war can inflict, as they were standing in a shell hole about 4:30 that afternoon, a German projectile exploded, felling Revere and eight of his twenty-man crew—some killed outright. Revere himself suffered several shrapnel wounds. Obviously in distress, he was taken to a gun pit, his wounds were dressed, and he was then transported to the 131st Field Ambulance Dressing Station over two kilometers away. From there, his injuries were recognized as severe, and he was motored to the 47th Casualty Clearing Station—a properly outfitted surgical unit— arriving about four hours after injury. His appearance immediately aroused concern. He was still conscious but clearly in shock. In a voice barely audible he bravely muttered to one of the attendants, "this will take me home."[40]

Immediately, American surgeon Harvey Cushing, dear friend of the Oslers who just happened to be attached to this field surgical hospital, was summoned and rushed to his aid. He called upon nearby fellow surgeon George Crile to help. Cushing was a first-rate specialist, new head of the surgical unit at the Peter Bent Brigham Hospital of Harvard University. Crile was, as well, the no-nonsense head of surgery at Case Western Reserve Hospital in Cleveland and a foremost expert on hemorrhage and shock. The sight of the pale, gaunt young man alarmed Cushing. "It could not have been much worse," he remarked. Revere was taken straightaway to the operating room. Upon opening the abdomen blood and feces spilled out. He was exsanguinating and had a macerated bowel. It was a wonder he had even survived four hours. So little blood remained in his veins and arteries that it seemed hopeless. Despite their efforts to stop the hemorrhage, Revere could not be revived. Not even two blood transfusions could reverse the damage. His surgeons worked frantically but, stunned by lack of blood, Revere's heart simply gave out. He died a few hours later. Of all the magic Cushing and Crile had worked on terribly mauled soldiers, they could not save the son of their dearest friend. It was crushing for both.

Whether premonition or not, Lady Grace had written Harvey Cushing only ten days before, knowing her son was in proximity to Cushing's surgical unit, "How badly you would feel if you should see him brought in wounded; but what a mercy it would be for him [to have you there]."[41] Now he was gone, buried, wrapped in an army blanket and covered by a worn Union Jack in a barren field in Belgium. The Oslers were distraught, stricken with grief. For a mother, she now witnessed the loss of all her children—her only two other babies died shortly after birth. "I always expected this to happen—but I never could be ready," she wrote Cushing a few days later. For the father, one of the great humanitarians of all time, he bore a broken spirit, far more damaging than any imaginable disease. "Our dear laddie has been taken!" he wrote his friend and Revere's former commanding officer at the Canadian hospital, Herbert Birkett.[42] Osler might had expected such tragedy as well. Such is the fate of men that fortune had blessed. "I have had so much and no knocks to speak of," he admitted to Birkett. "Call no man happy until he dies," he now felt, and understood the plight of the Biblical Job.[43]

It was the worst nightmare of parents. William Osler's spirit ripped asunder. For the man who had healed so many—corporally and spiritually—his own healing, if at all possible, would have to begin in the recesses of his heart. Outwardly few could tell. He brushed off sorrow and emotions with rather flippant remarks like "And if I laugh at any mortal thing, 'tis that I may not weep."[44] And, indeed, he wept often inside. There would never really be a full recovery for the man. He was a shadow of his former self. Bouts of solitude, weight loss, and reclusiveness followed. Yes, he would rise to the occasion and maintain his preeminence as a renowned professor, but Revere would always be close in his memory. His would be a pensive look, the eyes full of sorrow, the brow featureless as if joy had fled.

And Osler's spirit began to hemorrhage—the blood of affection. He would not recover. His wife wrote that he felt for the first time in his life he had nothing to live for. His appearance became gaunt. Weight dripped from him although he ate. He told Grace that "it is a broken heart," as if the burden was simply too much to bear. Grace mourned for him. She told a friend [I]sn't it awful—too too awful—Sir William never having that boy again? I can hardly endure it for him."[45]

In May 1919, Osler delivered his presidential address before the Classical Association at Oxford. He titled it "The Old Humanities and the New Science." Despite acknowledgment of scientific advances, he would not diminish his insistence on integration of body and spirit so essential to healing. In this address he acknowledged the tremendous achievements of science, but, devoid of humanism, it could have been responsible for the horrendous devastation of the recently finished Great War. "The extraordinary development of modern science may be her undoing," he suggested. Now, scientists should concentrate on the "secrets of life," not the "secrets of death." Turn again to the humanities, he urged. They are the essence of vitality. Humanities, like hormones "lubricate the wheels of life." They give meaning to the stark experimentalism of science, Osler implied.[46]

Osler's seventieth birthday celebration on July 12, 1919, in London included an audience of luminaries and friends—both British and American. Bound volumes of his essays were handed to him in commemoration of his contributions to medicine. Moved by such recognition, Osler managed to stammer out a speech barely able to hide his emotions in gratitude for such appreciation. At the dinner, though, a subtle cough developed, and on the way back to Oxford Grace worried he was coming down with another bronchial infection.

By late 1919 Osler looked ghastly. His eyes dark circles. October and November of that year were times of sickness and distress. Osler could not get rid of his cough and nighttimes were filled with paroxysms of hacking. Pneumonia and pleurisy were the culprits. He even thought he could feel the rub of his inflamed lungs against his chest wall. He fatigued easily and fever sapped any strength he could muster. Only drugs—probably morphia—could provide relief from his suffering. Some said he was dying of a broken heart. Perhaps, but perhaps not. Yet surely his grief over Revere punished his stamina and dampened his spirit. As December lengthened, he became riddled with infection. Fevers and pleurisy kept him down, and a broken spirit could not fight as one might fight to rid those lungs of infection. Empyema, lung abscess, surgery. To no end. More fevers, cough, and weakness took him on December 29, 1919, at age 70. Some suspected that he was another victim of the influenza pandemic sweeping England. One of the last words he spoke were those written by Samuel Taylor Coleridge in "The Rime of the Ancient Mariner": "He prayeth best who loveth best all things both great and small."[47] He slipped peacefully away, Grace at his side.

At last, aequanimitas. He had long preached it to so many others and now, perhaps, he had found it in his own soul.

The true healing that comes with peace.

C H A P T E R   T E N

~

Temptresses, Sorcerers, and Scientists

Women as Healers

Women know life. They give birth, nurse, nurture, and comfort. From conception their bodies deliver the very blood of sustenance. Their breasts suckle; their arms shelter; their sacrifice enables. They are domestic healers. Their simple remedies are legend. In history, "wives' tales" circulated—one household to the next—for pregnancies, birthings, and childhood illnesses. Yet a common misconception—among men, mostly—was that they were ill-equipped as true medical practitioners, considered instead, homebound, physically inferior, emotional, and volatile. So often, their caricature was portrayed as one of feebleness, manipulation, and seduction—a string of veritable Eves repeatedly offering the healing apple to an unsuspecting Adam—and by their sultry wickedness (as the male version goes) intent on the corruption of mores and intentions. According to psychologist Jeanne Achterberg, women as healers alternated "between light and shade," meaning materiality and myth. Even as science began to unravel the mysteries of the universe, Achterberg felt, "[m]en feared—and tried to bar from the new scientific worldview—women's intuitive nature, as well as their strong sense of the inherent link between humanity and the earth."[1]

Such might be the treachery of women unleashed on the helpless sick. Quackery. Incompetence. Deceitfulness. But beyond myth, were the very real struggles of women to apply their sympathetic instincts, keen intellect, and familiar dedication to the male-dominated realm of healthcare. Their unique perspective on illness and suffering allowed an equally unique perception of care and compassion. Medical respectability in a man's world, though, would be hard earned and a storied history.

It began as fables of temptresses, seductresses, and sorcerers.

133

The richness of Greek mythology again comes to life and tells enchant-
ing tales. Helen, Queen of Sparta, that seductress as fetching as Aphrodite,
had run away with the Trojan Prince Paris to his formidable citadel in Asia
Minor. She was a goddess herself among men, daughter, in fact, of Zeus and
Leda. Of her beauty, admirers would say "wondrous like is she to the immortal goddesses [Aphrodite] to look upon."[2] Homer's *Iliad* embellished her story.
She had ensnared Paris and was spirited off to seaside Troy by his consuming
love for her. It was lovely Helen, wife of the Spartan Menelaus, and Paris, her
lover, who caused that disastrous ten-year siege of Troy by enraged Greeks.
She begrudgingly returned to Sparta after her husband's warriors burnt Troy
to the ground. Her Paris had been killed by the marksman Philoctetes. Helen
had pleaded with his wife, Oenone, whom he had abandoned, to save him,
but she bitterly refused. Then, back in Sparta, Helen saw the grief war had
wrought on brave men who had fought to free her. Among them was the
courageous Odysseus, now lost at sea and feared dead.

How his comrades wept for him. So distraught were they that, as they
gathered to mourn, the resourceful Helen, a mistress of potions and remedies,
calmed them with her ministrations.

> "Then Helen, daughter of Zeus . . . cast into the wine of which they were
> drinking a drug to quiet all pain and strife and bring forgetfulness of every ill.
> Whoever should drink this down, when it is mingled in the bowl, would not in
> the course of that day let a tear fall down over his cheeks, no, not though his
> mother and father should lie there dead, or though before his face men should
> slay with the sword his brother or dear son and his own eyes behold it."

The drug $\nu\eta\pi\varepsilon\nu\theta\dot{\varepsilon}\varsigma$, "nepenthe," was an agent that erased sorrow—a
euphoric—likely something akin to opium.[3] Homer told that Helen had
been given the cunning drugs by Polydamna, wife of Thon, a woman of Egypt
where the earth bore the greatest store of drugs that, when properly mixed,
healed. Egypt, Homer said, was the seed of such richness that it brought
forth the greatest store of nostrums. According to the Hellenic historian
Herodotus, Egypt literally teemed with physicians—both men and women—
"the country swarms with medical practitioners, some undertaking to cure
diseases of the eye, others of the head, others again of the teeth, others of the
intestines." So widespread was this feeling, that Greeks considered Egyptians
the founders of medicine.[4]

At Troy, the attacking Greeks brought their own brand of female healing. The old and wise King Nestor of Pylos took with him his servant girl
Hecamede. The formidable warrior Achilles had seized her as a hostage when
he sacked the island of Tenedos guarding the Dardanelles. Achilles, in his

admiration for Nestor, gave him Hecamede. She was versed in the skills of a healer in that she knew many comforting nostrums for hurt and grieved men. When asked by Nestor to tend to wounded Greeks, Homer tells that "Fair tressed Hecamede mixed a potion [in her splendid cup] . . . with Pramnian wine, and on this she grated cheese of goat's milk with a brazen grater, and sprinkled thereover white barley meal; and she bade them drink." Pramnian wine, called κυκεον ("kukeon") was a well-known concoction with sedative properties—almost sacramental in significance as pleasing to the gods.[5]

Then, the marvelous ιατρος (healer) Machaon himself, that son of Asclepius, was wounded by an arrow to his thigh. And his brother Podalirius was nowhere to be found. Nestor's fair Hecamede responded:

> And the cry of battle was not unmarked of Nestor, albeit at his wine, but he spake winged words to the son of Asclepius: "Bethink thee, goodly Machaon, how these things are to be; louder in sooth by the ships waxes the cry of lusty youths. Howbeit do thou now sit where thou art and quaff the flaming wine, until fair-tressed Hecamede shall heat for thee a warm bath, and wash from thee the clotted blood, but I will go straightway to a place of outlook and see what is toward."[6]

In Nestor's household, with some knowledge of calming remedies, she was likely involved in the treatment of everyday ailments and child rearing—as many household servants were. Women were expected to handle the day-to-day issues of health, such as proper diet and exercise, and the treatment of minor disorders that required catharsis, purging, or application of various salves and plasters. Hecamede seemed particularly suited to this but did not have the educated τέχνη, the technical skill, of an ιατρος to pull embedded arrows as Machaon and Podalirius might. She dared not try. For that the Greek warrior Patroclus, perhaps coached by his friend, Achilles, in the care of wounds, laid Machaon down and, with his knife, cut out the arrow, washed the wound, and applied a "bitter root" that "slayeth pain." Perhaps, at that point, Hecamede's gentle bath would quiet the pained fighter. Homer tells that Machaon's wound mended, and he completely recovered.[7]

Interspersed with folklore in antiquity were real-life examples of legitimate female physicians. In first-century Rome, with a dearth of Roman-born male ιατροί, women were less viewed as sorcerers and more inclined to earn respectability as suitably trained healers—full-fledged *medici* (physicians). On an inscription uncovered in the Roman Forum there was found this engraved message: *ΤιΒεριω Κλαυδιω Αλκιμω ιατρω Καισαρος εποιησε Ρεστιτουτα πατρωνι και καθηγητη αγαθω και αξιω εζησε ετη πβ*, which, translated, reads: "For Tiberius Claudius Alcimus, Physician to Caesar, made by

Restituta for her patron and dear professor, good and worthy. He lived years ago." So, the presumed healer Restituta endeavored to honor her cherished teacher, who, as Hippocrates had felt, should be as valued as family and so recognized.[8]

In actuality, Restituta, the author of this message, was very likely a slave woman. "Restituta" meaning "Restored" was probably given to her following her assignment to a Roman household (much like the mythical Hecamede). She was perhaps freed by Alcimus, as she became his pupil.[9] Alcimus, almost certainly a freedman, may himself have been enslaved at some point as, being of Greek heritage, his healing talents soon became manifest. For this, Restituta, too, may not have been a freed woman but, clearly, she was also an ιατρινη, a feminized title of a male healer, an ιατρος. The fact that she acknowledged Alcimus as her patron and called him καθηγητης (kathigitís), her professor, implied that she was not merely a σωτειρα, or physician assistant. Restituta had a more formal relationship: teacher and student of τέχνη, the healing art.

But the more imaginative fables continued. Like the purported healer, Helen, in Homer's *Iliad*, thirteenth-century poet Gottfried von Strassburg's *Tristan and Iseult* featured two plotting shrews, Queen Iseult of Ireland and her lovely daughter, Iseult the Fair. The tale began with the Cornish knight, Tristan, on a mission to Ireland to bring back to his uncle, King Mark, a suitable bride—Iseult the Fair was his choice. But, unexpectedly, Tristan was met by her brother, Morolt, who challenged him to combat. It was in this brawl on both horseback and foot that Morolt slashed Tristan in the thigh. A survivable gash ordinarily but for Morolt coating his sword with a deadly poison gotten from his sister, Queen Iseult. She had promised that no physician could heal it. Incensed by this wound, Tristan fell upon Morolt and hacked him to death. In a fit of rage, he also took off his head.

Yet the wound of Tristan spelled doom. A doctor was needed. Making light of the gash at first, Tristan trembled when he heard the fateful verdict:

> Though they summoned the most skillful physicians from all the lands around, not one of them had skill enough to aid him, for the poison was of such subtle venom that they could not bring it from the wound, but it spread all over his body, and his color and his look were so changed one might scarce know him.[10]

Tristan knew, then, if he were to be cured it could only be at the hands of Queen Iseult who had given Morolt the poison. Only by her famous talents would this happen for she alone possessed *arzatliche meisterschaft*, "medical mastery."[11] Pretending to be a minstrel, he earned favor with the Irish people and soon was taken to Queen Iseult's chamber. She beheld his wound and judged him a victim of a poisonous weapon. No physician could help, he told her. It was beyond human wisdom. "I live, and yet I am dead," he stammered.[12] So impressed was she of this young, sick minstrel—now the pretender he knew he must be, for he had killed her brother—she vowed to him that if he would sing his sweet songs, she would heal him. She "set all her thought and her skill to work to see how she might bring about Tristan's healing." The wise queen tended to him night and day. After almost three weeks the poison had gone and the wound was healed.[13]

Her daughter, Princess Iseult, was of exquisite beauty. "She is so fair a maiden that all that we hear of beauty is but as an idle tale compared to her." Helen of Sparta (and Troy) held that honor once, but no longer. Iseult had supplanted that woman in all her radiance.[14] Yet once again, Queen Iseult displayed her devious knowledge of herbs and potions. She prepared one for Iseult the Fair to take with her as she sailed for Cornwall and a marriage with Tristan's uncle, King Mark. The compound this time was a love potion designed so that any man must love whomever he drank it with, above any other, whether he wished it so or not, while she must love him in return.[15] Indeed, it was not King Mark who drank this but, mistakenly, Tristan and Iseult, and the two commenced their adulterous affair, soon to be the death of them both. "Love, who never resteth but besetteth all hearts, crept softly into the hearts of the twain, and ere they were ware of it had she [love] planted her banner of conquest therein, and brought them under her rule." From that point forward, "both were one in love and sorrow."[16] Now, it would be not the mortal wounds of the flesh but the mortal wounds of the heart, this time not to be cured. Tristan, bereft of his lover, would jump to his death. Iseult lived out her life, loveless, with her arranged husband, King Mark.[17]

Such stories of sorcerers and seductresses—perhaps appealing to medieval romanticism—would be offset by the legitimate materiality of women practitioners of healing.

Twelfth-century mystic and visionary, Hildegard of Bingen (1098–1179) was no seductress. While puzzled, and at times frankly irritated by men, she had no designs on them. Her focus was the sick. She proclaimed spiritual and physical healing throughout medieval Europe that even permeated the palaces of royalty. Outspoken and forthright, Hildegard was the founder and first abbess of the Benedictine community in Bingen, a former Frankish settlement on the banks of the Rhine River. A polymath—versed in art, music, and medicine—she did not begin her scholarly compositions until she was forty-three, essays on Christian doctrines and ethics, cosmology, and a compendium encyclopedia of medicine and natural science. Visited by hallucinatory visions of the spirit world, she composed music and painted images, in part, guided by her apparitions. Her composition *Ordo Virtutum* (Order of Virtues) is considered the oldest known morality play. Outspoken in her rigid Catholicism, Hildegard was a public preacher of monastic and clerical reform. Yet her extrasensory perceptions earned her a sorcereress-like reputation with her contemporaries as "the Sibyl of the Rhine."

Hildegard was born into wealth and influence, daughter of a noble family of Bermersheim near Alzey, the tenth of ten siblings. With her patrician status, she had easy access to political and ecclesiastical power. When a member of a neighboring family, Jutta, a reportedly beautiful daughter of the Count of Sponheim, decided on a life of recluse, Hildebert and Mechthild, Hildegard's parents, offered the then eight-year-old Hildegard as a tithe—the tenth child—by placing her in Jutta's hermitage at the Benedictine monastery in nearby Disibodenberg. This was the custom, even among wealthy families, that the tenth child be offered up for service in the Church. For most impoverished families—but certainly not Hildegard's—this was a relief in the care and feeding of an extra mouth. Her parents, being devout Catholics, abided by the custom. In Jutta's tiny one-room cell, Hildegard studied the Bible, chanted the monastic office, and performed the rituals of solitary life. Her comprehension of biblical text astounded her elders, and she spent countless hours in solitude absorbing her Church's teachings. She then made a formal profession of virginity, and in mid-adolescence committed herself to the vows under the Rule of Saint Benedict—poverty, chastity, and obedience. Upon Jutta's death, Hildegard, a spiritual virtuosa, was the natural selection of abbess to succeed her.

The plucky Hildegard accepted but requested a move of her nuns from Disibodenberg to the monastery in Rupertsberg, near Bingen. She felt restricted by the overbearing monastic male presence—and a physically confining convent—and wanted more freedom for her community. The Benedictine abbot, Kuno, denied her petition—through her scholarly works she had brought him much prestige. So headstrong was Hildegard, though, that she went to the archbishop of Mainz, who reluctantly agreed. Abbot Kuno was understandably miffed at her insolence and still refused. Hildegard then was suddenly stricken with paralysis (or so she claimed) as punishment for disobeying God's instruction to move her nuns. Her disdain for what she considered a lukewarm and sluggish clergy did not help her impatience (and may have fueled her paralytic wiliness). Still skeptical, Abbot Kuno examined her himself, and behold, he was convinced her affliction was the will of God. Only then did he relent. Not surprisingly, with that news, Hildegard's palsy quickly disappeared. From then forward, Hildegard considered the Archbishop of Mainz her superior and freed her community totally from Benedictine control.

She never hid her disdain for the Abbot, however. Her contempt for monastic corruption erupted from time to time. At one point, when asked to submit to him some of her musical compositions, Hildegard responded to Abbot Kuno with a vicious condemnation of his perceived evil ways: "Why do you not examine your own heart and reject your unabashed lasciviousness? I am the One who brings the lost sheep back to the fold, the One to whom you should always turn, but you fail to do so, and thereby slap me in the face."[18]

With permission thus granted—devious though it might have been—in 1150, Hildegard and twenty nuns settled into their new convent at Rupertsberg where she began her mission of caring for the sick. Surrounded by the infirm, Hildegard studied their illnesses and became an avid student of health matters.[19] Five years later she experienced a series of vivid mystical revelations that led her to compose the *Scivias* (Know the Ways of the Lord) and begin her public mission as God's advocate on earth.[20]

Why the visions, some wondered. Hildegard had been a precocious child. In her own words, she admitted a peculiar temperament that lent to chronic ill health but also a propensity for revelations from early childhood. She would describe things that were invisible to those around her, foretell the future, and detail particular luminosities she saw around objects, as if there was an aura. In her auras, she witnessed a variety of figures—animate and inanimate. These radiances came and went throughout her life, for forty years until they seemed to coalesce into specific messages from God that she recorded—often with the aid of a scribe—as her visions.

Her God-ordained hallucinatory experiences began in earnest in 1141. As she later told, she received her prophetic call in the form of a fiery light that illuminated her whole heart and brain. She wrote, "And behold! In the forty-third year of my earthly course, as I was gazing with great fear and trembling attention at a heavenly vision, I saw a great splendor in which resounded a voice from Heaven, saying to me 'O fragile human, ashes of ashes, and filth of filth! Say and write what you see and hear.'"[21] So distinct was this experience that Hildegard, disturbed by this otherworldly message, wrote to a religious adviser, Bernard, Abbot of Clairvaux:

> Father, I am greatly disturbed by a vision which has appeared to me through divine revelation, a vision seen not with my fleshly eyes but only in my spirit. . . . I have from earliest childhood seen great marvels which my tongue has no power to express but which the Spirit of God has taught me that I may believe. . . . Through this vision which touches my heart and soul like a burning flame, teaching me profundities of meaning, I have an inward understanding of the Psalter, the Gospels, and other volumes.[22]

Hildegard seemed suffused with mysticism. In her specters, God permeated nature, and infused all living things in a manner that had no beginning nor end.[23] And God made all things in the heavens and on earth and gave them life. As for humans, God had infused a special grace. This he called the spirit. So vital was the spirit to mankind that its temperaments dominated the flesh. "The soul [spirit] is the mistress, the flesh the handmaiden." Spiritual essence ruled the body by virtue of giving life to it. Without spirit, the body would decay.[24]

She spared no effort to spread her convictions. As a Christian, Hildegard was constantly aware of the presence of evil and the dangers of complacency in spiritual matters. She wrote prolifically and sent her candid—and many times caustic—epistles to numbers of contemporaries, either admonishing or counseling or simply giving worship to God. Emperor Frederick Barbarossa, King Henry III, and Eleanor of Aquitaine, Queen of England were improbable recipients. To Eleanor of Aquitaine, she wrote: "Your mind is like a wall which is covered with clouds, and you look everywhere but have no rest. Flee this and attain stability with God and men, and God will help you in all your tribulations. May God give you his blessing and help in all your works."[25]

Perhaps this was her motive to heal. God cured the spiritual and the spiritual might cure the flesh. Her convent would be a refuge for illnesses,

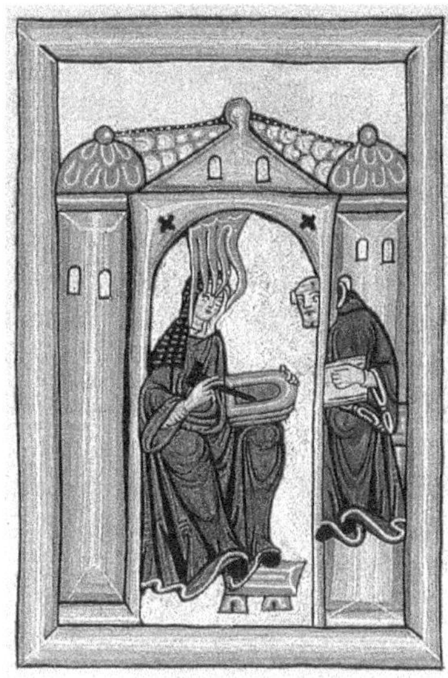

Figure 10.1 The medieval mystic and healer, Hildegard von Bingen. Miniature from the Rupertsberg Codex of Liber Scivias.

whether of body or soul. Certainly, even in the twelfth century, monastic medicine still flourished. In monasteries and nunneries, clerics cared for the impoverished ill, cultivated vast botanical gardens, and housed precious written records of academic interest. Hildegard was no different. She welcomed all sick into her nunnery and soon was immersed in their care. Her apparitions convinced her of the ever-present enmeshing of natural and supernatural in afflictions. There was a continuous refrain in her spiritual epistles that spoke of the corruption of body and spirit as causes of ill health. To heal, she seemed very much aware of the marvels of nature bestowed by her Creator, and rich in opportunities to unite physical with spiritual. She was intent on bringing together the apparent rifts promoted among religion, nature, and science. Her mysticism and artistic appreciation of music, painting, and poetry softened the realities of medicine for her—they blended into the circle of life. So, she considered physical and spiritual sickness as manifestations one of the other and their remedies equally interdependent. The supreme state of health, in her estimation, was perfection of soul through worship and service to God. This would inevitably reflect on health of the body.[26]

In Hildegard's major work on healing, *Causae et Curae*, she heavily flavored her precepts with spirituality. God has breathed a living wind into the body to give it life, she explained. The spirit, Hildegard implied, was the motor for the body, filling the veins with blood and infusing the stomach with vitality. The spirit filled lungs, heart, and viscera with juices (perhaps she meant the Hippocratic "humors") of life. The body cannot be without this vitality, just as the body cannot be without blood. The spirit illuminated the body as fire illuminated darkness, she explained:

> Therefore also every work which the body demands, the soul works in it, and therefore the soul is also the worker of the body longs, and the soul is more powerful than the body, since it fulfills its desire, nor does it itself make it possible without in the body of man there is thirst, which passes through and moves man, who is the work of God; and he would not be without a body . . . but the soul can live without the body, but no more than the body lives without the soul.[27]

As for disease, Hildegard followed Hippocratic orthodoxy, blaming disturbances of health on malicious acts of the spirit that created disharmony of the four humors. God allotted the humors, she thought, in different proportions to reflect the strength of Sampson or the prophecy of Jeremiah or the wisdom of Plato. When the humors were in their proper constituency, man was at peace.[28] At the core of it all, Hildegard believed, was the beating heart. From this organ temperaments radiated and humors percolated. Yet a vicious nature threatened with its fire, wind, soil, and moisture. The heart must be protected, and all innards converged to do so. In her construed physiology, the liver warmed the heart, the lungs covered it, and the stomach fueled it.[29]

At the same time, man's spirit was corruptible. Her medical writing was laced with carnal lapses. She spoke often in her visions of the perversion of the flesh and the ruination of souls from sensual desires and actions. It was almost as if a struggle within herself prompted such vehemence. She hated the "filth" of sin and stain of matter over spirit. She dwelt on sexual themes—both man and woman—in *Causa et Cura*. Her descriptions of male and female eroticism were graphic and hinted at personal familiarity—odd, especially considering her cloistered existence. In almost pornographic prose she wrote "[f]or the blood of man boiling in the ardor and heat of lust casts forth foam from itself, which we call seed, just as a pot placed on the fire casts forth foam from the water from the heat of the fire."[30] And for the man, sexual temptation was particularly loathsome, as if an innate tendency difficult to check. "Of the pleasure of the flesh," she added:

> [W]hich are in the liver and belly of the male, meet in his genitals. And when that delectable excitement comes out of the marrow of the male, it falls into his loins and stirs the taste of pleasure in the blood . . . he burns, so that in that ardor he forgets himself and is unable to control himself, without bringing up the foam of the seed . . . the fire of pleasure burns stronger, as in great waves.[31]

When the tempest of lust arises in the male, she continued, "it revolves in him like a millstone, because his loins are also like a fabric, into which the marrow sends fire, so that that fabric and the same fire in it spills over the male's genitals and causes him to burn strongly."[32] She wrote descriptively of female orgasm and the process of conception. So insightful were these portrayals it almost spoke of private recall:

> But when a woman is in the union of a man, the heat of her brain [builds], which has pleasure in itself, the taste of the same pleasure in the same union [that] brings forth from the male the shedding of seed. And after the seed had fallen into its place, the aforesaid strong heat of the brain draws it in and holds it and soon, the organs of the woman contract and all openings for the menstrual period close just like a strong man closes his fist. And then the menstrual blood will mix with the seed and incarnate it.[33]

Her solution for the male's lusty nature? She recommended dampening it with a summer concoction: dill, bachmenza, and lunchwurz. Whether it ever worked, she kept to herself.[34]

In a more practical light, Hildegard published a wide array of botanicals guaranteed to help. Her knowledge of herbs and plants appeared extensive, including various suggested concoctions of foods designed by her suppositions to aid in digestion, or to bolster weak blood, or to dampen man's evil desires. She had an extensive garden in which she mixed and matched her herbal remedies. To her, the plant world was another place where forces of good and evil clashed. Some herbs had in them by virtue of their potent aromas the power to fight evil spirits. Others purported to induce man to seek diabolical fortunes. The botanical virtues of her plants she matched to the human terrain of the sick to effect relief. Of course, all was accompanied by formulas of prayer to support the actions of her nostrums.[35]

In *Causae et Curae*, she produced an extensive inventory of diseases and therapeutics. She had studied well and was familiar with any number of herbal remedies. Included in her compendium were descriptions of headaches and melancholy, eye conditions, toothaches, "heart pains," lung pain (pleurisy perhaps), stomachaches, fistulas, ulcers, menstrual disorders, bloody flux (dysentery, *cholera morbus*), vomiting, hemorrhoids, erysipelas, cancer, scabies, jaundice, colic, leprosy, scrofula (tuberculosis), and periodic fevers such as malaria. She provided remedies for retention of menstrual flow (anise and febrifuge) rubbed on the belly and genitalia. For irregular menstruation, the woman should dip a cloth in cold water and wrap it around her thighs to cool herself internally. And for difficult labor, women should boil fennel and aspen, then press this concoction around her thighs and back, thus provoking opening of her womb. One must remember, a woman's health issues were, by and large, a matter of women's business. Pregnancy and labor were extremely taxing conditions, and men largely shied away from the bloody task of facilitating uterine function and the stressful conditions attendant to birthing. Yet she could not divorce her remedies from the supernatural, explaining that "for the aforesaid infirmities, the prescribed medicines shown by God will either free the man or he himself will die, or God does not want him to be delivered."[36]

Practical or not, Hildegard's religiosity rose above all and infused her interpretations of nature and healing. It applied to her sense of a spiritual awareness of the completeness of God and his diffusion into all of nature. Her God was a God found everywhere, a supreme force giving life to all animate beings and planting the earth and water for their sustenance. How could it be otherwise that healing evolve through a blending of the natural and supernatural? Healing? There was no compromise. The spirit must take precedence. If God is pleased, the body was sure to heal. For example, to Arnold, Archbishop of Trier, she admonishes, "Learn also to heal the wounds of sinners with penance in mercy, just as the supreme physician is to leave you an example to save the people." And later she added, "Whoever suffers vomiting from infirmity of his body, and longs for the body of Christ with all devotion . . . let him place the body of the Lord upon the head of the same man, and call upon God who sent the soul into the body, that he may deign to sanctify his soul with body and blood."[37]

Hildegard's writings were consumed by the influence of spirit over flesh and disease as punishment. Her reputation as a self-styled healer and critic led some to believe the Sybil of the Rhine was tainted, an imaginative moralist who rained down admonition on wicked mankind. She was the purveyor of visions and fanciful antidotes and persecutor of the sinful. A healer of the spirit as it perverts the flesh.

For most households, though, healthcare was the domain of the wife and mother. With little knowledge of Hippocratic principles, women governed issues of diet, activity, and sleep. Washing, bathing, and attention to bowel and bladder were some of the immediate concerns of domesticity. Wives' tales and recipes—informal prescriptions—were utilized by women to address common maladies of the home: headaches, stomachaches, constipation, diarrhea, fever, and vomiting—even matters of pregnancy. Little was written down. Most women were illiterate. Common peasants passed these informal strategies by word of mouth. Nevertheless, women carried the brunt of healthcare from birth to death. Still, they received little, if any, recognition for their role and were, in public, almost denigrated for intrusion into academic health matters.[38]

Change would be painful. Fast-forward to nineteenth-century America. Elizabeth Blackwell did not think women were irrelevant in health matters.

In December 1847, the widely read *Boston Medical and Surgical Journal* published the startling report of a certain Miss Elizabeth Blackwell, a young lady bold enough to consider herself worthy of a male-dominated medical education. It seemed she unashamedly "made her appearance in the lecture room about two weeks ago [Geneva Medical College, New York]." The article continued, "[s]he is a pretty little specimen of the feminine gender, registering her age at 26." But there was nothing coquettish about her demeanor, the report read. "She comes into class with great composure, takes off her bonnet and puts it under the seat (exposing a fine phrenology), takes notes constantly, and maintains throughout an unchanged countenance." Elizabeth Blackwell was the first female admitted to a United States medical school.[39]

The matter did not end there. In a backhanded endorsement of the whole affair, the *Buffalo Medical Journal* wrote that, "We should regret to see any innovations tending to lead woman from her appropriate sphere—the domestic hearth, and the social circle," the article misogynistically argued. "But we can perceive no good reasons why females whose duties are not prescribed by domestic or social relations, should be denied the privilege of obtaining a support," the anonymous author condescendingly put forth. And for those women so mindless of their traditional roles, such a medical education permitted them at least to "[exercise] usefully their faculties in the capacity of Medical practitioners under proper limitations." Yet the manner of their care was more that of nurse than doctor, the article implied, hardly hinting at their real potential contributions—those of a true healing nature:

> Poetry invests woman with the character of a "ministering angel" in the hour of sickness, and this idea almost ceases to be a figure of speech when we witness the labors of "sisters of charity" . . . devoted to the claims of the poor and friendless, enhanced by the sufferings of disease . . . [t]he poetical idea of a "ministering angel". . . or the more prosaic character of a "sister of charity", cannot suffer depreciation, but quite the reverse, by being associated with medical education.

Yes, the author magnanimously conceded, the duties of the medical practitioner were certainly not the "exclusive prerogative of the *lords of creation* [italics mine], but may be claimed as belonging equally to the softer sex." However, not to be labeled as feminist, the same writer was quick to distance himself (presumed gender) from the "metaphysics of woman's rights." Still, his point was made. For those irresponsible of "the domestic hearth," a medical education should (begrudgingly) be granted.[40]

Despite the antics of her male counterparts—almost sophomoric in their immaturity—Elizabeth Blackwell pushed on, not even shying away from the potentially awkward lectures on the reproductive organs amid blushes and even hysterical squeals of the male students. Not the least deterred, she kept a featureless face but had to stifle laughs at their comical behavior.

Elizabeth Blackwell received her medical degree in 1849. Her graduation ceremony had been a major news item. For the event, she dressed all in black for a crowd of women's bonnets and feminine faces eager to catch a glimpse of the controversial figure, called by many as "the Lioness of the day." Her gown was extravagant, but she recognized the moment and felt that she should not appear in any shabby gown that "would disgrace womankind." Her gratitude showed, though. "Sir I thank you," she responded to the bestowing of her degree. "By the help of the Most High it shall be the effort of my life to shed honor upon this [diploma]." And, indeed, she

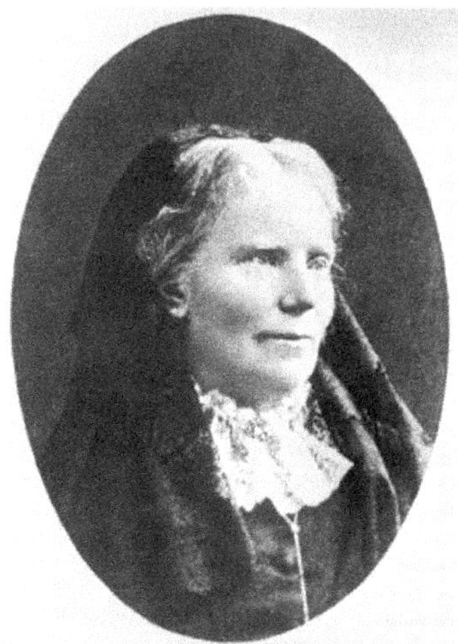

Figure 10.2 Pioneering American woman physician Elizabeth Blackwell. National Library of Medicine.

did so, serving the underprivileged sick both domestically and abroad, even after losing an eye to gonococcal conjunctivitis. "Very few understand the soul of this work. . . . My work is undoubtedly for the few. It is labor in the interlinkings of humanity," she said at one point. As for her profession, she felt stirrings at the need for a woman's medical college, an insatiable urge that led to her founding of the New York Infirmary where newly graduated female physicians could train.[41] Her persistent efforts in a male-dominated medical world led her to the finest clinics of Europe, experience at the side of European masters, and unfailing conviction of her usefulness in medical practice. She never ceased to consider herself the equal of men and a credible practitioner of the healing arts.

Blackwell was convinced women were needed as physicians. Midwifery—that historic and often maligned occupation of questionable quality—was the domain of women for centuries, but Elizabeth saw much more potential. So inflamed with conviction was she that in 1856 she published a pamphlet—more of a women's medical manifesto than whimsical thinking—promoting a radical concept: a women's medical college.

> Midwifery and medicine, which for so many ages were degraded by the grossest superstitions, are now open to the light of science; they have passed forever from the ignorant class—both male and female—who once exercised them, and are now presented as a noble art to the women of this age.[42]

In her mind, women were perfectly suited for the medical profession. They seemed much more in tune with the compassion necessary for true healing. "The grandest name of woman is mother—the noblest thought of womanhood is maternity," she said. But maternal instincts led to a deeper appreciation of the impact of disease. Maternity, in her estimation, "is far wider in its spiritual significance than in its simple physical definition. The great motherly spirit enters into all the interests of her children, and spreads her large loving wings over all existence."[43]

Imperative in all this, though, was a proper schooling in scientific integrity. "[W]hatever tends to widen the thought and enlighten the judgment of any woman . . . is the search for the truth. . . . The direct effect of this train of thought and study, is to create a truthful, earnest, and in the widest sense loving spirit," she reasoned. Blackwell believed, however, that science should not substitute for soulful attention. "In the womanly nature, scientific culture would produce a deeply religious spirit," she argued, cognizant of the spiritual interplay of visible and invisible.[44]

There was untapped potential in her gender, she knew. In a true Hippocratic tone, she emphasized that "[t]he study and practice of medicine, presents a noble field of exercise for the highest qualities of head and heart . . . to various classes of women, it should command our highest interest."[45]

But with regard to women's diseases, Blackwell saw not nobleness but ignobleness. On open hospital wards, female patients were literally stripped, poked, probed, and discussed in the open, with little regard for modesty or privacy. The senior male physician would gather his students around a half-naked subject, point out pertinent findings, and then lecture, all the while the humiliated woman lay there unrobed. Blackwell knew that women physicians would not behave so callously. To the obvious, she wrote, "honorable, intelligent and wise female physicians would be an immense blessing to society."[46] That could only happen if women were educated in a setting designed only for them. Male control of medical education allowed for no other option. And dignity for female patients demanded it. Only women doctors seemed to understand the compassion healers should provide.

Certain enlightened males agreed with her. There had been no more active feminist movement than the Religious Society of Friends—Quakers, for short—who acknowledged the vital role of women in family and community. Thought blasphemous by the Church of England, they fled to America in the seventeenth century where, there, too, they were viewed as heretics by evangelicals. Certainly, colonial Protestantism, while initially liberating women, had balked at the idea of expanding female roles in the public domain. Quakers felt differently. From the mid-nineteenth century, feminist movements championed by Quakers denounced traditional women's duties and promoted equality before God.[47] Abiding by that philosophy, the Women's Medical College of Philadelphia was founded by Quaker men in a refreshing burst of egalitarianism. "Why should not women have the same opportunities in life as men?" founding Quaker Benjamin Fussell had proclaimed in 1849.[48] Fussell garnered generous support for his idea, and, on October 12, 1850, the building at 627 Arch Street—then called The Female Medical College of Pennsylvania—admitted its first students. Quaker physician and co-founder, Joseph Longshore, an inveterate advocate of women's education, gave the inaugural address. He had already tutored his sisters-in-law in medicine, one of whom, Hannah Myers Longshore, was among the entering students. Longshore pointed out that in the inevitable advance of civilization it is only logical and just that women be incorporated into the healing profession. Moreover, it was not only logical, it was immoral that they not be privy to such studies:

> That the woman, from the acuteness of her perception, correctness of her observation, her cautiousness, gentleness, kindness, endurance in emergencies, conscientiousness and faithfulness to duty, is not equally, nay, by nature abundantly better qualified for most of the offices of the sick room, than man, very few will venture to contradict, and so far as the management of the ailments, and peculiar necessities of her own sex, and the disease of children are concerned, woman, by virtue of her superior natural qualifications should be vested with the entire prerogative.[49]

It was not a popular idea among medical professionals. Supporter Henry Hartshorne candidly wrote "[f]or a medical man to be connected at that time with the Women's Medical College required pluck."[50] Advocates for female doctors had betrayed an informal pact, that medicine was exclusively male, as if a secret cult had endowed membership based on gender alone.

Of necessity, the first faculty were all male, but in the inaugural graduating class of eight women, two were chosen for faculty positions. One, Ann Preston, was elected to the professorship of physiology and hygiene; the other, Hannah Longshore, was named instructor in anatomy. Preston, an extremely determined woman, impressed her peers with administrative acumen and was shortly appointed dean of the school in 1866. In a remarkable turn of diplomacy, she arranged that women from her school could attend clinics at the exclusively male Pennsylvania Hospital. Clinical material was meager at the Women's College and could not match in complexity the wide range of pathology seen at the all-male Pennsylvanian Hospital. On November 6, 1869, thirty-five women—now given the honorary title of "Pathfinders"—walked across town to observe surgery in its grand amphitheater. As later told by one of the female participants, Elizabeth Keller:

> We entered in a body amidst jeers and groanings, whistling and stamper of feet, by the men students, who had determined to make it so unpleasant for us that, from choice, we would not care to attend another. On leaving the hospital, we were actually stoned by those so-called gentlemen. An attempt was made to have us excluded from the surgical operations. Timely action of the directors, however, secured for us the privilege, which we are still enjoying.[51]

The *Philadelphia Evening Bulletin* gave a candid account two days later: "[r]anging themselves in line, these gallant gentlemen assailed the young ladies, as they passed out, with insolent and offensive language." When they actually entered the amphitheater, the paper reported, "they were greeted by yells, hisses, 'caterwaulings', mock applause, offensive remarks upon personal appearance." Even after exiting the building, the women were hounded on their way back by a growing street crowd of like-minded gangs.[52]

The male students were not the only ones dissatisfied with coed classes. Little more than a week hence, after a lengthy diatribe on all the wickedness of "mixed classes," the faculties of the Jefferson Medical College and the University of Pennsylvania fired a letter to Dean Preston: "the undersigned do earnestly and solemnly protest against the admixture of the sexes at clinical instruction in medicine and surgery, and do respectfully lay these their views before the Board of Managers of the hospitals in Philadelphia." Preston quickly fired back: "in common with medical men . . . science is impersonal, and the high aim of relief to suffering humanity sanctifies all duties." She would not back down. Women would continue to attend, but the Board of Managers bent to the will of its masculine members and insisted the sexes be segregated.[53]

The Philadelphia tempest was not an isolated circumstance. In May 1867, that same *Boston Medical and Surgical Journal* which two decades before had startled the medical world with Elizabeth Blackwell's classroom entrance, now published a caustic article by an anonymous author titled "Female Practitioners of Medicine." Admission of women to medical school was ill-advised, the author began. His reasoning was steeped in myth, misinformation, and more misogyny:

> [A] physiological obstacle has often been alluded . . . menstruation. . . . During the menstrual period . . . the woman is an invalid . . . and thus amounts to an impediment. . . . [During menstruation] [s]he is often perverse in her feelings, her views of things are liable to be distorted, and her judgment to be less reliable than usual.

But there was more. One must dispense empathy grudgingly. Men are much more adept at this, the author thought. Women overflow with sympathy and "[it] stands in the way of [their] efficiency as a physician. . . . The tendency of uncurbed sympathy is toward impatience of the slow action [or total ineffectiveness] of remedies, towards frequent changes, and toward redundancy in the employment of them."

This mystery author was not done yet.

The female intellect was also problematic. "[T]he feminine intellect is cast in a different mold from the masculine." How so? He explained in flawed logic that the female mind was intuitive and given to impulsive conclusions, and not the "careful collection, sifting and comparison of evidence indicative of the [male] judicial mind." Even beyond that preposterous reasoning, the "fairer sex" should be shielded from the graphic displays of sexuality. "To initiate [women students] into the ghastly mysteries of the dissecting-room and dead-house, must blunt their natural refinement." To expose them to the delicacies of the male and female generative systems, including venereal diseases "we believe would unsex them." So, the forthcoming conclusion was predictable. "We do not believe that women are adapted to the study and practice of medicine."[54]

The *Boston Medical and Surgical Journal* did not let up. In their not-so-subtle crusade against women physicians they published a couplet allegedly penned by Sir Andrew Douglas Maclagan, the poet laureate of the periodical *Edinburgh New Town Dispensary* in 1873, predicting:

An' when the leddies git degrees
Depen' upon 't there's nocht 'll please
Til they hae got oor chairs an' fees,
An' there's an en' o' you an' me.
For a' that ken the woman craitur
Maun own it is her foremost faitur
To tak' to lecturin' by natur';
An' hoo she'll do 't ye sune 'll see.[55]

What compelled such misogyny? Was it that the medical profession was *their* space—a professional locker room of exclusivity, freedom of behavior and liberality of speech? It was not for women. Women belonged in the home. Household duties and child-rearing were instinctive and best served by the fairer sex. Were women medically competent? Yes, but as one female doctor mused, "A man, it seems, may be intellectually in complete sympathy with a woman's aims. But only about ten percent of him is his intellect—the other ninety is emotion."[56]

Women half-believed all that. In 1882 physician and social reformer Mary Putnam Jacobi wrote that people do not ask if a woman physician is capable, but "will she upset our ideal of womanhood . . . and the social relations of the sexes? Can a woman physician be lovable; can she marry; can she have children; will she take care of them? *If she cannot, what is she?*" In particular, child-rearing raised concerns. "The care of children, particularly those under the age of four or five years of age, is the point at which feminism is most open to attack." Feminist Henrietta Rodman wrote in the 1920s.[57] Even by 1961, some male physicians editorialized that even the small percentage of spaces allotted to female medical school applicants should be eliminated, since male doctors were more productive. Although, he condescendingly allowed, there was the occasional "shooting star in skirts."[58]

Still, even the enlightened twentieth century buckled under the weight of male chauvinism. From the *London School of Medicine for Women Magazine* in March 1917, an anonymous female surgeon wrote of her frustration barred from the front lines of the Great War because of her gender. Well trained and willing, such female physicians and surgeons were kept away when mankind suffered terribly and wounded lingered in understaffed hospitals. This woman surgeon, confined to the home front, railed at the injustice in her poem titled "A Lament":

I wish I were a doctor bold,
Adoctoring at the front!
But as it is I'm feeling sold,
And want to do a stunt.
My friends who're at the front by now
Are wreathed in happy smiles;
A halo rests on every brow –
You see the shine for miles.
No horrid doubts disturb their rest,
A gentle peace surrounds,
They operate with happy zest,
Or keep the germs in bounds.
My job's their work in circles tame,

A far inferior lot,
And if you think it's all the same,
I firmly say it's not.
Then do you wonder if I scold,
Or yearn to do a stunt?
I wish I were a doctor bold,
Adoctoring at the front![59]

Nevertheless, through it all, with obstacles still imposed by male members, women fit well into the profession of healing. Yes, there were the particulars of divided time between child-rearing and medical practice. Women understand, as some men do not, the impact of disease and suffering on the psyche. Yes, as even anti-feminists of the 1860s pointed out, women do have an intuition for empathy, and where is empathy more valuable than in healing practices, where sensitivity is as vital as drugs and knife? But whether man or woman, healing never fails to be a connection of one mortal human to another. No, as a woman physician put it, "[p]atients don't really want their doctors weeping by their bedside; there is usually a job to be done. But there are times when all that our patients require of us is to be ourselves."[60]

Howard Spiro, former director of the Yale Program for Humanities in Medicine, put it succinctly. In 1975 he wrote, "[W]hat are generally seen as psychic characteristics of women should be just what American medicine needs at present . . . [n]urturing . . . along with tenderness, caring, and empathy. So what is wrong? Women come along at a time when medicine needs these qualities."[61]

CHAPTER ELEVEN

Alexis Carrel

A Search for Miracles[1]

As the Belle Époque inched toward the twentieth century, there seemed a diminution in the role of spirituality in the healing process. Beliefs in the dream-like beneficence of Asclepius and the charitable philanthropy of Jesus faded in comparison to the astounding discoveries of the scientific age. To many, natural law was sufficient to explain permutations of disease. For them, deciphering the unexplainable was, in all likelihood, merely a factor of research and time, not petitions to the heavens. With advances in medicine, ailments would topple before relentless innovations of man—not gods—and the worried mind would quiet. Perhaps civilization was entering philosopher Auguste Comte's (1798–1857) third realm of knowledge: the "positive" age, when all theological and metaphysical forces were discarded in favor of explainable physical relationships. The modern age, then—this unfolding twentieth century of discovery—was to be the age of positivism.[2] Would the emotional response to disease—the spiritual illness—become irrelevant and suffering merely dissected as cleanly as the organs, muscles, nerves, and arteries that it impacted?

The mechanistic age prevailed. Vitalism, the belief in "some sort of immaterial 'vital force', which has many names—*anima*, soul, *archeus*, vital principle, life force, *entelechy*, *élan vital*—all of which point to an essence in and of the living that is not material," so popular in preceding centuries, was on the decline and some felt relegated to historical interest only.[3] The ψυχή and *pneuma* of Plato faded into the background.

Alexis Carrel

Young Alexis Carrel was a complex man. He had chosen the path of the scientist, yet his heritage was spiritual. His selected profession was medicine—the art of healing. It was a fascinating field, rich in tradition and scientific exploitation, but in late nineteenth-century France, distinctly atheistic. For Carrel, though, its logic and pragmatism had become an irresistible urge. So engrossed had he become that his focus was not just the usual obsessions with diagnosis and therapy. He had undertaken the laborious pursuit of the minutely detailed and methodical skills of surgery. Carrel's analytical and mechanistic mind would eventually clash with the transcendent convictions of his childhood.

He was born Marie Joseph Auguste Carrel Billiard on June 28, 1873, in Sainte-Foy-les Lyon, a small village perched on one of those sentinel hills overlooking Lyon to the southeast. Nearby was the Fourvière, an elevation rising from the River Saône, and the site of the original Roman settlement of Lugdunum. During Roman times, Christians were martyred there in abundance, liberating dozens of saintly souls to heaven.[4] In more placid times it hosted convents and monasteries so numerous as to be called "the hill that prays." Not far were the confluence of the Rhône and Saône Rivers that defined the metropolis of Lyon, a sprawl that was hopelessly French in all manners and customs.

The household in which he was raised was one of comfortable affluence, although not, by usual standards, luxuriant. His family enjoyed the presence of three servants and stabled two horses for errands and journeys into town. His father Alexis François Marie Carrel Billiard, was a textile maker, characterized as "robust and jovial." His mother, Anne-Marie, was described as a petite figure and pleasant features framed in auburn hair. Auguste, the oldest, had a younger sister Marguerite, and brother, Joseph. For a time, childhood seemed idyllic, the home full of life with loving parents. Rather suddenly, fortunes changed. Auguste's father, ready to open a large factory in Alsace, was taken with pneumonia. Despite a constitution known by all as "strong as an ox," the young man, just thirty-three years old, worsened quickly and succumbed to his illness. Auguste was not quite five years of age. His mother, only twenty-five at the time of her husband's death, was stricken with grief. She was now saddled with the rearing of three young children. Her mourning was profound, yet her oldest child provided immeasurable support and comfort. And in return, she filled his head with what she felt was the best of herself. Her influence on him was substantial. Her religion played a substantial role in family life, and Catholicism was no better practiced than in the holy grounds around Lyon.[5]

Even at his young age, Auguste, being the oldest, assumed a dominant role with his widowed mother. He had become "the man of the house." By age nine, he was simply called "Alexis" no doubt in honor of his father. It was by that name, Alexis Carrel, he would be known forevermore. An independent and adventurous child, he was also quiet and meditative. Alexis, with his observant and curious mind, drifted toward the sciences; his brother Joseph to music; and Marguerite, the trappings of a typical bourgeois girl of the time.

Although now living by thrifty means, relegated to smaller accommodations, his mother Marie nevertheless scraped money together to send young Alexis to a Jesuit secondary school. The Catholic religion was obviously of value to the family and they conducted themselves in a faithful manner, the fabric of religiosity ingrained in Alexis' consciousness from an early age.

In the nineteenth century, Jesuit secondary education focused on traditional aspects of contemporary Christian (and Roman Catholic) thought. The classics (Latin and Greek) were stressed as were the analyses of ancient philosophers such as Aristotle. Of course, science was an integral part of Jesuit investigations, particularly in the realm of mathematics, physics, and natural philosophy. Still, Jesuits had a superb record in preparing secondary students for the *grandes écoles*—higher education. Categorically, Jesuits were opposed to much of the secularism of French attitudes, claiming to hold true to the Ignatian philosophy of finding God in all things, including science. Jesuits did not argue whether God exists. It was a foregone conclusion. God simply is; it is the task of humans to find Him. Positivism held little place in their philosophy. Instead, as claimed by historian John Langdon, "[Jesuits] offered their students the belief that by-gone days were preferable to the present." And importantly, from a clerical standpoint, "that a return to the monarchy [and a cozy relationship with the Church] would be better than a continuation of the Republic, and that Christianity in France was under siege from all sides in a war of extermination [or at least irrelevance]." It was not a popular position. Jesuit education was an implicit threat to the Third Republic.[6]

In this climate of religious cynicism and scientific positivism, it is no wonder that, by the age of twenty, Carrel had begun to question his faith—and doggedly pursued his education. In 1889 he completed his *Baccalauréat en lettres* (Bachelor in Letters) at the University of Lyon—one year later he was awarded his *Baccalauréat scientifique* (Bachelor of Science). Not long after, in 1893, he admitted he had "[t]errible difficulties with religious problems." Organized religion, in all its historic pomposity and anticlerical opposition, weighed on him. He was appalled at the fate of the destitute, seemingly vulnerable to the authoritarian power of Christian morality.[7] "[I]t is pitiful to exploit people under the pretext of curing them," he said at one point.[8] Yet the mysticism of his faith had been inexorably ingrained in him. He wrote in his journal at one point that "I feel myself inevitably drawn towards a figure, that of Christ."[9]

Despite its perceived abuses, for Carrel, religion and science could coexist. Still, in his mind, science held sway over man's ability to interpret nature. Science was "certain" knowledge. Knowledge that could be seen, measured, reproduced, analyzed, and verified. He was, above all, a scientist. But the supernatural was different. It was, unlike science, unknowable. God and the spiritual lay distinctly outside the realm of science—even philosophy, Carrel believed. It defied explanation by the intellectual, but was as easily felt as "the heat of the sun or the kindness of a friend."[10]

Following his bachelor's degrees, he began his medical education, serving in hospitals around Lyon. By 1900, he had earned his doctorate from the University of Lyon.[11] Carrel seemed to excel in his manual dexterity. Fellow classmate and friend René Leriche remarked that "he had certainly, along with Jaboulay, the best surgical hand that I ever witnessed in a career which allowed one to watch most of the greatest surgeons in the world."[12]

And Carrel had an insatiable mind for discovery.

On June 24, 1894, the president of France, Sadi Carnot, during his visit to Lyon, was stabbed by an Italian anarchist by the name of Sante Geronimo Caserio. Caserio plunged his dagger just below the right costal margin and into the liver. A second wound to the portal vein occurred when Carnot recoiled from the blow. He soon collapsed. An operation, performed by the renowned surgeon Léopold Ollier, was futile. The portal vein had been severed and hemorrhage was uncontrollable. The bleeding veins were ligated but to no avail. Carnot died the following day.[13] Carrel witnessed the bloody operation and frustration of Ollier. It annoyed Carrel that Ollier and his contemporaries had little stomach for the meticulous approximation of delicate blood vessels. And he was not quiet in his displeasure, perhaps feeling that such brilliant minds should arrive at a practical solution for injuries so imminently fatal as the disruption of vital vascular channels. Carnot could have been saved, Carrel argued, if surgeons were able to directly repair the severed veins. Then just twenty-one years of age, his critique as a very young house officer of such a distinguished dignitary as Ollier was a point of perceived insolence that would not put him in good stead with his superiors. But what defined Carrel was his curiosity and ingenuity. At the fin de siècle, Lyon was the silk capital of the world. Carrel sought out Madame Leroidier, a silk embroiderer, one of the finest in Lyon (his mother had embroidered as well, and Carrel, as a child was enchanted with the process). Madame Leroidier taught him the use of tiny needles and fine thread. The culmination of his work appeared in the journal *Lyon Médical* in 1902 as two research articles. Each detailed his method of an end-to-end anastomosis of dog jugular vein to external carotid artery using fine Alsace cotton thread and equally dainty Kirby straight sewing needles.[14] This ingenious work would win him the Nobel Prize in Physiology or Medicine for 1912.

But his ingenuity did not explain the spiritual. With this his brilliant mind quarreled.

"Does God exist?" Carrel wrote in 1896. "Certainly, although it is difficult to prove it. Besides, it is also impossible to prove [His] non-existence. It is therefore possible, and, in the end, it is most prudent to behave practically as if [He] existed."[15] It was lack of that evidence, so crucial in the experimental sciences, which bedeviled him. Despite all, he did not fail to embrace his faith and his God. "If God wanted me entirely, I would rush to Him, and without measure, I would devote myself entirely to His service, because He is the only truly great Master, the only one who is worthy of absolute devotion," he entered in his journal that same year.[16] Yet he was hounded by his belief that "truth" could only be found through science. As for religion, perhaps it was time to seek the truth there. No longer was docility and passive acceptance of Church teachings acceptable. Such behavior frightened him. To believe, then, Carrel must investigate. He must somehow seek the proof of God's existence as he had with scientific principles of physiology and medicine. What could be more meaningful as a certainty of God's existence than a miracle, an event that defies natural law, as if its occurrence was the work of a supernatural force. "God acts on men . . . only through the intermediary of physico-chemical and physiological factors," he wrote. Analysis to him was central to believing:

> When I got into the habit of analyzing and criticizing things and people, and especially asking myself what life was like, what to do with it, and finally examining the question of existence of God and of Christ, I thought I was simply indulging in an entirely intellectual game. Without realizing it, I was caught up in it and now it would be impossible for me to take my eyes off [God].[17]

There must be a way to verify the supernatural. Miracles. The miraculous deeds that defied natural explanation could provide proof of God's existence and His involvement in natural activities. Did not the biblical Jesus himself work miracles as demonstrations of His divine power to wipe away human suffering?

The Drama of Lourdes

And so began Carrel's quest for proof, his pursuit of the miraculous. What better place than the French village of Lourdes. For decades reports abounded of unbelievable events. Decrepit victims suddenly cured by the waters of the shrine where, reportedly, the Virgin Mary appeared to an impoverished peasant girl, Bernadette Soubirous. So frail and impressionable young Bernadette appeared to be and so fanciful were her tales of apparition that many questioned her validity and even her sanity. Would this be a site for scientific study? Could Carrel investigate, examine, observe, and conclude as he might do at the bedside, in the operating room, or in his laboratory? His Catholicism was ripe with the miraculous. Perhaps he could at length blend the natural and supernatural as one continuum of a divine design for the universe and, according to Christian teaching, the certainty of an everlasting existence. In their review of the Lourdes cures, Bernard François, Esther Sternberg, and Elizabeth Fee concluded that exposure to the Lourdes waters and prayer had the peculiar effect of producing remarkable cures for any variety of diseases, from tuberculosis to blindness to paralysis. Thus science was pitted against the spiritual, each camp proclaiming certitude that their respective beliefs in fact hold true. Religion claiming divine intervention, science insisting on as yet undiscovered natural explanations. But here, too, the authors ultimately subscribe to that which Alexis Carrel had voiced a century ago, that the Lourdes phenomena are of considerable interest to science, not from an atheistic point of view, but from extraordinary circumstances demanding investigation.[18]

Was the Lourdes experience commercially driven and designed to appeal to the most gullible of nineteenth-century pilgrims—women? Was this another manipulation by Church authorities? The secularists surmised rather cynically that the so-called cures were simply the permutations of a hysteria heavily influenced by outward stimuli meant to strike at the heart of an emotional fragility only too ready to accommodate. And hysteria was a phenomenon distinctly viewed as feminine, perhaps a derangement of female substances arising from their infamous uterus. Women were considered emotionally vulnerable, more susceptible to the fanciful hallucinations of religious fervor.[19]

Yet intensification of inquiry by the end of the nineteenth century, kindled by the tremendous backlash of secular skepticism, prompted deeper and deeper unraveling of the miraculous, subjecting such happenings to the scrutiny of established scientific norms, probes, and conclusions. In fact, historian Jason Szabo sought to attribute the probing analyses of cures to efforts by the Roman Catholic Church to exonerate miraculous dogma for the sake of the faithful and even the survival of the Universal Church.[20] However, spillover liberalism of the nineteenth century, sparked by revolutionary thought, discredited the possibility of miracles. Materialism took hold as the primary plausible path of belief. As contemporary philosopher G. K. Chesterton remarked, "In their doubt of miracles there was a faith in a fixed and godless fate; a deep and sincere faith in the incurable routine of the cosmos." God became irrelevant.[21]

"Miracles" must have an explanation beyond the divine, then. Not that influence of mind over body was unheard of in the nineteenth century. Skeptical psychologists such as the English physician and psychologist Daniel Hack Tuke (1827–1895) could skillfully outline numbers of cases where "cures" were reported and, for the most part, attributed to poorly understood effects of mind over matter. The state of the mind—including emotions and even volition—Tuke seemed to conclude, exerted a tremendous influence on bodily function that, perhaps, gave rise to so-called miracles. "Imagination, Expectation, Faith, Hope, and Joy" he implicated in these cures, but soon excluded "Imagination and Faith" as evidence.

The influential French novelist and naturalist, Émile Zola, scorned romantic theories of unseen influences and focused on the observable and scientifically provable. He was, then, as no surprise, the supreme sceptic of Lourdes. He had spent fifteen days there in 1891 and again for a national pilgrimage in August 1892. The immensity of suffering and hope struck him. "I interviewed a number of people at Lourdes, and could not find one who would declare that he had witnessed a miracle," Zola recalled in the preface of his novel *Lourdes*.[22] The residents of that remote region of Lourdes "were superstitious, devout, and simple-minded" enraptured with trees which sang, stones oozing blood, and horned beast ready to pounce if magical words were not uttered, he wrote.[23] The teenaged Bernadette Soubirous, one of the impressionable—"poor-blooded" and "slight of build"—had a special devotion to the Virgin Mary. Her existence was one of squalor, her lodging abominable—dirty, cramped, decayed. It was no wonder, then, that the appearances of the girl in white at the Grotto of Massabielle, Zola argued, was a figment of her imagination.[24] Even the extraordinary declaration by the apparition that she was the Immaculate Conception failed to stir total belief in witnesses, many claiming the impoverished Bernadette only too eager for relief from her miserable existence. Others were convinced of the divine, however proof of God and His heavenly kingdom. And the throngs of pilgrims now, begging, pleading, praying for a cure flocked to the Grotto and Basilica, their upturned eyes and faces—the crippled, disfigured, cachectic—beseeching the Virgin to rid them of their miseries. The waters of the Grotto soothed, refreshed, and ministered. For some, like Zola's fictitious Marie de Guersaint in *Lourdes*, miracles lifted them from their wheelchairs and pallets and restored animation and vitality. Of course, as Zola pointed out, Marie's illness was more akin to hysteria—subject to the powers of suggestion—than an identifiable organic disorder (despite her emaciated appearance). For others, like Marie's childhood friend, the priest Pierre Froment, nothing of the kind. His illness is one of the spirit, a conflict between vocation and desire. The Virgin would not help him. Dejection and disappointment. In this dichotomy of joy and sadness erupted sorrow, jealousy, and anger. None of the attributes of a holy spirit. In Zola's *Lourdes* such was the breadth of emotions among the faithful.

Yet "the same cries, the same words—gratitude, thankfulness, homage, acknowledgment—occurred again and again, ever with the same passionate fervor . . . proclaiming the everlasting devotion of the unhappy beings whom she [the Virgin] had succored."[25] It was all a "hallucinatory intoxication of dreams," Zola wrote.

Just like Zola, the scientist-physician Jean-Martin Charcot, neurologist at the famed Parisian Hôpital Salpêtrière, embodied the positivist skepticism of the *fin de siècle*. Moreover, he was obsessed by the contemporary phenomenon of what was considered hysteria.[26] In *La Foi Qui Guérit* Charcot insisted that the faith healing is nothing more than a reflection of the evolution of science. "Evolving science does not claim to explain everything," he wrote.[27] Miracles, in time, seem to disappear with discoveries and new conquests of the unknown. Such occurrences seemed localized among religious shrines, and the driving force a hysteria that mimics numbers of organic disorders, even certain manifestations of cancers, he goes on to claim. In Charcot's estimation "so-called supernatural healing under the guise of faith healing obeys natural laws . . . the suddenness of the cure is much more apparent than real."[28] Even rigid (hysterical) contractures bend to the psyche and resume normal motion. "The influence of the mind on the body is effective enough in producing healing from maladies that ignorance . . . of their true nature, made them considered incurable."[29] Hysteria had become, thanks to the promotions of Charcot, the great mimetic, elusive, mysterious, but always lacking the tangibility of derangements such as inflammations, degenerations, or neoplasms. In some shadowy way was it truly mind over matter?

Or did physicians of Charcot's ilk sense the incessant encroachment of religion on the medical field, misleading expectations?[30] Was this a counteraction of science against the intrusive presence of clerical ministers despite efforts by the Third Republic to suppress the Church? Would there be no ridding science of angels?

In their somber practicality one could not fault the rural peasants of nineteenth-century France. Impoverished and imprisoned in their miseries, French commoners were a dejected lot, eager to grasp any sign of redemption or hope. Even the seemingly irrational seemed plausible. For that reason, perhaps religion existed—to placate the masses, to furnish faith to the disadvantaged and ignored. Perhaps escapism in the form of miraculous happenings provided that glimmer of relief from everyday existential anxieties and some justification for their religious convictions. As one historian noted:

> Miracles . . . appear to distil the irrationality discernible in unorthodox medicine. . . . They almost always involved the sudden restoration of health, usually after a pilgrimage to a religious shrine, and were seen as a celestial reward for this devotion.[31]

In that case, miracles flourished in the context of need and misery, "as an affirmation of the inadequacy of the existing order."[32] So, such events as the Lourdes cures (and there were numerous other examples throughout France) provided a relief from their material lot, a ray of hope that existence had merit, that their lives had worth, if only in preparation for the world to come. God was the thread that connected all people and prepared a better home than the desperation this one offered them.

The Voyage of Louis Lerrac

Alexis Carrel did not share the cynicism of Zola or Charcot. He may have wanted to intellectually, but his heart rebelled. Childhood religion had been deeply instilled, and he was nagged by doubts. So, it is no wonder that the miraculous—and especially those happenings at Lourdes—captured his attention. When Carrel wrote his account, titled *Le Voyage de Lourdes* (*The Voyage to Lourdes*), is unknown. His widow found the manuscript among unpublished papers and submitted it to the Parisian publishing house Plon, which printed the work in 1949. Harper and Brothers then reproduced the English translation in New York in 1950. It is a fictionalized story of Carrel's experience at Lourdes and his witness to a miraculous cure. There is no question that Carrel, by way of his *nom de plume* Louis Lerrac ("Carrel" spelled backward), is writing about himself, the details of his journey, and his examination of the deathly ill Marie Ferrand (in real life Marie Bailly). With amazement, he recounted her spectacular recovery from almost certain death after exposure to the waters of the shrine. He had been there at her side to witness the seemingly miraculous. In the end, his tale was not fiction. It was fact.[33]

What brought him to the shrine? Carrel was admittedly fascinated by the rumors of the place. Catholic periodicals shamelessly promoted the "cures" that had been endorsed by Prosper Gustave Boissarie, physician and head of the Lourdes clinic. Even the supreme skeptic and agnostic Émile Zola had witnessed strange events. Yet Carrel, despite his religious convictions, wanted a firsthand experience. As a scientist, he thought it reasonable to investigate firsthand the miraculous affairs. His aim was to apply scientific methods to tell whether the supernatural was at play or the wonders simply misinterpreted illnesses and extreme psychological impulses. "Almost nothing was known, biologically speaking, of such phenomenon," Carrel's young Lerrac reflected. An objective examination should resolve the perplexing conditions reported by others. If unexplained cures occurred this would be of most profound importance to the scientific world and, personally, to himself and his mind plagued with the complexity of religious and scientific overlap.

Carrel's central figure in the story, Marie Ferrand, was a young, cachectic woman riddled with tuberculosis. Hers had been a life of seclusion in one tuberculosis ward after another. Now, on the train to Lourdes, she was near death. Consumption, as it was also known, had overtaken her abdomen and threatened to kill with peritonitis, her swollen belly now exquisitely tender. "The death of a believer . . . was a peaceful death," Lerrac reasoned. The solace of eternity to those who hold hope in God's presence. "A longing now swept over Lerrac to believe." He, almost instinctually, prayed for Marie. At Lourdes, Marie was taken to the Grotto and the blessed water was poured on her abdomen. Lerrac was sure she would die in the process, her breathing and pulse rapid, her skin the color of a cadaver.

And then it happened. Lerrac looked at Marie again and noticed a change: her skin less ashen, the shadows on her face gone. He leaned over her. The pulse was slower, the breathing less labored. Then, "Look at her abdomen!" It was flattening. "How do you feel?" Lerrac asked. "I feel very well," Marie responded. Before long, her condition improved to the point that she was scarcely recognizable. Then he had to admit: "[i]t was a resurrection of the dead; it was a miracle!" He had seen it with his own eyes. Two other doctors in attendance examined the girl. "She is healed," one declared. The other agreed. "It is a great miracle." Neither could explain the events by natural means. One, "Dr. C.," said to Lerrac "[i]t is a great miracle. . . . Will you convert, Monsieur Lerrac? I have prayed for you."

"This young girl is completely healed," Lerrac said to himself. "It is a manifestation of the impossible," he reckoned. Wondering if he had made an incorrect diagnosis, he retraced his examination. No, he concluded. Surely, it was tuberculous peritonitis. Of that, he had no doubt. This is the miracle that could not have been more perfect. For him to hear and inspect and to see firsthand the wonders of the waters, there was only certitude that the unexplained was present, the mysticism of religion, defying all that was scientific, had appeared as surely as the Virgin herself. As valid as any laboratory experiment, he could not deny what he had observed, supernatural or otherwise. Now his embedded faith crippled by years of scientific skepticism, spoke. *"Does God exist?"*

A shaken and baffled Lerrac could only mutter to himself as a scientist might, "[w]ait a year or two to see if she had truly been healed by the Virgin." As the mystified Lerrac pondered the events of Marie Ferrand, he found himself in prayer, beseeching the Virgin herself:

> Sweet Virgin, caring to the unfortunate ones who implore you humbly, protect me. I believe in you. You wished to answer my doubt by a shining miracle. I don't know how to interpret it, and I doubt again. But my greatest desire, and the highest goal of all my aspirations, is to believe, to believe hopelessly, blindly, never more to discuss or criticize.[34]

In fact, the dossier on Marie Bailly—the real Marie Ferrand of Carrel's fiction—described an event almost identical to Carrel's Lerrac—surely it was the same experience. Prosper Gustave Boissarie, then director of Medical Investigation at Lourdes, had scrupulously recorded the events of Marie Bailly's case. Upon entering the waters of Lourdes there was a dramatic change in Bailly's condition, heretofore moribund, almost terminal. Pain disappeared; a calmness overtook her. It was a feeling she had that she was cured. Within an hour, her respirations had slowed and a rosy tint spread over her face. Soon her swollen abdomen relented and assumed a more flattened, normal configuration.[35] It was an unusual case, Boissarie noted, in that a certified doctor, one of impeccable credentials (referring to the young Carrel), had witnessed the whole event and faithfully recorded developments almost minute by minute. His findings as reported to Boissarie mimicked almost exactly the narrative portrayal in his novelette by the fictitious Lerrac.

Alexis Carrel could not let go of his Lourdes experience. The perplexing miracles there were indisputable. What remained elusive was an explanation, any rational explanation, that would involve a deduction from hypothesis to understandable permutations of the natural order. How could something as sublime as faith, as mythical and fantastical as an invisible supernatural power, influence the biochemistry and physiology of the human machine in ways science could not decipher? He could not totally subscribe to it all, his analytical mind would not let him. Yet he was far from dismissing it. It was not that the religion instilled since childhood could not be extracted and discarded. It was that the power of faith and of prayer—of a divine influence on human affairs—was so seductive, so integral to a world swept up in inconsistencies, hardships, and suffering. And then with his own eyes, right in front of him, he saw a manifestation of that intrusion—the unseen world into that seen. Was there not a time when what appeared to the naked eye was to be held as irrefutable proof? The world was flat, the sun revolved around the earth. The liver was the soul of life. Was not science wrong then and might it not be wrong now to deny a dimension outside of the measurable, the scrutable. And so, he traveled again and then again to his mysterious Lourdes and the healing grotto where happenings unfolded as spectacular as those of the historical Jesus Mark the biblical evangelist portrayed.

While his analytical mind tried to separate natural from supernatural, a compelling urge brought him back, time and again, to intangibles of the divine. God and the spiritual lay distinctly outside the realm of science—even philosophy, Carrel believed. It defies explanation by the intellectual, yet for the senses, it is as easily felt as "the heat of the sun or the kindness of a friend." His curiosity of faith was unrelenting and not the deprecations of a new agnostic or atheist. "There would be no religion if certain phenomena had not been observed," he wrote in his journal in October 1929. How else to know there is a world that cannot be seen, felt, or touched. At the same time, Carrel believed that prayer could produce material results. "It is the response of a very powerful and good being."[36]

He was flawlessly hopeful. In fact, of the two realms of existence, natural and supernatural, both required intense discernment. Of the natural, the scientist God was a form of mysticism, divorced from carnal pursuits and materiality. Religion provides a different interpretation of death from that furnished by science. For the faithful, death is not the end of life but the beginning. The spirit, now separate from the decaying flesh, ascends to realms that, unaltered as in earthly life, unites with God.[37] Not that he behaved as a devout Catholic. In the 1930s, while in New York, Carrel rarely went to Mass. It caused, Carrel claimed, an inner discomfort for him, even though the man often visited Manhattan churches to listen to Gregorian music—that exercise, on the contrary, he felt was soothing and even essential to the soul. To Carrel it seemed spirituality and religion were separate.[38]

It was this spiritual core, though, that Carrel realized needed nourishment. He thrived on periods of solitude and quiet, insisting that such times allowed him to contemplate, energize, and engage in the mysticism that, to him, was inescapable. Carrel identifies a superior power—God, in Christian terms—as a form of mysticism. Religion, Carrel believed, assumed various forms. "In its more elementary state it consists of a vague aspiration toward a power transcending the material and mental forms of our world, a kind of unformulated prayer, a quest for more absolute beauty than that of art or science. It is akin to esthetic activity." Rituals, so elementary to the Catholic faith, did not hold him. He preferred to wander outside them, to direct his curiosity to the mystical, the intangible entanglement of man with God, the hope that, by cultivating his spirit, he was preparing for a life outside death.

For Carrel, one must prepare for faith. In his thinking, it was an offering of one's self, as "the canvas before the painter or the marble before the sculptor." Only in such a sterile setting can true faith enter. "Leave the children alone, and do not forbid them to come to Me; for the kingdom of heaven belongs to such as these." The uncluttered soul—like that of a child—accepts readily the perplexities of faith, the Christian Jesus said. Carrel now believed the supernatural could truly influence the natural in healing processes. He later concluded:

> [Miracles] prove the existence of organic and mental processes that we do not know. They show that certain mystic states, such as that of prayer, have definite effects. They are stubborn, irreducible facts, which must be taken into account. . . . The miracle is chiefly characterized by an extreme acceleration of the processes of organic repair. . . . The only condition indispensable to the occurrence of the phenomenon is prayer. . . . They show the reality of certain relations, of still unknown nature, between psychological and organic processes. They prove the objective importance of the spiritual activities.[39]

Carrel, overwhelmed by his experience with Marie Bailly, returned to Lyon. Totally in awe, he spoke of his encounter with the supernatural, proclaiming Bailly's cure as the most striking miracle ever to occur on the pilgrimage. Marie Bailly named him as a witness, as published in the local press, *Le Nouvelliste* June 3, 1902. "A Cure at Lourdes," the periodical proclaimed. [40] Then, second thoughts crept in. Whether concerned about his reputation among Lyon scientists or whether true doubt intruded, Carrel tried to backtrack only days later, hoping to distance himself from the distinctly unscientific happenings at Lourdes and maintain his credibility in the academic community.

> In the story of Mlle. X [Bailly], only one point is beyond dispute. This young girl who was seriously ill at one in the afternoon of May 26th was cured at seven in the evening and remains so to this day. Beyond this certain fact

everything else in vague . . . it is impossible at this moment to draw from that observation the conclusions that you have presented [a miraculous event].[41]

Editors at *Le Nouvelliste* would have none of it and refused to publish his retraction. Now, it was too late. Carrel's marginal status in the community deteriorated further. He was to be labeled as a sympathizer to the Lourdes cult of believers, and not a critical analyzer of fantastical hypotheses. Rejected by his compatriots, Carrel fled to Canada and then to the United States. Only later, during World War I, would he return to France, again criticized; this time, for deserting his homeland.

Conviction

Carrel went to Lourdes again in 1912. Perhaps, despite vacillations about miracles, his heart spoke louder. He remained curious, even hopeful, the miraculous to him proof of the divine. Unbelievably, on that very visit, a blind child of eighteen months recovered his sight. Carrel was there to witness the event. Truly, he felt, another miracle. How to explain such a phenomenon with science. A blind child, too young to fake this handicap, now with sight. That evening Carrel, wandering the grounds, encountered a woman who he recognized as the one carrying that small child. She was Anne Marie Gourlez de la Motte, and he would marry her in 1913. He was then forty, she thirty-seven, a widow. Her late husband, Henri Jarret de la Meirie, had been an officer in the French Army and had died quite unexpectedly at age fifty-eight shortly after retirement, some years before. She had a son with him, Henri, on whom she doted. Anne Marie was the daughter of Alfred Gourlez de la Motte, proprietor of the grand chateau on the border of Brittany and the Vendee. Carrel, in turn, would dote on her. They were to have no children of their own, but conjugal life was one of his most cherished blessings. He felt at home with Anne Marie. She was a spiritualist much like himself, and deeply religious. In her, he found a comfort that the mysticism for which he so eagerly searched resided in his lifelong companion.

And that spirituality guided him throughout his later years. It should influence human behavior, he wrote. Faith is a powerful human surge to "cultivate virtues of courage, endurance, and moral strength."[42] It is the engine driving creative effort. And that was at the core of humanity.

In December 1940 Carrel wrote an article for *Reader's Digest* titled "Prayer is Power." In this essay, Carrel maintained that "[p]rayer is the effort of man to reach God, to commune with an invisible being." The article was translated into French but Carrel, not satisfied with the translation, wrote an

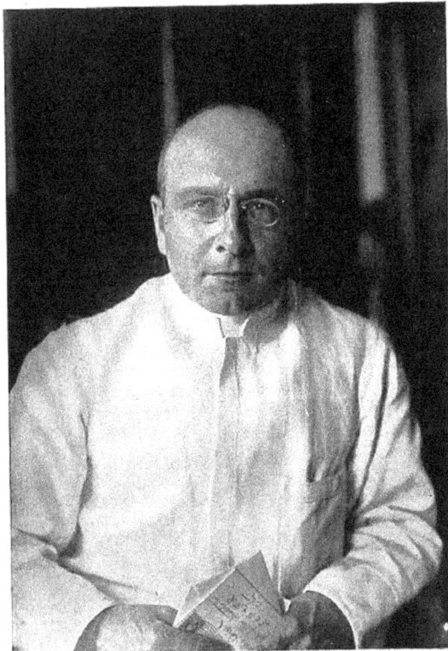

Figure 11.1 Miracle seeker and Nobel Laureate Alexis Carrel, 1912. The American Museum journal" (1900).

amended version in 1944, *La Priere*, his final published work. His sentiments regarding the divine left no room for doubt as to his belief in a higher power. His faith seems to have been restored:

> Everything happens as if God listened to man and answered him. The effect of prayer is not an illusion. We must not reduce the meaning of the sacred to the skepticism felt by man in the face of the threats, which surround him and the perceived mystery of the universe.[43]

That there were powers at work, whether from within human physiology or without, were now indisputable. He had witnessed two. Was it an unknown effect of neurohumoral changes invoked by prayer or simply an overriding of natural mechanisms by supernatural influence? That he could not rectify. But he pondered the question throughout his life. His actions, including his fondness for a like soul in Anne Marie, speak to that. His writings on the subject never stopped. He almost seemed preoccupied, if not obsessed, with the matter. And there is little doubt that prayer was a constant companion. Faith to Carrel became a personal issue, one that related directly to his God, irrespective of organized rituals of orthodox religion. This interactive mysticism appealed to him. It made some sense, despite its immeasurability. In his mind, at the end, Carrel seemed comfortable with nature and soul as two universal constituents of man's complex composition—one definable and the other, by its very character, not. Yet the physical—the φυσικός— and faith are not mutually exclusive. Carrel now knew that. They intertwine in a medley of the knowable and unknowable that forms the mosaic of life.

"Should we accept the answer of science or that of religions?" he mused. "Should we be guided by reason or feeling?" The mind—and by this he includes the spirit—exists outside the jurisdiction of science. It is impossible to know all, to understand how the spirit could be separate from the body, but spiritualists insist that apparitions—and, he added, there were large numbers of cases of indisputable authenticity—proved it so. Science provides only a sterile and finite definition of life. Scientifically, death ends all. For the religious, death provides an incentive to live life to the fullest, to develop consciousness in its highest form, to strive for the eternal. "Religion," Carrel wrote, "brings to man the answer his heart desires."[44]

Miracles? Who is to know? In the words of Eleanora Gordon, "We cannot . . . analyze those 'miracles' which defy a rational explanation: the sudden and total disappearance of crippling physical disabilities, the restoration of speech, vision, and hearing . . . or the instant regrowth of an amputated tongue. Nor should we try." They are wonders that may never be explainable, even to the most educated in the arts of healing.[45] As historian Sebastien Normandin concluded

> [T]hus we are left with life. Life constantly ordered, organized, constrained, systematized, analyzed, institutionalized, disciplined, prescribed, described and, sadly at times, senselessly destroyed. But despite these factors, life is a constant reminder of the small, essential truth of vitalism.[46]

Hence the undefinable spirit, the essence, the mysterious. Hence, then, perhaps the metaphysical, even the supernatural. And hence, enigmatic healing.

~

CHAPTER TWELVE

Humanism

The Bostonian

Twentieth-century science was driving a wedge between healing and spirituality. Natural laws and natural mechanics were reason enough. Anatomy, physiology, pathology, psychology, morality, depravity: all are consequences of mankind's unique composition. What is uninterpretable will soon be. It was the philosophy of humanism.

The eighteenth-century German philosopher, Emmanuel Kant (1724–1804), believed, in his theory of transcendental humanism, that the human subject is at once, together with all of creation, a part of nature, subject to its laws, but on the other hand, an autonomous, rational being who, through his elaborate cognition and curiosity, is one who transcends nature, incompletely bound to its laws and, in fact, on occasion the author of those laws. In many respects, then, humans have agency independent of any divine influence. One must respect that autonomy—both physical and spiritual—in the search for truth and knowledge.[1]

Had a fascination with human autonomy, then, taken the place of the metaphysical? The modern concept of humanism excluded the need for supernatural influence. Mankind could promote morality by virtue of its own reasoning rather than mandates issued by divine decree. The end objective of humanism is the controllable, engineered welfare of human beings instead of unassailable supernatural directives. The individual person then is all-important, their needs, their wants, and their interactions with society as a whole—irrespective of divine influence. According to humanist Andrew Copson, humanism can be interpreted as "a certain set of linked and interrelated beliefs and values that together make up a coherent non-religious worldview." Human beings, then, have the responsibility to give meaning and shape to their own lives. Man can weigh values, gain knowledge, and consider decisions based on sensual input. This does not completely exclude a less defined spiritual component of their internal discourse. In a humanistic way, the spiritual does not imply the supernatural but pertains to those aggregates of mental and emotional networking that gives personality, temperament, and character. As much as the physical, the spiritual and all the convoluted workings of the mind contribute as essential components of health maintenance.[2]

The English philosopher Matthew Arnold (1822–1888) considered man not through the lens of religious metaphysics but "through the everyday experience of ordinary human beings, of all classes and both sexes." He was one who promoted secular individuality, not conformity with ordinary individuals "acting out a bloodless theological paradigm."[3] Of course, his atheistic tendencies were front and center. "People . . . will use the germ of curative power which lies in Christianity, because they cannot do without it," he once wrote. Humanism, for Arnold, existed independent of religion. As for the supernatural, it was all a myth, as fantastical as the quarrelsome gods of Mount Olympus, he supposed. There was no will of God, only the will of mankind.[4] Then, one might conjecture that the true humanist is skeptical of divinities and of miracles, at least until they need one. Certainly, though, one can be a humanist and a person of faith simultaneously. Each man and woman have an autonomously functioning will which must be addressed irrespective of divine influence. So, for the religious—even those acknowledging the holistic, individualistic being—miraculous healings of faith supersede technology and are as possible as knife to skin. To them, the missing component of humanism is a benevolent and merciful God.

Yet for others, by minimizing religiosity, has a humanistic trend rearranged traditional notions of healing? Does this, in fact, represent the evolution of health care: from the divine to the metaphysical to, now, the human-centric? Is the supernatural sphere of reference to be disregarded? Have we decided that spirituality is simply a matter of biologically fueled neural networks and not some mysterious *pneuma* inserted at birth and destined, perhaps, to live on forever? Are we no longer a part of a universal force that guides a more perfect union? The humanism of modernity seems to counter traditional beliefs of mankind as spirits encased in corrupted flesh, imperfect derivatives of deities. Ignore the supernatural, humanism is inclined to preach. There is no internal struggle of a purifying mind on animal instinct, vying for eternal salvation. There is only cause and effect on ourselves and each other.

In fact, humanism appealed to the healing arts. No longer might abstractions be necessary to explain the complex physiology and pathology of human nature. Scientists had begun to lean heavily toward technology and seemed more occupied with the machinery than the mystical. And the darling of the healing specialties as the twentieth century unraveled was surgery. There was no better demonstration of man's ability to heal than the sudden, dramatic reversal of fortunes many surgical procedures could produce. Such technical finesse delivered a cult of pragmatism. Put aside a troubled spirit, worry instead about corrupted flesh. Corporal healing will promote spiritual healing. There is no better claim to joy than eradication of disease. At the turn of the century, surgical virtuoso William Steward Halsted of Baltimore (1852–1922) led the charge in his devotion to research and his own amazing technical finesse. Be flawless in technique, not so much compassion, his practice seemed to say. Healing was of the flesh and not the intangibles. His unique training paradigm produced equally competent technicians who would populate medical centers of North America with newfound skills. Their rugged, matter-of-fact character assumed the mantle of healer in a more profound manner than any other physician. For they had not only scraped the outer veneer of man but also sliced through to enter the deepest and most intimate recesses, so deep inside that some consider them close to the soul itself.

Despite their often-perceived callousness, surgeons, more than any other practitioner, fostered an unavoidable and unique intimacy with their patients. They touched and explored and massaged the most precarious and cherished of bodily anatomy: brain, heart, liver, gut—those organs the ancients considered the core of humanness, the essence of life. "The history of surgery . . . is partly a history of touch: technologically extended and transformed by the invention and refinement of surgical instruments," wrote art historian Suzanne Biernoff.[5] And even today, superb technical surgeons like transplant surgeon Nancy Asher of San Francisco still understands the bond of practitioner and patient. She admitted to a deeply emotional connection to her subjects in a television documentary of her cutter's art, that there is nothing more intimate than surgeon and patient when one has their hands inside a living human and brings them back to life.[6] For this reason alone, believers or non-believers, religious or atheists, surgeons had to confront the elusive component of humanness—the human spirit; the spirit which meandered through those organs of animation—that sped the heartbeat and wrenched the gut and tortured thoughts. Were surgeons cognizant of the consequences of their knife on those abstracts? Their operations were not universally successful. Many ended in abject failure, a suffering patient, unplanned disabilities, dashed hopes, and, perhaps worst of all, death. Could one simply walk away from their failures? Could one look their subjects in the eye and admit shortcomings, errors, poor judgment? There must be a connection besides knife to skin and fingers to tissue. Surgeons more than anyone needed to address the sorrowful spirit beneath the blemished flesh. The technically gifted neurosurgeon Harvey Cushing pointed out that "three fifths of the practice of medicine depends on common sense, *a knowledge of people and of human reactions.* . . . [Medicine] is an art and can never approach being a science." In all their reputed flashy elegance surgeons would do well to remember this.[7]

Yet in the words of one non-surgeon in 1896, "[s]urgery has run wild and there has been a great deal more of operative work than was needed."[8]

So, in the midst of this exponential growth of technology, perhaps surgery needed a softer side. Perhaps it needed a William Osler.

Edward Delos Churchill (1895–1972) rose to the occasion. His passion was not only perfection of technical performances but also, in those same patients, care of tender sentiments so easily rattled by disease. Churchill would be the holistic practitioner of humanism. He grew up in Chenoa, Illinois. His grandparents had settled there in 1805, probably some of the earliest settlers to do so. They were typical of the westward movement, first homesteading in Connecticut and Maine in the 1640s before moving to Illinois. The family business was in grain, haltingly successful but so much toil that Churchill's parents encouraged their offspring to move elsewhere. That the youngest son, Edward, did by entering the small Methodist college of Northwestern University in Evanston, Illinois. Majoring in biology, Churchill spent an extra year at Northwestern earning his master's degree before entering Harvard Medical School in 1917. Because of his academic brilliance, Churchill was accepted as a house officer on the West Surgical Service of the Massachusetts General Hospital his senior year in medical school, a notably prestigious appointment. He would spend two years as House Officer ("House Pupil" was the local term used) and two years as House Surgeon (or "Resident Surgeon"). Unlike the rigid Johns Hopkins program, his training was inconsistent and at the whim of visiting attending surgeons, many of whom failed to prioritize education. The Massachusetts General Hospital, despite its renown, did not have full-time teaching faculty, far different from the new Peter Bent Brigham Hospital under Harvey Cushing. Cushing had managed to muscle across his belief that faculty should be "full time" and not the itinerant practitioners who flooded Boston. While perhaps practical from a healthcare standpoint, Cushing claimed that visiting faculty was an educational risk and not desirable as a teaching model. Moreover, supervision of residents suffered, indirectly jeopardizing patient care. Aside from lack of proper education, residents were tasked with almost total management of ward (charity) cases for whom busy community surgeons had little time.[9]

It took, then, an extremely bright and motivated individual to thrive in that environment—basically, to self-teach and glean what he could from a preoccupied attending staff. Churchill proved to be one of those. While he was aware of Cushing's system across town, he did not apologize for his curriculum. At the Massachusetts General Hospital few senior surgeons knew any better. "They [the attending surgeons] had been conditioned as apprentices to the standards of the generation that preceded them," he later wrote, referring to his time in training. Still, he acknowledged it was a tradition laden with dangers. Young residents were deprived of the opportunities to ponder, investigate, research, and discuss challenging clinical problems. They too often avoided difficult cases for fear of failure and lack of experienced support. In particular, that most vital of surgical education, mentoring, was unavailable. While there were exceptions most attending surgeons of "Brahmin Boston" stepped in and out of their lives almost by day of the week. "What a wastage of the vigorous and creative years of [their] youth," Churchill wrote.[10]

Despite perceived shortcomings of his surgical training, Churchill was a standout. His quiet, calm composure and self-effacing personality charmed quickly. In fact, he was so well thought of that, when there was talk of him leaving for the University of Pennsylvania, Dean Linn Edsall of Harvard Medical School offered Churchill the Mosely Traveling Fellowship as an enticement to stay in Boston and join the Harvard faculty. Churchill accepted. He prepared for his year abroad (1926–1927). He would call it his *Wanderjahr*, his "wandering-year," a whirlwind tour through the big academic centers of London, Berlin, Prague, Munich, Zurich, and Heidelberg. Besides, there had been a quick resurgence of German surgical ingenuity following World War I, and they were eager to demonstrate it. Of the German system of training, he would write this:

> They were men who had at most . . . one or two years of so-called house-pupil experience. Then they began as an assistant or apprentice to an older surgeon, and if they happened to line up with a very busy surgeon, they would get his point of view exclusively. There was a great contrast between what might be called the poorly trained surgeons under whom I had been brought up, and men who had spent years as assistants under a master surgeon in Europe. The later were more scholarly.[11]

It was that interminable loyalty and subservience that the German surgical virtuoso Theodor Billroth (1829–1894) fostered. So ingrained were those assistant-apprentices that they knew nothing else but the master's methods. Yet he was put off by the German doctor-patient relationship. Churchill felt the Germans treated their subjects merely as clinical material. Few words of comfort emanated from the mouths of professors. Their speech was clipped, technical, their subject catatonic in silent terror—hiding a soul fearful and worried. It was a professional attitude bred from centuries of Teutonic hierarchy, and now surgeons welded their knives as knights might have done, adorned in the armor of their newfound skills. A steely determination was all that was necessary to rid their patient of illness. It was much too militaristic for Churchill's blood.

But he was on a heady ascent of his own. Not more than a year after his return from Europe, the thirty-five-year-old surgeon was named the John Homans Professor of Surgery and soon, Chief of Surgery at the Massachusetts General Hospital, a remarkable achievement for one so young and relatively inexperienced.[12] While his clinical interest was in thoracic surgery, he was keenly aware of the dismal condition of graduate surgical education at the Massachusetts General Hospital. He knew it must change. Yet he did not have the enthusiasm for the Johns Hopkins system as did Harvey Cushing. In truth, Halsted promoted surgery an investigative science and, through the mere redundancy of his training method, instilled an unswerving set of principles to his residents. But his training was impractical. Too few curried the favor of Halsted and finished the program, and the length of time for that to happen was exasperatingly indeterminate. Those cast off by Halsted or Cushing, while maybe finding other learning opportunities, might be lacking in matters of knowledge, judgment, or technique. "Half a surgical training is about as useful as half a billiard ball," Churchill once said.[13] Communities deserved more skillful practitioners, Churchill believed. Halsted's method would not fill that need. "[T]he traditional manner by which the practical art [of surgery] was passed down from dominant master to docile apprentice [must undergo] conversion to an interchange of knowledge between teacher and pupil," he wrote of that period, realizing that Halsted had not altered that relationship but actually *intensified* it.[14]

Edward Churchill, whom his friends called "Pete," was not an imposing figure. His manner was far from that. Churchill exuded gentlemanly reserve and thoughtfulness, but not intimidation. A man of medium build, trim, with no dominant features, Churchill was orderly in his appearance but not fastidious—one who did not necessarily stand out in group photographs. He exhibited a kindly face more fatherly than scholar, more inclined to smile than frown, more listener than talker. Polite at first encounter, Churchill seemed almost shy as he engaged. He would lower his head just slightly when conversing as if to catch every syllable spoken like a shortstop anticipating a sacrifice grounder. Yet he seemed to read people between their utterances as if words were mere interference to distract from inner ruminations. By dodging them like so many darts, he could figure the true measure of a man. Churchill was not content to accept the apparent, rather he was more inclined to gently crack the surface and peer inside. It seemed intuitive to him that fearful solitude was inherent in any person, and often was the true driver of curious and disparate behavior.

He was a fan of Rudyard Kipling, who was an unabashed admirer of surgeons. Like Kipling, he aspired to compassion for the endless line of patients

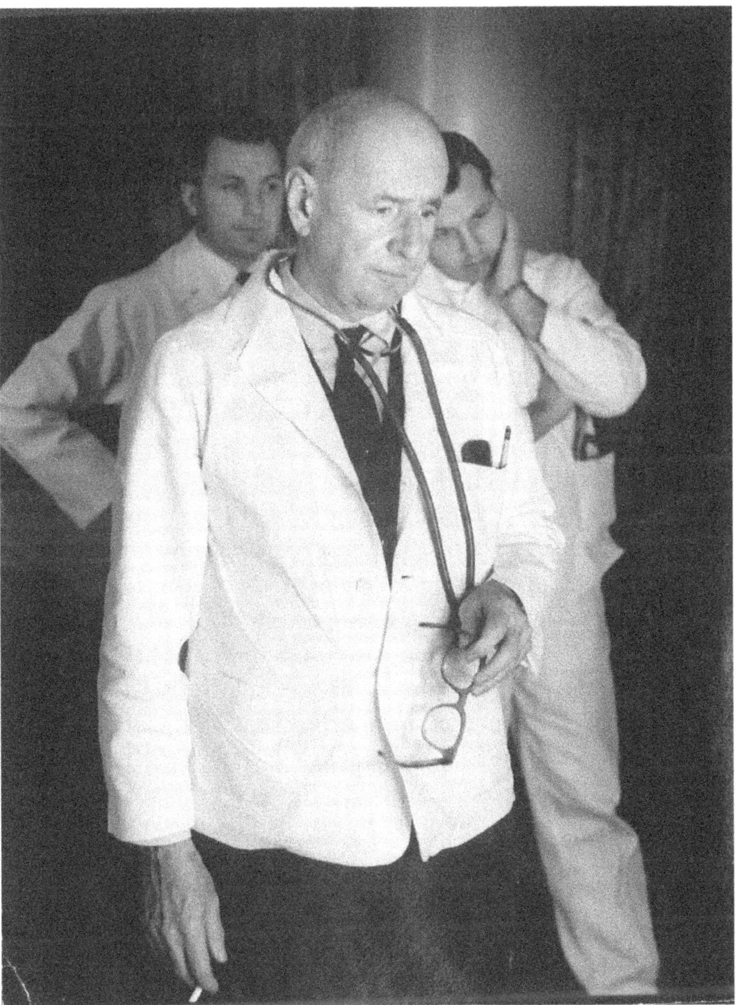

Figure 12.1 The humanist Edward Delos Churchill of Boston. Countway Center for the History of Medicine.

seeking physical and, perhaps, spiritual redemption. In speaking to an assembly of British surgeons, Kipling had once said of their profession: "[i]s it any wonder, gentlemen of the College of Surgeons, that your calling should exact the utmost that man can give—full knowledge, exquisite judgment, and skill in the highest, to be put forth, not at any self-chosen moment, but daily at the need of others?" He called their lives ones of "single-minded devotion."[15] Like Kipling implied, for Churchill, healing was not just a matter of the reunion of damaged tissue and restoration of bodily integrity. Healing encompassed a deeper commitment to massaging bruised emotions, bestowing hope, and taking a measure of suffering onto themselves by words or touch that might momentarily lighten the burden of illness for their patients.

Churchill had an equal dedication to shaping hands, minds, and hearts of the young surgeons of the future. He believed that American surgical training was woefully unstructured and unsupervised. To William Halsted's seemingly endless grinding agenda of honing one surgeon of many candidates—the so-called pyramid system—Churchill proposed equal training for every student—his alternative "rectangular" system—and limited the time of training to a more reasonable five years.[16] It would be a complete reshuffling of graduate medical education.

Even deeper, though, than the mechanistic training of surgical skills, Churchill, the humanist, knew there were aspects of practice that were distinctly unscientific and pertained to the sensitive, compassionate side of surgical dealings. The human constitution was no mere machine. The underlying spirit—however it might be thought of—permeated all aspects of vitality. Whether one supposed it was of divine origin or a mere result of hopelessly complex neural networks, intellect and emotions in some inexplicable way gave impetus to life and were inseparable from the blood-red organs that sustained them. What impacted the body, impacted the spirit. "How much greater the satisfaction of him who practices scientific medicine, tinctured with a love for the suffering humanity placed in his care," he wrote in 1949.[17] To address this complexity, Churchill's idea of the surgeon was a blending of both technical wizardry and empathetic support. Surgeons could not be emotionally illiterate. He urged a blend of scholarship and spirituality. He often quoted the legendary chemist and historian, George Sarton (1884–1956) who contended that

> Many men of science, even among the most distinguished ones—the very ones
> who are called the greatest authorities on this or that—are so uncultured, so

ignorant outside of their specialty, so lopsided, that their claims of leadership are preposterous.[18]

Churchill aspired to nothing of the sort. So different from the callous cutters of a century ago he preached a different philosophy, one of charitable proficiency. Charity, the "compelling force of Humanism," he orated, "is the most precious possession of Medicine." In fact, to those so enraptured with the rigidity of German science, he admonished, "[m]edicine is too close to the needs of humanity, and is too loyal a friend of mankind in times of fear and trouble, to cast aside abruptly its heritage of Christian ethics for what has been called the 'moral irresponsibility' of Science." The German-like system of Halsted, he felt, was too impersonal and inflexible and terribly deficient in morals:

> Exploitation of these hands [of young trainees] by neglect of the minds and ideals that must be developed to guide them will repeat the evils of the undergraduate proprietary schools of the last century, when "the teaching of medicine was, directly, in cash, and indirectly, in prestige, a profitable business."[19]

In line with his caring nature, the transformation of postgraduate surgical training would be Edward Churchill's most enduring legacy. Indeed, he was the consummate surgeon: grounded in the sciences but aware of the unique privilege to shape not only the human body but also the human soul—both in his students and his patients. It was imperative, he believed, that each generation pass on those indispensable building blocks upon which the profession ascends. Before the American Surgical Association in 1947, he echoed the Oath of Hippocrates when he said: "I will impart this Art by precept, by lecture, and by every mode of teaching."[20] As he pointed out in his new design for surgical training, the art was more than $\tau\varepsilon\chi\nu\eta$, the skill acquired through learning. "[I]t transcends Technology in the desire and responsibility to find safe application of these technics to the needs of humanity."[21] His "Content of Surgery" encompassed not only "hand work" but humanism, science, and empiricism. "The surgeon worthy of the name combines in liberal measure the love of humanity, science, and craft," he declared.[22] As Halsted and Cushing impressed, the surgeon was no longer ringmaster of his own sideshow—adept at speed and slash—he was now methodical and precise. Operations had become quiet affairs—almost secretive—no longer intended for the amphitheater.[23] No, the surgeon has transformed, Churchill believed:

> If technical training dominates these years of a young surgeon's life, he will emerge as a pure technician. It is very essential that he be taught to understand the nature of the tools that he is using, and develop a critical judgment in regard to new procedures and new tools, not merely attain proficiency in existing techniques.[24]

In fact, as a man devoted to history, Churchill, like the medievalists, understood the intensely personal nature of surgery. Foreshadowing others of his profession, Churchill knew that the surgeons' handiwork required intimate contact—touching—of their subjects, thus keeping the surgeon close to the physical ills and suffering of humanity. The humble character of surgery demands seeing, feeling, even smelling disease. It is this that binds the surgeon to the patient and family. This was in direct contrast, he pointed out, to the historical evolution of "Internal Medicine" that hopelessly indulged in "metaphysical speculation that threatened completely to separate its practitioners from the patient." For this reason, he felt that, over the centuries, surgeons closely served humanity and, as a result, they have developed a high moral and ethical sense, that, while science may have disclaimed moral responsibility, surgeons have stepped in to act as middlemen between virtuous and dispassionate behavior. He held in small regard the academic bent of aloof scholarly types in favor of the proletarian nature of the surgical craft, as if he and his colleagues were better suited to "blue jeans than academic gowns."[25]

At a deeper level, Churchill's humanism touched on the supernatural. He was of the belief that medicine and religion were inexorably entwined. However, science had produced a rift in this alliance. This division of responsibility "left the soul and the nurture of man's spiritual life to religion and defined the mind and the body as the province of medicine."[26] Yet Churchill knew—as many physicians did—that "effective therapy is as often as not based on and dependent on the interpersonal relations of doctor and patient." It is the doctor who must tend to the spiritual as well as the corporal. There can rarely be a clean distinction.[27] His mannerisms put patients at ease, so adept was he in recognizing the worried anxieties of the seriously ill. Friend and fellow surgeon Michael De Bakey wrote him in 1951 about a personal referral, "I am certainly grateful to you for your considerable attention to Mrs. T-. I realized that she presented a tough psychological problem . . . and I was confident that you were best able to cope with it."[28] To communicate with human beings under the powerful emotional stress of illness "is no easy matter and not infrequently requires the heart as well as the head," Churchill had said.[29]

He was a man of faith. In his chosen religion of Christianity, he embraced Christian doctrine, which guided his thinking and integration of medicine into personal philosophy. Christianity was based on the miracles of healing attributed to the Great Physician Jesus Christ. It was a healing religion. And religion, Churchill felt, is consequently a psychological matrix that surrounds one's life from birth to death, "sanctifying and enclosing all its ordinary and extraordinary occasions in sacrament and ritual." He went on to elaborate, "[t]he image of the healer was ever a constituent of man's religious matrix. Small wonder that man is now seeking out the physician for symptoms that arise in frustrations, loneliness, and uncertainty."[30] The paramount accomplishment of Christianity, he felt, was the evolution of the hospital. The Christian attributes of charity, compassion, and mercy have found fertile ground there and full expression, he wrote. There, the troubled spirit of the ill could find comfort, understanding, and nurture. It was a place of total healing—body and spirit.[31]

There is an immediacy to surgical healing that Churchill understood. An attack on human tissue, once begun, must be finished. Once, raging in pain, the howling of victims prompted speed. Now, with anesthesia, such radical rearranging of parts demanded resolution and repair. Surgeons' actions aimed to heal, if not in the moment, then surely in the recovery. Outwardly, it had become technical. Inwardly it must remain humane. Patients react to physical sickness with fear. Self-preservation is instinctually threatened. Their behavior might not be what one would logically assume, but may be rooted far deeper in sentiments not initially anticipated. He rightly noted in 1954 that "illness is an emotional event that demands value-judgment, and that in the face of suffering and death, logic and rational thinking are quite regularly tossed out of the window."[32]

Halsted was right insofar that he considered surgery a clinical science, not just manual skills but a thorough knowledge of the biological disciplines. Churchill saw more, though, and advocated for the additional dimension of *caritas*—that singular passion for human welfare. In the words of one historian, by the early twentieth century, surgery had changed from the "heroic, daring, fast and energetic . . . [to now] fastidiousness, gentleness, conscientious and slowness were the ideals." New methods emphasized control, decisiveness, precision, thoroughness, and refinements of technique that required a quiet, patient proficiency. As radical disruptions of anatomy and physiology became commonplace and anesthetic techniques necessary to countermand surgical invasiveness evolved, a deep familiarity with those basic human workings were essential for survivability. But it was not everything. Surgeons and their technical wizardry must come to the rescue of the inner spirit, to calm the nerves of anxious subjects. There must be a deeper connection. Echoing the words of Churchill, "A surgeon must have humanity, understanding, and love of people," surgeon Walter C. MacKenzie said in 1966. In short, the modern surgeon must now be anatomist, physiologist, pathologist, and artist, a true scholar, sculptor, *and* savior. Or, as one thoracic surgeon later said, "[t]hough science must be applied to give good patient care, a good surgeon need not be a true scientist." Hence, a good surgeon must also be a humanist. It is the surgeon who must repair not only a damaged, disordered frame but also quench the inner fires that have been stirred by the phobias of fate. There was no one else so intimately attached once the stolid exterior of skin—the visible armor of indifference—had been penetrated.[33]

How did Churchill feel about the impending mortality of each human? There was no escaping it. Even the most skillful of physicians could not forestall it indefinitely. He told a professional audience at one point,

> Death, as the senior practitioner, is bound to win in the long run . . . but it is your business [as physicians] to make the best terms you can with Death on our behalf; to see how his attacks can be longest delayed or diverted, and when he insists on driving the attack home, to see that he does it according to the rules of civilized warfare.[34]

With retirement, Churchill spent his time at the family farm in Vermont, tending his trees and blending into the local community, much as he had tended his patients and trainees. It was consistent with his perceived role as caretaker of the world within his grasp. On an August afternoon in 1972 he went for his customary walk through the hills of his farm. In a fashion entirely consistent with his modest and humble character, Edward Churchill collapsed somewhere in that countryside, alone and without fanfare. When he did not return, his wife called friends and began a search. He was found lifeless some time later.

Churchill was a man for the ages. A student of history, he interpreted his contributions as one of many in a line of healers extending from ancient Greece and before into an unfolding future. While insisting on a scientific foundation to medicine, he felt an irresistible bond with antiquity and with humanity. His guiding principle of charity was never far from his lips. As he spoke as President of the American Surgical Association in 1947, "Charity in the broad spiritual sense—the desire to relieve suffering for its own sake . . . is the compelling force of Humanism." And that charity—that love—aims for the complete healing of human beings.[35]

CHAPTER THIRTEEN

A Certain Brutality

Healing and Cancer

In Western culture the female breasts have been viewed as the epitome of womanliness and, for men, lustfulness. Yet there is a dark side. Monuments of femininity, the bosom is too often a woman's curse. The silent specter of cancer may be growing within, turning her life-giving glands into appendages of terror. For those ancients who rationalized earthly events by mimicking the divine, it was as if the treasure of Aphrodite—her voluptuous bust—too often became tales of mourning sung by the mythical Muse Melpomene; the allure of her offspring, the Sirens, leading woman, in her voracious beauty, to calamity.[1] Yet, in reality, it took little imagining to grasp the impact of the disease. The revered Hippocrates is said to have written "[a] woman in Abdera had carcinoma ($\kappa\alpha\rho\kappa\acute{\iota}\nu\omega\mu\alpha$) on the chest and through her nipple a bloody serum flowed out. When the flow was interrupted, she died."[2] He well knew the danger of breast cancer. An affliction of women, it decimated them. Hippocrates went on to write:

> In the breasts hard tumors form, some larger, others smaller; they do not sup-purate, but become continually harder; then hidden cancers form there. . . . The nipple is dried out, and the whole body is emaciated. The nostrils are dry and blocked, they do not stand straight; breathing is shallow; the sense of smell is extinguished. . . . When the disease has arrived at this time, it can no longer heal, and it causes the death of the patient.[3]

Women suffered disfigurement, smells, ghastly appearances, and, at the end, agonizing pain. Treatment, even if possible, was radical. It would take a certain brutality to heal. The wise Galen advised, "[i]f ever you attempt to cure cancer by an operation, begin your excavation by purging the melancholic humor, and . . . cut away the whole affected part." The Alexandrian surgeon Leonidas, in the second century CE, sliced into the cancerous breast deep, above and below, down to the chest muscle and then burned the gaping cavity with cautery, a suffering akin to crucifixion for the unfortunate victim.[4]

History has sympathized with women in their anguish of this disease, both physically and spiritually.

Such was the fear of this cancer and the mutilative surgery sure to follow, that Christians turned to heaven and appointed a patron saint, Saint Agatha of Sicily. Agatha earned her martyrdom in 251 CE, during the persecution of Emperor Decius. She had attracted the attention of the local Consular of Sicily, Quintianus. A brutish sort of man, he featured lusty designs on the comely and virginal Agatha, sure to succeed, he assumed, because of his perceived irresistible stature. She was of Christian bearing, but certain to acquiesce to his fetching charm, he judged. Yes, she would be an alluring prize for his boudoir. Nothing of the sort, Agatha insisted. Her devotion was to Jesus Christ. Incensed by her refusal, Quintianus seethed at the brazen Christian, and, suspecting some sort of witchcraft from this bizarre sect, tossed her, first, into a seedy brothel, but failing to break her that way, imprisoned her in his dungeon. She did not waver in devotion to her Lord. Further enraged and no doubt obsessed with her lovely, veiled bosom, Quintianus decided to rid her of those possessions and, in a pitiless display of violence, stripped Agatha naked and tore off both breasts with iron shears. Taken back to her cell, raw flesh aflame, her breasts were miraculously restored that evening with a visit from Saint Peter and the Christ child—as the legend is told. Never released from her prison, though, Agatha died a peaceful martyr's death before any more violations. However, because of the curative powers of her devotion to Jesus, she has become the patron saint of breast diseases. Over the millennia, women facing a similar fate at the hands of an equally malicious scoundrel named cancer have sought her aid, and prayed for miraculous restoration—if not breasts, then their serenity.[5]

No better description of the plight of breast cancer victims in preanesthetic days was the story of the petite English novelist Frances Burney d'Arblay. In Paris, in August 1810, d'Arblay—her friends called her Fanny—was troubled by a fleeting pain in her breast, steadily becoming worse from week to week. Fanny was at the height of her success. Her 1778 novel *Evelina*, a satirical play on dissipated British aristocracy, had been critically acclaimed as a masterpiece of literature. So engrossed had she become in the art world of Paris by then, that it was easy, at first, to ignored her pain, feeling it must be of little consequence. The writing had become wildly popular with her stories of English aristocracy told in satirical fashion, sometimes poking fun at the well-heeled of British society. Framed in conventional love stories, her heroines were sometimes victims of England's rigid societal principles. Now, at fifty-eight years of age, this bothersome breast pain began to worry her. See a surgeon? She revolted at the idea. Surely care and warmth would conquer this modest inconvenience. Months passed. Her husband finally urged her to have an examination. "I thought their fears groundless," she retorted, and would not hear of such nonsense. Finally, after friends warned her of the possible consequences of neglect, she agreed "painfully and reluctantly." Did she by then feel the lump? A physician was summoned. Worthless advice, she realized. Her pain did not improve but only got worse. Another doctor visited. More medication. Another month. Another visit. Now he began to placate her. She, disturbed by his ramblings, began to suspect the worst. Hushed mumblings away from her only heightened her anxiety. Her physician sought to tranquilize her with his words, but "his looks were shocking, his features, his whole face displayed the bitterest woe." A small operation would be needed, he said, "to avert evil consequences." Yes, her pains were becoming even worse, and the hardness of the "spot" increased. Now the heart pounding began, the nights of sleeplessness devolving into pure fright.

It was then that the name Larrey was mentioned, "a surgeon of great eminence." In her fear, she gathered strength from friends and acquaintances who flooded her apartment with well wishes. Yet, despite her naturally rebellious nature, she melted to the great Dr. Larrey. He exhibited for her the warmest of tendencies. With tears in his eyes, he described his surgery and offered the advice of fellow physicians as well. No, she said. If he could not save her alone, she would have no hope of salvation elsewhere. Still, he insisted, even consulting Baron Antoine Dubois, obstetrician to the Empress Marie-Louis, wife to Napoleon Bonaparte himself. His consultants agreed with her doom should surgery not be done. Cancer would be a death sentence, she feared. The breast and tumor must be removed. Cancer, it surely was. After this sentence was delivered, she "was in hourly expectation of a summons to execution." But it was a full three weeks before the date arrived. Larrey visited from time to time but was always melancholy. The iron-willed surgeon, who had stalked the bloody battlefields of Napoleon in search of mortally wounded men to repair, now faced the tenderness of beauty and prepared for mutilation. His soul, too, was deeply troubled. Yet Fanny was drawn to him and had the fullest confidence in his ability to rid her of this cancerous evil.

This Baron Larrey was the premier surgeon of his day. His illustrious career as Napoleon's own preceded him, legions of wounded warriors bowed to him.

Yet he remained humble, a reticent hero of the empire. Maybe his upbringing taught him humility. The son of a hardscrabble shoemaker, he knew early the value of honest work. Dominique Jean Larrey (1766–1842) was born of modest means in the village of Beaudéan in the foothills of the Pyrenees in 1766. So frugal were his beginnings that the dwellings of Beaudéan straddled a single narrow street. Along that road his family home was situated, a rather unpretentious two-story structure of stone-colored plaster. Sadly, his father died when Dominique was only three. His mother carried the burden from then on, piecing together a workable life for her family. At some point in his childhood, Larrey came under the spell of the local Catholic priest who kindly taught him the classics and instilled an indelible moral compass—or, perhaps, simply brought to light one already there. Whether he ever was a deeply religious man, he certainly carried a sympathy for the religious life and the morality it avowed. But, sadly, his mother did not last, either. He was orphaned at age thirteen. He left Beaudéan to live with his uncle, Alexis Larrey, in Toulouse, some one hundred miles away. His father's brother, Alexis, had moved away years before, intent on hand work of a different nature. He was an up-and-coming surgeon in Toulouse. So impressed with his uncle was young Larrey that he fell into a passion for the healing arts. His uncle was a dutiful preceptor, ushering Larrey as an apprentice through the halls and wards of the Hôpital Général Saint-Joseph de La Grave in the heart of Toulouse. It all served to whet his nephew's medical appetite. After completing elementary studies at the college de l'Esquile Dominique, not yet twenty-one and certainly with the help of Alexis, decided to continue studies in his newfound profession in the capital city of Paris.

There he worked in the surgery clinic of the famous Pierre-Joseph Desault at the Hôtel-Dieu. He sharpened his skills on the victims of the brutal French Revolution. Under the master Desault, he perfected care of dastardly injuries, the probing and carving techniques of *debridement* that forestalled ugly gangrene. His dexterity earned him a position with Napoleon Bonaparte, accompanying the armies across Europe and developing a novel method of casualty care, his *ambulance volantes*, or "flying ambulances"—speedy, cushioned wagons to carry the wounded, poised just behind the skirmish lines. Soon Napoleon appointed him surgeon-in-chief, and would not go into battle without him. So distinguished was his career that, in 1809, he was made a baron. The shoemaker's son was now of French nobility.[6]

Through it all, Larrey remained a humble man, cherished by the troops as one totally invested in their care, and respected by his peers. His looks, though, spoke otherwise. In his prime, he presented a rugged, forthright figure, one of common sense rather than given to speculations. A strikingly attractive individual, his looks no doubt contributed to his image as a bold, fearless, and determined military surgeon. Later in life, his angular features softened and he assumed the slightly corpulent bearing of middle age, the chiseled face now with some pudginess of the jowls. Nevertheless, his countenance still exhibited the forthright, but kindly demeanor of his younger years. Now, he languished in Paris, Napoleon's arduous Austrian campaign at an end. It was here that he dabbled in writing and lectures, and the numerous lessons of war he had absorbed. This was where Fanny found him, one of the most sought-after of French surgeons.[7]

But butchery on battlefields was one thing; the butchering of lovely Madam d'Arblay was quite another. On September 30, 1811, it was to be done. The accomplished Larrey arrived at her home. She was apprehensive he could see. The lovely Madam d'Arblay bravely submitted, her rosy complexion now the color of alabaster. She lay supine on a couch in her own home and undressed, breast exposed. As he positioned her, arm straight out, bosom uncovered, he could even smell the fear her glands were releasing. He might have used on the young lady what he had given to those about to undergo amputation: extract of opium combined with camphor, both of which were agents promoting drowsiness and dissociation from pain.[8] It would be decades hence before the amazing report of Henry Jacob Bigelow of Boston in 1846 described the use of ether to produce insensitivity to pain during surgical procedures. For now, there was only the hope of twilight narcosis.[9]

Larrey's face was drawn. There was no escaping the vicious wound he was to inflict. He understood the trepidation wrought by his skill; he had seen it in the numbers of soldiers from whom he was about to separate arm or leg. The master was assisted by three other black-frocked doctors—including the distinguished Dubois—and two students.

A case contained his surgical instruments. Most likely, it was the same case used by military surgeons. Knife, saw, fine metal probes, scissors, and hooks with which to encircle larger blood vessels to ligate with suture. Foremost among them, though, was his stainless-steel scalpel, a one-piece instrument with broad handle and exquisitely sharpened blade. These were the pride of every surgeon, some with curved blades that folded into the handle, others with elaborate tortoise-shell handles, still others with double blades and a blunt end for dissecting.[10]

He would use his scalpel first. By holding it as a pencil or pen, he could define his ovoid incision around the breast and exert enough pressure that the steel cleanly split skin, now marked with a thin red line of divided skin and then, exerting more pressure, enter the fatty tissue under the skin. Bleeding was sure to come, controlled by an assistant pressing against tissue with cloth compresses. There must be, at this point, an assurance of technique. Hesitation would only heighten the obvious pain for the patient. Down through breast tissue until the hearty red strips of chest muscle was encountered. He had learned his technique well, from fellow surgeons in Paris. The entire breast had to go, perhaps muscle, too. All around, his knife sliced through, until the breast remained as a fleshy island on top of pectoralis muscle. Then, pulling up on the breast, he carved it from muscle until the whole mammary gland was free. It was then, perhaps, that he applied his camphor solution to staunch the flow of blood from a myriad of small bleeding points along the chest. The hemostat, that ratcheted clamp so universal in later surgery to stop bleeding points, was probably not used by Larrey. He relied on firm pressure and the body's innate ability to clot blood. More likely, purified nitrate of potash was used to effect cauterization of small bleeding points, as Larrey mentioned in his memoirs.[11]

For Fanny, only a thin veil placed over her face separated her from the workings of her surgical team, so thin that she could clearly see through it. The sensation of Larrey's work was stomach-turning. She could feel him literally carving her bosom off her ribs, much like slicing apart a turkey breast—at times paring skin from fat under the skin—"cutting against the grain." He did not pause in his work. No time to stop them. Her cutaneous nerves must have been exploding in staccato bursts of pure agony. Another swipe. Then another. There was no alternative. Be quick or the exercise would become pure torture. This evil tumor had to be gone. It would have eventually eaten its way through her chest anyway, and that pain would have been unrelenting. In a letter to her sister sometime later she vividly recounted the awful event:

> When the dreadful steel was plunged into the breast—cutting through veins—arteries—flesh—nerves—I needed no injunctions not to restrain my cries. I began a scream that lasted unintermittingly during the whole time of the incision—& I almost marvel that it rings not in my ears still! So excruciating was the agony. When the wound was made, & the instrument was withdrawn, the pain seemed undiminished, for the air that suddenly rushed into those delicate parts felt like a mass of minute but sharp & forked poniards, that were tearing the edges of the wound—but when again I felt the instrument describing a curve—cutting against the grain if I may so say, while the flesh resisted in a manner so forcible as to oppose & tire the hand of the operator, who was forced to change form the right to the left—then, indeed, I thought I must have expired.[12]

At least twice she fainted dead away. Rattled, too, was the surgeon himself, eager to complete the cruelty. "Pale as ashes," Fanny recalled in a brief glance. The effect of a screaming subject, spurting blood, and raw flesh would undermine even the steadiest of hands and will. Only resolute determination would have carried him through with his task. All, of course, wished for a blessed syncope, the patient finally lapsing into unconsciousness. There was no way to tell, however, how dangerous swooning might be. No sphygmo-manometer had yet been devised to use in such circumstances. The pressure of blood flowing in the arteries to bathe the heart and brain was merely conjecture at the time. Only a finger on the pulse at the wrist gave any indi-cation of the nature of the heart and its vital beating. Fast or slow, bounding or thready were the only qualities appreciated. That state of syncope was precarious. Some slipped further so that cardiac activity ceased. Larrey knew from conversations with his colleagues that the likelihood of dying during the procedure was roughly one in ten.[13]

The operation in all its violence lasted but twenty minutes. The wound left behind, that oval of crimson, took over two hours to repair and bandage. Fanny would lay there on that couch for three hours.

She was lifted from the table to bed, her features "utterly colorless." She saw Larrey, the poor dear, pale as she, his countenance streaked in blood, a look of "grief, apprehension, and almost horror."

Larrey's students must have wondered what they had signed up for, not yet equipped with the necessary hardened indifference such brutality demanded. No doubt blood drained from their faces as well. It was a vivid display of the craft with which they had conspired to join. Would they someday be like the great Larrey: seemingly emotionless, decisive, detached? No wonder surgeons were looked at as monsters. It was licensed manslaughter. And the magnifi-cent technician Larrey. Would he numb himself with brandy that evening to shut out the distress of the Lady d'Arblay or the barbarism he was forced to employ? After days like this sleep would be troubling. He would write some years later about such matters:

> The misfortunes of others affect my strongly. Serious disasters afflict my soul and plunge me into the deepest grief; I often think I can do something to help, and even attempt to remedy the situation. But such is my nature that I am thrown off balance and reason is no longer in control.[14]

Was it now the manner of the dashing surgeon who, quick to rescue the gravest of wounded—sturdy young men in the prime of life, struck down during the noblest of pursuits—could not reconcile the suffering of the most delicate gender and the frank mutilation of the hallmark of femininity? The howls of dismembered women echoed in his head and mixed with the cries of his own trepidations. What dastardly dealings this surgery business was. Meant for wartime, it now fell more and more on the innocence of peacetime. He longed for the days of combat, where the honor of bravery under fire was reward enough for the defacement of cannon and flintlock.

For Fanny, weeks in bed were needed for proper healing, the pain electric with even slight movements of her arm. She would not speak of the event for months. Each time she remembered, the sting struck again, so that she refrained from even a thought. As for the tumor, was it ever cancer? She died almost thirty years later of unrelated causes. A cure? And how much of those years did Fanny spend in anxiety—the darkness of night giving birth to demons of worry. Would she fall victim again to a cancer's persistent presence as it slowly grabbed her in elegant suffering? No doubt she had seen others in the throes of wasting, begging for more opium, gasping for relief, their gaunt faces drawn in total fright. And what was worse? The pained soul suffering in advance, as if each day it reckoned with the stealth of death slowly approaching. Were her last days unrolling? Was this ache or that a malignant warning? Such was the nightmare of cancer, then and now. Such was the mind persecuted even though the body might be healed.

Larrey was well aware of the disease; all surgeons were. Mammary cancer—cancer of the breast—was a nemesis of medicine. The ugliness of neglected lesions as they grew to imprison every fiber of sensibility, drove women mad with pain and doctors enraged with frustration. All cancers were that way, it seemed. The Greeks had labeled such maladies καρκινος, "crab" like growths with tentacles extending under, around, and through healthy tissue. Even removal was no guarantee. Lumps reappeared a distance away—telltale signs of further mischief—or swellings of glands under arms or in the neck heralded a return of the silent assassin. Unbeknownst to physicians of Larrey's day, in its organic roots, cancer is really a disorder of the genetic material deoxyribonucleic acid (DNA). DNA is that replicating molecular spiral giving rise to life itself. In the process of replication (renewal), mutated sequences of nucleic acid alter cells in such a nefarious manner that normal cellular behavior is replaced by wild and unpredictable growth, spread, and destruction, as if an intentional maliciousness had taken over. And too often, the body defenses—those immune functions critical to fight off outside invaders—stand impotent in recognizing the villains of this disease, so closely aligned are they to normal anatomy. Accordingly, the process of growth and invasion continues unabated until sicknesses appear or, even more terrifying, hard tumors are felt and the normality of everyday life ceases to exist.

Get it all out, surgeons insisted. From any experience with this affliction, they knew that relapse of tumors along the chest was a sentence to exquisite and long-lasting torture. Women would first feel the hard nodules along their scar, then see them growing and ulcerating. As they coalesced and invaded sensory nerves, the agony began, never to cease. Carcinoma *en cuirasse*, the French called it—"cancer like a breastplate." The malignancy eventually eats through skin and tissue underneath until the entire chest wall is encased by stiff legions of stinking sores. The pain and difficulty breathing it caused literally encased the victim in malignancy. Doctors like the French anatomist Alfred Velpeau shrank from the specter of creeping cancer that drove their patients inconsolable with pain, watching their bodies devoured by this ravenous monster:

> It involves a single area, or sometimes several isolated small areas of subcutaneous tissue and skin. The involved area feels hard, rough, stiff, and thickened. It has an abnormal reddish color and stippled appearance, [t]he skin looks as if it had been tanned, or as if a portion of stiff leather had replaced the natural skin. . . . Despite their [initial] benign appearance these spots are cancer of the worst kind . . . they eventually fuse together, forming plaques of larger and larger size and finally a true cuirasse [breastplate].[15]

Mammary cancer was a universal malady. But its first appearance seemed so innocent, so minor, that many women dismissed it as merely a sore or harmless lump—or they were simply embarrassed to share such intimate findings. The New World of the eighteenth century was awash in strict Christian fundamentalism. Women were of a weaker nature, more libel to the charms of Satan and must, therefore, be kept under wraps. While sex was encouraged in marriage, bodies of women in public were well concealed beneath swaths of clothing. Blemishes and illnesses were kept private, sometimes not even the physician was privy. Only witches flaunted their breasts and only to suckle the devil, Puritans believed. Examinations of the female bosom by doctors were likely few and far between.[16] Doctors, informed by their patients of the various rashes, ulcers, and tumors of breasts, lacked decisiveness for fear of threatening modesty. Victorian scruples compromised male physicians in any dealings with female patients. American physician Charles D. Meigs, who fancied himself an expert in female diseases, cautioned his class of medical students even as late as 1848:

> All these evils of medical practice spring not, in the main, from any want of competency in medicines . . . but from the delicacy of the relations existing between the sexes. . . . It is, perhaps, best, upon the whole, that this great degree of modesty should exist even to the extent of putting a bar to researches.[17]

The horrid disease was equated with death and only divine intervention would save those afflicted, so the feeling was. So monumental the diagnosis, that the dual torture of physical mutilation and mental foreboding devastated not a few women. Only God could stop their cancers and restore peace of mind. Even the necessary savagery of surgeons like Larrey seemed unable to stop the spread of this malignancy. Few of their subjects would survive to old age and some would suffer horribly. Body and mind would both fall victim. And so, they turned to Jesus, Agatha, and prayer. To add insult to injury physicians speculated that these cancers were brought on by personal temperament. Grief, worry, rage. sudden reversal of fortunes, or overwork seemed likely culprits. Doctors counseled that women full of emotions be damped down, that they "avoid overtaxing their strength and bear the ills of life with equanimity." Those with apparent benign tumors of the breast were encouraged to be cheerful and refrain from the stronger emotions of distress.[18]

As for physicians of the day, it seemed a terrible affliction, the palpable tumor usually ignored for a time by the patient until pain became unbearable or, more ominously, ulceration occurred. The gifted William Osler, in his first publication in medical school in 1871, reported on a patient at the Montreal General Hospital with "carcinoma mammae." His patient had noticed her breast tumor about four years ago, gradually enlarging to the size of an egg by the time she sought advice of physicians. Now, there was severe pain with the tumor as it began to grow more rapidly. "These circumstances excited her fears," Osler reported. Indeed, it was the pain that made her seek medical attention. The surgeon, in a rather mechanistic fashion, removed the breast down to chest muscle—this time with the patient blissfully asleep under chloroform. There was little science to his method, and no heed made to the warnings of Petit that glands around the breast might harbor the malignancy. After surgery, as so many wounds did, the incision inflamed and began discharging infected material. She endured a painful recovery, her incision healed slowly, and she was sent home from the hospital "cured" not until almost a month and a half later.[19]

The enigmatic, but dexterous William Halsted of Baltimore would begin to change all that. A man of complexities, his brilliance was dampened by very human vices. The talented physician had taken a position at the new Johns Hopkins Hospital in Baltimore in 1889 and had immersed himself in the experimental planning of daring surgical operations. He had seen similar feats performed on his visit to Europe in the surgical amphitheaters of Theodor Billroth and Emil Kocher—two of Europe's foremost surgeons. Their operating techniques were impeccable, and he soon modeled his behavior after them. "He worked with superhuman energy and with the strength and endurance of ten men," colleagues would say. He was a bold, yet careful technician, full of confidence and curiosity. When not at the bedside, clinic, or operating room, he wrote. Scientific publications flowed like spring water. Work consumed all in a manner that could be construed as almost manic. He was in love with the precision of his hands and the artwork of which he was now capable. How else to recover health, he might have imagined, than to banish the scourge of disease? If not the mind, he fancied himself a healer of the flesh—it would be his singular trademark.

Halsted's downfall would be the personal demons of his own—and the new drug cocaine. Cocaine was an amazing agent; it anesthetized sensory nerve branches making procedures once considered inordinately painful, painless. Halsted had learned of its powers from one of his German acquaintances, Carl Koller of Vienna, who described its wonders with eye surgery in Heidelberg in 1884. Halsted was enchanted with it and used it in a range of operative cases. In the process, he was aware of its psychogenic properties: a certain exhilaration occurred, a feeling of enhanced enthusiasm. It was intoxicating, even adding more impetus to his work schedule. Sleep seemed no longer required. Mental capabilities skyrocketed; his mind limitless and indefatigable.

For Halsted, his dependence soon became painfully obvious. His conversations were frenzied. He would deliver rambling discussions so disjointed as to be embarrassing. Ironically, Halsted even wrote a paper about cocaine in 1885, titled "Practical Comments on the Use and Abuse of Cocaine" and published as a first installment in the *New York Medical Journal*.[20] A second installment was to follow, presumably addressing the "abuses" of the drug, but by that time, Halsted was so rattled by his addiction he could barely function, and the whole matter was dismissed. A close friend, William Welch, advised institutionalized treatment. Halsted agreed but the regimen was demonic. Doctors substituted morphine for cocaine as an attempt to wean Halsted from the drug. Their plan failed. Shortly he was addicted to both. Cocaine to soar, morphine to settle. It would last a lifetime.[21] Was it that his sane mind could not handle the assaults he inflicted on his patients; that he had to numb his thinking or rev it into high gear in order to dive into the heretofore uncharted recesses of living humans?

Nevertheless, his dangerous addiction was brushed aside in favor of his technical wizardry, and he returned to his duties.

He began to focus on breast cancer. Halsted contended that "most of us have heard our teachers in surgery admit that they have never cured a case of cancer of the breast." Most would say in private conversation that they only did surgery for the moral effect on the patient, that they felt operating shortened, rather than lengthened life. In those women who did manage to survive for years afterward, it fell into the realm of the miraculous almost.[22] Halsted felt differently. His solution was a firm belief in the wonders of the scalpel. Radical surgery. Like his European colleagues he cut wide and deep. In one grand swath he could remove the whole mass of mammary tissue and pectoralis muscle from ribs beneath. Under the arm of his anesthetized subject, he stripped away all vestiges of glandular tissue which enveloped vein and nerve there. His meticulous performance seemed almost microscopic in expanse, careful teasing out of nerves, arteries, veins, and glands in a magnificent demonstration of human anatomy. Doing anything less, as one English surgeon had said, was "a mistaken kindness to the patient." When finally finished the huge mass of breast, lymph glands, and muscle was lifted away and sent to the pathologist.[23]

As opposed to his predecessors, Halsted claimed that his "radical mastectomy" almost eliminated the risk of cancer resurrecting in the hollow scars of mastectomy; that cancer of nightmare proportions called by the French carcinoma *en cuirasse*. He declared that in his patients less than one in ten would fall victim to this. So impressed were his colleagues that they eagerly referred cases to him for mastectomy, now assured that surgery was no longer hopeless butchery but could, in fact, cure.[24]

Yet it was still a surgical disease. The only hope for cure was the defacement of femininity.

A transplanted New Yorker named Cushman Davies Haagensen (1900–1990) would carry Halsted's radical surgery even further. Haagensen was a tall, lanky man with stone-cut face, broad smile, and oversized hands. No stranger to illness, he himself had weathered an episode of tuberculosis that had kept him out of medical practice for two years. There is no better teacher of compassion, it is said, than illness itself. Perhaps that is what drew him to breast cancer victims. One could not ignore the emotional insecurities of breast cancer and the necessary sympathies to gain trust. At New York's Columbia-Presbyterian Medical Center, he incorporated the science of tumor pathology into his operative technique. Even more meticulous than Halsted, his results were amazing, and his practice blossomed. Haagensen's soft mannerisms, his easy conversations and his intimate understanding of women's emotional toll appealed to his patients:

> Fear is the most important of the factors that deter women with breast disease from seeking medical help. It has two aspects. The first is fear of mutilation ... she will lose her breast ... [the second] fear that terrorizes women with

breast disease is that they will not be cured of the cancer that they suspect they have.[25]

With his understanding of the emotional turmoil of their disease, he knew that his radical surgery and mutilation of womanliness needed the key element of trust in him from his patients.

> The main reason why the mental preparation of patients for breast surgery is so much neglected is that it can be done only by one person—the senior surgeon in whom the patient places her trust . . . [t]he responsible attending surgeon who has the patient's confidence should sit down with her . . . and explain her problem to her as simply and as truthfully as possible.[26]

Like Halsted, Haagensen tried to cure with his knife. Chest muscles—down to ribs—and gland tissue under the arm all came out at once. He removed so much breast skin—nipple and all—that very often a skin graft on bared ribs was necessary to cover the wound. With all that might come a cure. In his patients in only one in fifteen did the malignancy reappear at the surgical site, he claimed.[27]

Yes, it was defacement. Few women easily looked in a mirror again. The woman was left, after surgery, with a hollow contour to her chest and shoulder, and a visible rib cage under her likely skin graft, that was a badge of certainty about her diagnosis. His radical method garnered severe criticism in the professional and public spheres. Mutilative. Deforming. Not always curative anyway. Some began abandoning his technique in favor of less radical operations: simple mastectomy or "modified" radical mastectomy—leaving the chest musculature which gave a shoulder contour back for fashionable

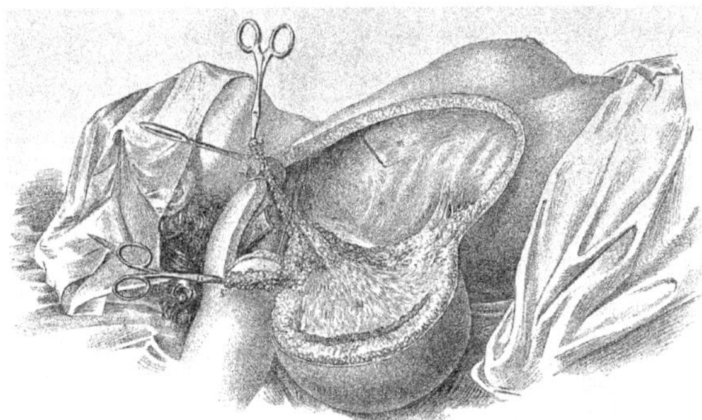

Figure 13.1 Halsted's mutilative radical mastectomy. William Stewart Halsted Surgical Papers Wellcome Library Images No L0004968.

dressing. Haagensen disagreed. He retorted that "surgeons had not learned how to select patients for radical mastectomy," and "many surgeons are unwilling to devote the time and patience required to do the operation well."[28] He even demurred at the idea of restoring breast contour, as if surgeons were later day visitors of Saint Agatha. Leave the site well enough alone, he maintained. "In opposing breast reconstruction, Dr. Haagensen said he believed that cancer could be spread by another operation, that the cosmetic results he had seen were not esthetically successful and that if there was enough skin left to do an implant, the surgery had not been radical enough and the patient had less chance of survival," the *New York Times* reported.[29] Damn the cosmetics; cure the disease was his opinion.

Women might have wondered, though. While removing a breast promoted cure from cancer—and, in the process, perhaps eased the fear of death—it had terrible psychological effects. The culture of the breast had become engrained in American life. Plastic surgeons fed into this by encouraging breast augmentation as a way for women to be "more feminine," the so-called bosom mania of the 1950s and 1960s. One prominent patient wrote of her mastectomy surgery in 1970:

> Losing a breast made me feel dewomanized. I'd been proud of the way I looked. I was well built and my designer clothes showed off my body. Now I felt the surgeon had taken the part of me that made me feminine and attractive. . . . I'd like to chop off parts of *that* doctor.[30]

Then, was such fanaticism really necessary? Despite his protests, Haagensen's radical surgery was fading in popularity. Scientific study groups like Pittsburgh surgeon Bernard Fisher's National Surgical Adjuvant Breast Program showed convincingly that a modified form of radical mastectomy was just as effective. Surgeons would leave in place muscles of the chest—the pectoralis muscles—that gave the upper chest and shoulder a normal contour. Fisher was able to enroll numbers of hospitals and dozens of surgeons from across the country. Women who volunteered—and almost 1,700 did—were assigned to either traditional radical mastectomy or modified radical mastectomy (plus radiation treatments afterward). The results seemed conclusive. Rates of local recurrence were no different in either group, meaning radical mastectomy was not necessary for what doctors felt were potentially curable cancers of the breast.[31] Fisher's research group was eventually able to show that even less surgery—now called 'lumpectomy'—could be sufficient for cure.

It was a truly monumental medical and societal achievement for women, dispelling at least one fear—that of breast mutilation—and quieting some trepidation regarding that perceived "death sentence" breast cancer carried. Fisher himself admitted that his greatest contribution to medicine was his laboratory and clinical work that "altered our understanding and treatment of breast cancer," and, once and for all, dispelled "the Halstedian principles [radicalism], which governed the treatment of breast cancer for almost a century."[32] Even discounting Haagensen's detailed microscopic findings, Fisher maintained that cancer cells did not progress in such an orderly fashion from primary tumor to lymphatics to blood stream, that malignant cells were sloughing off into blood from the very start. He believed that, even at the outset, breast cancer could be a body-wide (systemic) disease. So began the era of adjuvant therapy: radiation, chemotherapy, and hormonal treatments. Of course, progress in healing will always be that way. One must not discount the past as primitive and imperfect, especially not in the realm of cancer. Author Siddhartha Mukherjee rightfully supposed, "[w]ith cancer, where no simple, universal, or definitive cure is in sight—and is never likely to be—the past is constantly conversing with the future."[33]

Yes, the disease was understood better, but the illness? Women still reeled at the news. Many still faced Saint Agatha's fate: mastectomy. Their choices were antithetical. They were between a rock and a hard place. "I certainly didn't want any additional mutilation, but I wanted to live," one victim finally reasoned.[34] Young, active females in the prime of life were suddenly faced with their mortality—and loss of female dignity. Cancer had become a metaphor for "the fatalistic, the catastrophic, the disastrous, and the evil."[35] The mastectomy scar was a scourge, not a badge—almost the new "Scarlet Letter" of the times. Women hid their deformed chests and hid the nasty secret that cancer had visited them, as if a curse bestowed for shameful behavior. Soulful healing still lagged far behind scientific progress. Breast cancer crusader Susan Love understood:

> Once you are diagnosed with breast cancer you become an outsider. You no longer belong to the world of the "temporarily immortal" but have joined the world of the "defectives". This world includes the disabled, chronically ill, mentally ill, homosexual, and everyone who dwells on the tails of the bell curve.[36]

Psychologists know well the impact of breast cancer on the psyche. It is unsettling and disheartening. One patient confessed "[I]t just shocked me so. I mean all I could think of was dying. You know, 'I'm going to die. I've got cancer now.'" Even after curative surgery, she was still not placated. "I can't explain it except all my thinking is different . . . planning and the way I kept house, and the way I dressed. It's all different. I can't just get up and go on. It's like I'm waiting for this thing to come back." She tried to get those stubborn thoughts from her mind. She wished she could open her head and stick it under a faucet to cleanse the vile notions out.[37]

And as for the defacement of breast cancer surgery? Mutilation and the stripping of their femininity was a common perception still. It is a multidimensional effect. Breast cancer was not only a disease, it was a stigma. Ideals of womanly beauty, be they internal, peer-related, or cultural, may be dashed—that they are now flawed, insecure, inferior, lopsided, and unattractive—not to mention the very real physical hardships of adjuvant breast cancer treatment. Weakened emotionally and physically, they are prey to perverse thoughts that can very likely lead to mental health issues. One study showed that "[t]hree types of psychological distress—anxiety, hostility, and concern about the body—were consistently greater in women with breast cancer than women in the other [non-cancer] groups" and those miseries "interfere[d] with both intra- and interpersonal functioning," mental health professionals reported. This damage to psychological well-being did not improve even after one year of follow-up.[38] Other psychologists agreed. Almost one-third of long-term breast cancer survivors under the age of fifty reported significant depression. Over one-third of women admitted using alcohol or prescribed medications to help with coping. Doubts about treatment, nervousness about future follow-up, and concern about self-image were leading burdens. More than one in ten stayed depressed for years to come.[39] It is inescapable that the disfigurement of breast cancer surgery—whether it be conservation surgery, mastectomy, or even breast reconstruction—poses a significant challenge to patients and requires a concerted effort to rise above cultural psychosocial ideology. One cannot ignore the internalization of this disease on women's psychic health. That their quality of life can improve over time is a testament to the resiliency of woman's spiritual nature, even among young breast cancer victims and even after bilateral mastectomies.[40]

For the healer, what can be said of all this? That the disease has been kept at bay? That their sharpened steel and invisible rays and toxic drugs have attacked and attacked until cancer vanishes in defeat? And even now, with mastectomy, a vague semblance of breasts can be restored with the marvels of plastic surgery—mounds to fill out the figure. But what of the spirit, what has the healer done? Indeed, surgeons have set upon this disease with the gallantry of Lancelot, yet far more remains beyond their determination and educated wit. "No man can ever understand what such a mutilating operation does to a sensitive woman," one victim wrote.[41] The broken soul cannot be sliced, dissected, or burnt. It is not physical, it is metaphysical. It is reached through the spirit of the healer. Empathy, compassion, hope: the qualities of the shaman are now needed. It is emotional opium: soothing, reassuring, comforting. Walk with them, celebrate with them, suffer with them. That is part of the healing, too.

CHAPTER FOURTEEN

Sabina Spielrein, Healer of the Soul

The human spirit itself, the soul—the ψυχή of Plato—is not immune to its own diseases, too often as destructive as bodily afflictions. Even more so, perhaps, as the mind is a morass of instincts, feelings, emotions, and ideas that remain ill-defined, invisible, and mysterious. Yes, organic changes—tumors, degenerative diseases, physical trauma—could transform perception and cognition, but more often subtle alterations of thinking and sensing are without discernible lesions. Schizophrenia, hysteria, depression, psychoses, and neuroses plague individuals and rob victims of the *joie de vivre*—the joy of life. They affect health. The insane in their delusions, hallucinations, fears, and anxieties have perplexed caregivers and given birth to wild speculations. History is replete with examples. In antiquity, animistic concepts prevailed. These mysterious forces of nature—mythologic, demonic, or theological—were thought the cause. In ancient Greece mental derangements were supposed either divine reward or divine punishment. Only occasionally did the wise offer any meaningful enlightenment. Hippocrates, for one, acknowledged that an unhealthy brain was central to madness—not malevolent spirits, and advocated efforts to balance the humors he was sure were in disarray (melancholia, he felt, was an accumulation of an excess of black bile). Yet despite theories of a few learned men, the populous too often fell prey to religious exorcisms, rites, and amulets designed to ward off diabolical possession. Did such methods heal? Many have argued that they did. Biblical references are numerous. Jesus and his disciples were very much concerned with the muttering, convulsing castoffs who seemed to respond to their healing voices and touch. In parallel, however, healers struggled to understand the imbalances of the mind that tortured the insane, with little success. In fact, organized religion hampered progress in mental disease.

Far from ameliorating the stigma of the insane, Christianity fueled a paranoia of satanic conspiracy intent, it feared, on taking over God's souls and too often relegated the insane to dungeons, asylums, or burning at the stake.[1]

Tormented thinking. These were storms of the soul lashing against sanity's coastline; whirlwinds of doubt snapping confidence, floodwaters of guilt drowning virtue until the landscape was nothing more than stripped dwellings of reason and stagnant pools of recurring nightmares.

And women were particularly suspect. They were easy targets in a masculine world, relatively powerless and subject to intense moral scrutiny. It was inviting to assume women's aberrant behavior was the work of the devil—or worse yet, intentionally devious witchcraft in all its supernatural magic—drawing innocent man into a maelstrom of immorality. Detestable witches, women could be. The bane of male salvation, the logic went:

> What else is woman but a foe to friendship, an unescapable punishment, a necessary evil, a natural temptation, a desirable calamity, a domestic danger . . . an evil of nature painted with fair colors. . . . A woman either loves or hates, there is no third grade.[2]

In some respects, it was no different than in antiquity, where women were viewed as seducers and corrupters of male morals and sanctity. By the nineteenth century, gentler attitudes triumphed, but understanding, much less effective therapy, faltered. How do the experiences of infancy, childhood, adolescence, and adulthood—some barely remembered—feed into the universe of the insensible and augment, diminish, or distort the clash of conscious and unconscious thought? These mental "dis-eases" destroy well-being. Sufferers feel unwell. Physical complaints often follow: anorexia, fatigue, headaches, cramps. They are ill. The weight of their distress isolates them as they turn inward to their troubles. They are no less as sick as those with organic illness. Life is upended, defamed, frightful. Nights become as sleepless and gut-wrenching as victims of cancer. In their madness these sufferers of the spirit yearn to be understood. They yearn for compassion. They yearn for soothing. They yearn to be healed.

Enter Sabina Spielrein: fellow sufferer, psychiatrist, psychologist, lover, healer.

And, at her end, martyr.

She was the archetypical mender of the troubled spirit, a true *ψυχιατρική* (psychiatrikē)—a *ψυχή* (soul) *ιατρός* (healer). In particular, Sabina was an early voice for women, that they were a unique, self-contained gender and not just budding witches or receptacles and passive mirrors for men's desires. She probed, inquired, dissected. She analyzed. She understood. She was the champion of her gender. Woman is uniquely equipped to assume the suffering of others; to bring inside another's distress and assume the role of comforter, nurturer, even healer.

> The woman's biological roles, as mother and as governess of the human race, are roles which make such great use of the gift of sympathetic feeling that fundamentally the woman can rearrange only a comparatively small part of her feelings in her objectivization.[3]

But Sabina understood better than most hurricanes of the soul. She, as a young woman, entered her chosen profession not as a student but as a patient. Her earliest exposure to psychiatry was to that of the startling, if not controversial, field of psychoanalysis.

She was born of Jewish heritage, named Sheyve (Yiddish for Sabina) Naftulovna Spielrein, in 1885 in Rostov-on Don in the Russian Empire. Her family were traditional orthodox Jews. In Rostov-on-Don they prospered, as part of the "merchant guild class" entitling them to property and the right to trade abroad. However, she would use the name Sabina Nikolayevna Spielrein on official documents (her father had changed his name from Naftul to Nikolai when the family moved to Rostov-on-Don from Warsaw, Poland). She was the oldest of five siblings, all of whom were highly intelligent. Her three brothers were all scientists.[4]

Sabina's father was a disturbed individual, given to bouts of rage and depression, at times even threatening suicide. Sabina described him as intelligent, imaginative, moody, and at times, cruel. He was inclined to embarrassing discipline, even, reportedly, lifting up Sabina's skirt to spank her on her buttocks. Nevertheless, Sabina seemed fond of him and, in his complex behavior, her ambivalent feelings no doubt simmered in a sea of love and disgust. Whether there was ever a truly incestuous relationship is a matter of speculation. Her mother did not add to stability or even offset her husband's erratic behavior. She was a nervous woman, childish in nature, and given to extravagant spending.

At age eleven Sabina gained admission to a prestigious high school, the Yekaterinskaya Gymnasium, where she focused on languages and the classics. She was fond of music as well and sung and played the violin and piano. For some reason, following her *bat mitzvah* at age twelve, Sabina lost her belief in God and her religious tendencies. At around that time she also developed an interest in science.

Sabina's adolescence was peppered with love and loss. She had a series of love interests including a crush on her history teacher countered by the death of her dear grandmother and her sister Emil. These seemed to precipitate a decline mentally with various psychosomatic complaints—abdominal pains, headaches, and withdrawal from friends. It had become clear to her parents that Sabina would not recover at their hands, that she was seriously mentally ill and needed specialized help.

With all her buried issues and all her fitful deportment, Sabina was taken to the halls of the emotionally crippled, labeled as a hysteric and subjected to treatment, largely fruitless. She fell prey to a besieged mind. Her sickness stemmed from an environment fraught with parental manipulation, threats, indecent discipline, and erratic behavior. Her parents were narcissistic, focusing on their own interest and hinting at sexual overtones for their aberrant actions. Public punishment and spankings led to repression and substitution of pleasure with pain. She had been so unsuccessful at compensating that her internal conflicts surfaced as bizarre actions of her own. As if she might truly have been like one of those unfortunate beings from antiquity, twitching, blaspheming, and convulsing at the mercy of invisible demons. She might have been one who was tended by shamans, priests, and even Jesus the Christ himself. She might have been the benefactor of intense rituals of exorcism designed to drive the devil out.

But nothing so unorthodox would benefit her. Hysteria was her diagnosis.

Hysteria belonged to the peculiar realm of the neurotic, sometimes even the psychotic. The illness spoke of unresolved conflicts. Unaware conflicts. The unconscious battling the conscious. Suppress. Repress. Bury. Only burials of the mind can never be deep enough. Memories seep through cerebral barriers to resurrect at the edge of twilight. Then, in half awareness, the clash begins again. Dreams. Nightmares. Terrors. In Sabina's case daytime was no protection. The slightest reminiscence of her childhood set in motion the rebellion of her body. The tics and fury and profanity of her outrage took center stage. She was warring against herself but her violence struck at all around. In 1904, according to Carl Jung's recollection, when she was admitted to *the Psychiatrische Universitätsklinik Zürich*, more informally known as the Burghölzli Psychiatric Clinic, of which he was newly hired faculty, Sabina was an unmitigated mess. In fact, records from the Burghölzli Clinic on her admission by psychiatrist Carl Jung indicated,

> Tonight at 10.30 patient is admitted. . . . Pat. [patient] laughs and cries in a strangely mixed, compulsive manner. Masses of tics, rotating head, sticks out her tongue, legs twitching. Complains of a terrible headache . . . she could not stand people or noise.[5]

⁓

The Austrian neurologist Sigmund Freud (1865–1939) considered hysteria one of the great neuroses. Its cause lay in the buried memories of unresolved emotional trauma. Freud believed in repressed memories—usually of a distressing or painful nature—lodged in his so-called unconscious mind that conflicted with the conscious mind. Of course, a troubled unconsciousness stemmed, in his opinion, from some type of repressed sexual encounter. Psychoanalysis, as he and his mentor Breuer developed it, was talk therapy aimed at identifying and bringing to light these repressions so as to confront and accommodate them in a conscious manner. It was as if a deep-seated cancer, growing and fomenting, was finally found and, in the best cases, extirpated as a healing ritual. While Freud attributed some hereditary factors to this (see below), he also heavily flavored his theory with sexual overtones stemming from young childhood. He would write:

> The core of a hysterical attack, in whatever form it may appear, is a memory the hallucinatory reliving of a scene which is significant for the onset of the illness . . . the content of the memory is a rule of psychical trauma which is qualified by its intensity to provoke the outbreak of hysteria in the patient or is the event, which, owing to its occurrence at a particular moment, has become a trauma.[6]

He had written extensively about neuroses beginning in 1886, those conditions of mental stress and conflict that, while disturbing, do not necessarily detach from reality. Heredity must play a role, he argued, almost an indispensable one. Yet heredity alone was not sufficient. There were specific causes that add to an inherited tendency. While a healthy person might not be bothered, those same inherent traits lend a susceptibility to "neurosis, the development of which in intensity and extent will be consistent with the degree of that hereditary condition." In addition, he felt that other agents could provide additional stressors: "moral emotions, somatic exhaustion, acute illnesses, intoxications, traumatic accidents, intellectual overwork." The basis for such conflicts, Freud asserted, was sexual. The trauma of sexual seduction at an infantile age, when their sexuality was still dormant, fomented in the unconscious. These so-called incompatible memories forming the core of repression were sexual memories, Freud believed.[7] "Sexual wish-feelings from the infantile life experience repression," he would write in 1899, and are revived as part of the sexual constitution. "They thus supply the motive power for all psychoneurotic symptom formation." The repressed memory of the sexual trauma became pathogenic at puberty, Freud felt.[8]

He then had written, concerning hysteria:

> [T]he solution of the etiological question is surprisingly simple and uniform. I owe my results to the use of a new method of psychoanalysis (*psychoanalyse*), to the exploratory process of J. Breuer, a little subtle, but which cannot be replaced, so fertile has it been in shedding light on the obscure paths of unconscious ideation.[9]

His mentor in Vienna, Josef Breuer (1842–1925), had introduced Freud to this unorthodox "talking therapy" as a way to explore the nuances of hysteria. Both believed that there was an analogy between the pathogenesis of common hysteria and traumatic neuroses. With the latter, "the cause of the illness is not the trifling physical injury but the affect of fright—the psychical trauma," Freud contended. The same applied to hysterical neurosis. The cause of the hysterical symptoms was once again psychical trauma. "Any experience which calls up distressing affects—such as those of fright, anxiety, shame, or physical pain—may operate as a trauma of this kind."[10] For those upon whom they tried their new talk therapy, even without the suggestibility of hypnosis,

> [W]e found, to our great surprise at first, that each individual hysterical symptom immediately and permanently disappeared when we had succeeded in bringing clearly to light the memory of the event by which it was provoked and in arousing its accompanying affect, and when the patient had described that event in the greatest possible detail and had put the affect into words.[11]

The aim was to allow the patient to be a collaborator in the process of analysis. With ongoing explanation of the psychical processes, the subject could view him or herself as a co-investigator, breaking down defensive resistance. Once drawn to the confidence of the therapist, it was hoped the patient would probe, talk, and self-analyze their innermost feelings. It was talk therapy.

The therapist functioned as an elucidator, as a teacher, as the trusted guide to a frightful and confusing internal world, ready to sympathize, to understand, even to absolve. Like a confessor, he or she could pardon and restore salvation—much as in the priestly confessional. The doctor served to provide the patient with human assistance in the mental catharsis of literally vomiting forth the stored unpleasantries that have acted, presumably, as hidden toxins to sanity. Cleansing of the mind, then, was the primary focus of talk therapy, confronting and neutralizing potential emotional poisons that, left unattended, would disrupt the neural pathways of rational, healing thought.[12]

Later, in the 1920s, Freud would expand his theory of psychoanalysis, breaking down the human persona into a battle of Titans: a barraged "Ego," a moralistic "Super-Ego," and a brooding, passionate "Id." The unconscious self would most identify with the Id, which would batter the conscious Ego with innate desires and wishes, while the Super-Ego would counterpunch with guilt-ridden condemnations. In his picture of the psyche, Freud paints a confused, frayed Ego as arbitrator for conflicting powers of base instinct and worldly influence. It is this chaos that, in Freud's opinion, the psychoanalyst must unravel, interpret, and guide a troubled patient to comprehension. "Psychoanalysis," he would write, "cannot transfer the essence of the psyche into consciousness, but must regard consciousness [Ego] as a quality of the psyche which may or may not impact other qualities."[13]

The young Swiss physician who admitted Sabina to the Burghölzli Psychiatric Clinic was Carl Gustav Jung (1875–1961), a fervent disciple of Freud and a recent hire to the staff. It was there that he was introduced to Freudian theory of the unconscious, repression, and psychoanalysis.

Jung later explained Freud's concept of the repressed. "The basis and origin of the various symptoms grouped under terms hysteria and neuroses lay in unfulfilled desires and wishes, unexpressed and unknown to the patient for the most part and concerned chiefly with the sexual instinct."[14] According to Jung, "Psychoanalysis is the name given to the method developed for reaching down into the hidden depths of the individual to bring to light the underlying motives and determinants of his symptoms and attitudes, and to reveal the unconscious tendencies which lie behind actions and reactions and which influence development and determine the relations of life itself."[15]

He was a staunch believer in the healing power of psychoanalysis. Whereas before, mental anguish—wounds and conflicts of the soul—was outside the realm of scientific endeavor and left largely to religion and metaphysics, now, Jung believed, "this same assistance that surgery has given to the physical body, psychoanalysis attempts to give to the personality."[16]

⁓

She was a difficult case at first, rebellious to authority and uncooperative with instructions. She had declared she would never obey and never wanted to get better. She assured the assistants that she would behave badly.

> Her condition had got so bad that she really did nothing else than alternate between deep depression and fits of laughing, crying, and screaming. She could no longer look anyone in the face, kept her head bowed, and when anyone touched her stuck tongue out with every sign of loathing.[17]

So traumatized had she become by events of her childhood and adolescence that she seemed to break with reason and dwelt in fantasy worlds far removed from the confines of reality. Of course, conventional wisdom attributed hysterical symptoms to sexual frustration—the disease of virgins, nuns, and old maids. But by the termination of the nineteenth century the science of specific disease etiology prevailed—anatomy, pathology, and functionality were thought closely linked—and the hunt began for pathogens as a cause of psychiatric illness. Freudian theory of a hereditary predisposition, constitutional susceptibility, and extraordinary physical or emotional trauma served up reasonable explanations for such bizarre behavior. Some even wondered if, in the absence of anatomic changes in affected hysterics, that there might be some alteration of nervous networks caused by repeated psychological trauma. Perhaps Sabina qualified as a highly sensitive person, one whose sensory-emotional reaction to social, personal, even environmental stimuli is exaggerated or altered leading to overarousal and, without resolution or rescue, to withdrawal of emotional response, a so-called shutdown.[18]

Key to rehabilitation at the Burghölzli under director Eugene Bleuler was separation of Sabina from the outside world and, in particular, her family, the source of her repeated trauma. Jung started talk therapy and uncovered the source of her hysteria by allowing her to recover the memory of her abuses and provided opportunities for an emotional catharsis. According to Jung, her mother could be vicious as well. She tried to beat her in front of her brothers and her brother's friends. She would, when threatened, run away and try to harm herself, dowsing herself with cold water or running to the cellar to catch her death of cold. At age fifteen, she tried to starve herself, all this to punish her parents for tormenting her. Out in the open, her need to somatize repressed—unconscious—feelings gradually lessened. She was highly intelligent and remarkably motivated and seemed to improve rapidly with Jung's probing techniques of psychoanalysis. By the following year, in the spring of 1905 and while still an inpatient at the Burghölzli, she enrolled as a medical student at the University of Zurich. Not surprising, her focus was psychiatry. Who better to confront the nuances of psychological disease than one who had survived the illness? Sabina was so immersed in the field that she received top honors in psychiatry following her final examinations in January 1911.[19]

⌇

In her saner moments, Sabina was convinced she had an extraordinary destiny. And she was obsessed with science. "To me, life without science is completely senseless. What else is there for me if there is no science. Get married? But that thought fills me with dread: at times my heart aches for tenderness, love; but that is but a deceptive, passing, external display that hides the most pitiful prose. . . . And how stupid," she continued, "that I am not a man, men have it easier with everything" (diary entry April 25, 1905).[20]

Yet her female status did not deter her. "I remain defiant, because I have something noble and great to create and am not made for everyday routine . . . no pain is unbearable to me, no sacrifice too great, if only I can fulfill my sacred calling!" she wrote in her diary January 19, 1911.[21] On the brink of her professional career, she was twenty-five years old. Yet she could not completely unravel the mysteries of her own personality, entwined as they were with her sexual nature and expressed in her illness so frequently as sexual outlets. Sabina was consumed with the idea linking sex and death and how it might transform understanding the human mind. Were sex and death so fundamentally human as to hold hostage self-preservation?

And for women was it even more obvious that the sexual instinct consume unconscious thought, unlike men who could transfer their sexual energies—orthodox or unorthodox—to a female receptacle?

Then, yielding to her sexual nature, she fell in love with her psychiatrist, Carl Jung.

It was transference. Her sexual-romantic emotions so long repressed and distorted she now redirected to her therapist, a man of seeming compassion, understanding, and insight. He was her confidant, her mentor, her sympathy. He had rescued her. He had become her savior; her knight in shining armor. Jung had driven from her mind the demons that besieged her. He had, in a metaphysical sense, *healed her*. He was everything a man should be to a woman. Why would she not want to love him? Although married, he fell for her, too. Her lingering dependency, sexuality, and allure spoke to him. Of course, he was torn emotionally. Wife and children would soon pull him from her.

Yet it is likely that her feelings for Jung would help awaken in Sabina the unique quandary of women. As Sabina reasoned, women sublimate themselves for their lover. Is it simply dominance and submission or a far more primitive complexion? That their sexuality was not merely a libidinous nature—of whatever origin or construct—but tied inexorably to the barely hidden drive to procreate and nurture—to further the species. This was a drive in competition to their conscious awareness for joy and self-preservation. This was a drive that could disassemble them, even destroy them. Certainly, transform them. In all its permutations, love might annihilate self.

In her magnum opus, titled "Destruction as a Cause of Coming into Being"[22] and published in 1912, Sabina defined a new theorem: that human procreation must be a selfless instinct that invariably clashes with the ego, the instinct for self-preservation. Sexuality, then, not necessarily the libidinous drive of Freud or Jung, must disregard survival and focus solely on advancing the human race beyond the moment. She envisioned death as a possible sequala to impregnation, conception, and birth. She thus believed that the preservation of the species was more important than preservation of an individual.

In Sabina's theorem there were only two chief instincts: self-preservation and species preservation. Equally simply, she postulated only two psychic structures: the ego (roughly, conscious thought) and the unconscious. The ego, the "I," equated to self-preservation and individuality—to resist unwanted change. Moreover, the ego had differentiated itself from the unconscious. The unconscious was collective, expressed in communal, impersonal symbols and was indifferent to the fate of the individual. According to Sabina's postulate, the energy of the unconscious came exclusively from sexuality as it was intimately tied to species preservation.[23]

Sabina creates the female psyche. She defines the female unconscious and the conscious. But it is an unconscious fraught with anxiety that creates conflict with the innate tendency to sexuality shared by all women. In "Destruction" she wrote her observation that:

> In young women, I find that a feeling of anxiety is normal and moves to the forefront of repressed feelings when the possibility of fulfilment of the wish [for erotic activity] first appears . . . the enemy is within; its characteristic ardor compels you . . . to do what you do not want to do.[24]

She quoted Jung as stating, "[t]he passionate yearning . . . has two sides: it is the power which beautifies everything and under certain circumstances destroys everything."[25] Of this observation she agreed. That a male person could also appreciate the "danger" in eroticism indicated to her that it is not just social in character but instinctual in humans. For women, she was quite aware of the repression of sexual feelings that clash with the soon to be perceived enemy: her own "love heat" that compels her to do what she does not want—procreate and regenerate. She must escape. Sexual activity leads to destruction, transformation, and reconstruction. The life-cycle. Death.

Unlike Freud who based all pleasure on infantile sexual experiences, Sabina submitted that the unconscious is more complex than that. She emphatically maintained that the conscious, the "*Ichpsyche*," the "Ego," as well as the unconscious are governed by still deeper (more primitive?) "movements" that consider conscious feelings irrelevant.

As for love, Sabina lamented the plight of women. Women must change so that they become more the nature of their love interest (man) than themselves. Woman might only like herself when she was being like her lover. Man, the subject, she wrote, loves the object—woman. Woman, on the other hand, desires to be loved and transforms into the beloved and becomes the object. For the female, the ego—that bastion of individuality—has been taken over by the unconscious. By love. By the ultimate need for species preservation. Woman's sexuality of the unconscious wants children and is ready to sacrifice the ego to get them.[26]

At one point she quoted German philosopher Friedrich Nietzsche who said, "We must sometimes take a rest from ourselves by looking at ourselves from a distance and in depth, and with the same detachment as the artist, and by laughing at ourselves or weeping over ourselves, we have to discover not only the hero in us but also the madman."[27]

And even more poignant, she wrote, "we see our own pain in the soul of the other, that is objectively—hence the relief."[28] Indeed she could empathize from her own experiences. Sabina herself admitted that women lacked the ability to objectify their experiences and thus were handicapped in artful pursuits. Regarding the male ease of objectification, Sabina noted that

> Women's ability to do this is much less, for as a rule it is outweighed by a counter-mechanism; a woman conjectures about other's experiences in ways which correspond with her desires or fears and makes them her own, she frees herself from her feelings, mentally goes through these experiences for herself anew. . . . It is in this ability to live through another person that a woman's great distinctive social significance is to be found.[29]

For years, Sabina would examine the disturbed conditions of the mind through the prism of her own love-sick conundrums. She would struggle with her feelings for Carl Jung, and, even after their intimacy had cooled, she would write long, elaborate letters detailing her thoughts and self-analyses. She hoped for some connection still with him, that he would deliver messages that spoke yet of his profound love for her, but these types of responses did not come. So frustrated was she in waiting for a meaningful reply that, at the end of one of her 1918 letters she almost screamed from the page, *What do you think of all this?*[30]

Jung replied in a sterile, clinical fashion: "You are orienting yourself by everything around you, by the visible world, so the inner world is chaotic. The inner world . . . will take possession of you [eventually]. You will experience a remarkable transformation."[31]

Sabina grappled with the two clashing instincts: passion and spirit (*die Leidenschaft und der Geist*). In all her ruminations, once again the subconscious drive—call it passion—collided with the rational and intellectual ego, the spirit. Of course, all was flavored by her love for her mentor, Carl Jung, and his eventual rebuke of her desires. "I cannot allow you to defend yourself by humiliating me," she finally wrote. Her unrequited love, she knew, would turn her to solitude. "It is then that I realize how alone I am . . . the dark powers of destiny use us as they see fit, without worrying the least about the person's own wishes."[32] Perhaps, once again, just as she had succumbed to her biological parents' narcissistic tendencies, so with Freud and Jung in their narcissistic manipulations of her she fell victim to her need for love and attachment.[33] Yet she was at the heart of the psychoanalytic movement, along with Freud, Jung, and Bleuler. She understood the silent dialogue of the subconscious and its biting intrusion into the conscious. She had been there and was taught to converse with it, to reconcile even. She trusted the technique in bringing forth in her patients understanding of their emotional suffering. The catalyst for these psychic conflicts differed among the four—Freud, of course, rooted all in sexual frustration—and served to eventually cause a rift in relations between Freud and Jung, but the technique itself—more a craft than science—found major proponents in this tightly woven group.

~

After graduation from the Zurich school Sabina moved to Munich and began working in earnest on her paper, "Destruction as a Cause of Coming into Being." Then she moved to Vienna where in November 1912 she presented her paper, "Destruction as the Cause of Coming into Being." Her emphasis on the sexual nature of the unconscious mind was more in line with Freudian thought than Jungian, perhaps to reconcile her sexual frustration over the failing relationship with Jung. From Vienna she located to Switzerland, first at Lausanne and then Geneva. In Geneva she worked at the Rousseau Institute with psychologist Jean Piaget who might have stimulated her interest in child psychology.

Her thwarted relationship with Jung, whom she viewed as her soul-mate, and her imagined product of their union, a fantasy child she named Siegfried, seemed to fuel her near-obsession with love as a spark for destruction. "Why does this most powerful drive, the reproductive instinct, harbor negative feelings in addition to the inherently anticipated positive feelings?" she began in her thesis "Destruction as the Cause of Coming into Being." "Passionate longing," she continued, "is the power that beautifies everything and, in certain cases, destroys everything."[34] Is her dilemma how to reconcile this most essential of human emotion—this urge that most humans experience and which has the potential to not only destroy individuality, but also sanity—with the too often heartbreak that it engenders. Yet she insisted on a continuing relationship with Jung. He was not only her lover but also her mentor and father figure. He was her chaperone into the depths of psychoanalysis.

In a letter to Jung on January 6, 1918, Sabina seemed to anguish about the purity of psychoanalysis and its ability to contaminate any beauty of the subconscious by its impartial dissection:

> Analysis does not aim to completely eliminate all repression. A certain amount of repression is needed . . . to make [one] capable of functioning. . . . Depending on the personality of the patient and more especially that of the doctor, analysis of the "unconscious" can rob the analyzed material of its energy or "saturate it with blood."[35]

She was enamored with it. To Jung she implied that psychoanalysis should be fitted to the particular personality of the patient at hand. Too much or too little probing might actually harm recovery. Despite theories put forth by Freud and Jung, Sabina pointed out—rightly so—"[i]n actual practice things never work out the way one decides in theory that they should."[36]

Yet Sabina's concept of unresolved conflicts—the so-called neuroses— continued to manifest a love-struck theme. That neuroses are a consequence of fixation or regression, she attributes both. Everyone is an architect of their own fortunes, she believes, citing falling in love as a prime example. To punctuate her argument, she put forth, "What, in the last analysis, prevents a normally developed person from fulfilling his life goal?" Fear of life and feelings of inadequacy, she submits. In her case, she was almost infantile in her reluctance to engage in music. She was afraid, she admitted; afraid of putting forth those intimate feelings and desires necessary to achieve her goal—as a music composer. In Freudian psychoanalytical terms, she equates, to some extent, the "libido" with not just infantile sexual feelings but that instinctive component of personality: the unconscious, the soulful.

In effect, Sabina heralded the advent of feminist psychoanalysis. She decidedly argued that women and men were inherently different, that women were personalities of their own and not some "subject" under male dominance. That mothering was a different form of love than men experienced and that women alone carried the banner of procreation mixed intimately with their sexual nature, regardless of its existential threat.

Current psychologists like Nancy Chodorow have elaborated on Sabina's feminist arguments by reducing Freudian concepts as undesirably representative of a "normative masculinity, masculine bias, devaluation of women." Psychoanalysis, she points out, is intimately connected to gender and sexuality, flavored by "experiences, identities, cultural constructs, and personal enactments."[37] Chodorow interprets Freud as considering women clinically and theoretically as psychological subjects and objects. As Sabina pointed out, Freud ignored the important distinction of women as mothers, considering their sexuality one-dimensional and subject to interpretation by male conjecture.[38]

Despite probing the intricacies of the mind, she was frustrated by her inability to extirpate those troublesome issues of the subconscious. She even acknowledged a supernatural influence on it all that added even more mystery to her analytical "science." In a diary entry of January 19, 1911, she wrote:

> As the descendant of several generations of religious men I believe in the prophetic powers of my unconscious. One can actually get so close to this "God" that one can speak with Him and learn what He wishes. . . . If one's little bit of conscious strength meant anything, I ought to be wishing for happiness, and I cannot understand why I am so terribly depressed, as if there were no hope of salvation for me. . . . Either the gods are too weary and therefore not very productive, or my conscious mind is too critical to take in anything of beauty.[39]

For Sabina, the psyche was hopelessly entwined with experiences, traumas, instincts, and natures that sought repression but also expression. Were dreams the channel for recognizing the influence of hidden influences? "Practical experiences of dreams . . . teach us that our psychic depths harbor ideas that do not conform to our modern conscious thought process. These ideas cannot be directly comprehended."[40] In that, women were particularly susceptible and conflicted. From those antagonistic subconscious tendencies hysteria, in all its perplexities, was bound to surface. She felt for women. She understood them as she had tried to understand herself.

Sabina spent two years in Moscow where she attached to the State Psychoanalytic Institute and, shortly, became increasingly involved in pediatric psychiatry. She turned her attention to child psychology and the developmental patterns of mother–infant relationships and the social origins of language. She continued to be a major advocate for psychoanalysis, yet believed Freud was incomplete in his appreciation of only personal motives and not those of the social environment. Her view of child development was ambivalent, harkening back to the destructive nature of procreation. "I perceive the child as a dangerous, in itself, deadly disease. . . . [I]t is a common occurrence that a woman imagines a new being as something that grows at the expense of the old one. It is interesting that we react sometimes with lust, sometimes with anger, or at least with displeasure, to those images of destruction," she had written in 1912.[41]

She served at the Children's House, which functioned as an orphanage— but in practicality a boarding home for children of communist elite—and also an experimental school to study child development. Sadly, political unrest and political battles spilled over to the Children's House. Vladimir Lenin had died. Leon Trotsky, who was a major supporter of the project, was in decline. He was exiled to Turkey in 1929, and Joseph Stalin was forging a new view of communism, one of despotic control. In fact, too much ideologic protest fomented by the faculty forced a liquidation of the school and jeopardized the entire future of psychoanalysis in the Soviet Union. Stalin's anti-Trotskyist antagonism to psychoanalysis essentially killed it as a professed technique in psychiatry and quieted Sabina's public stance on the technique, even though she was convinced of its value.

Sabina returned to her hometown of Rostov-on-Don in 1925. Her motives might have been astonishingly simple. She reunited with her estranged husband Pavel and their daughters and attempted a reconciliation of family life. In that sense, her need for emotional connection and fulfillment overwhelmed any professional goals she might have had. It was as if she had returned home, to the source of her anguish, finally, perhaps, to set her past right. She had turned her attention to children and the peculiar psychic developments of childhood. Perhaps it was a final effort to understand herself and how her youngest years had shaped her disturbed unconscious. Sabina's last publication was in 1931. She presented her research on children's drawings with eyes open and shut, reflecting on the effect of the unconscious on mental imagery. Perhaps she aimed to unravel the mystery of her childhood imagery in terms of visual representations instead of mere words. Of interest, she dedicated this publication to her father, who likely provided the opportunities for much of her mental malice.[42] Aside from this last publication, little was heard from her. She seemed to have completely divorced herself from the avant-garde psychologists of western Europe—perhaps fearful of the popular Soviet skepticism for Freudian thought. By the 1930s, her stepdaughter, Nina, observed that Sabina had suddenly aged. "She looked like an old woman, although she wasn't that old. She was bent, wearing some old, black skirt that reached to the ground. . . . It was obvious she was a broken woman."[43]

And then Germany's invasion of the Soviet Union in 1941.

Sabina apparently survived the brief period of occupation of Rostov-on-Don by Wehrmacht troops in November 1941. However, Russians who retook the city could not hold them off, and Germans reoccupied the town in July the following year. Soon, the killing squads appeared. Many Jews had already fled the area. Sabina and her daughters had not. It is not clear why. Any record of her life at that point was destroyed. She must have sensed the danger. Was it a commitment to her people of Rostov, that ageless commitment of healer to the unhealthy? *Einsatzgruppe* D under *SS-Brigadeführer* Walther Bierkamp accompanied the Wehrmacht into the city and began to round up "dissidents" and Jews, registering them and compelling them to assemble that August. The Final Solution was at hand and *Einsatzgruppe* D wasted no time. Between August 11 and August 13, 1942, Jews were herded together and quickly transported to the place of execution. Time was of the essence so as not to alarm those not yet corralled. They were trucked to Zmievskaya Balka, a ravine just outside the city, undressed, and shot by the *Einsatzkommando*. Sabina was last seen amid the gathering of Jews on the street corners of Rostov, waiting for transports to carry them away. She was in the company of her two daughters.[44]

General Otto Ohlendorf, who preceded Walther Bierkamp as commandant of *Einsatzgruppe* D, upon questioning, candidly explained how the murder of Jews of the Ukraine, and presumably those of Rostov-on-Don, took place:

> After the registration the Jews were collected at one place; and from there they were later transported to the place of execution, which was, as a rule, an antitank ditch or a natural excavation. The executions were carried out in a military manner, by firing squads under command. . . . They were transported

to the place of execution in trucks, always only as many as could be executed immediately . . . [they were shot] standing or kneeling. . . . [For any still alive] [t]he unit leaders or the firing-squad commanders had orders to finish them off themselves. . . . The bodies were buried in the antitank ditch or excavation.[45]

What might Sabina have felt at the moment of death, at the inevitability of it, when rescue was no longer possible, when healing was done, when the body, in whatever radiance remained, faced termination? Was it a peace that prevailed as some had said? Or was it a profound sadness that all the great fears and dreads, all the magnificent gestures and words and deeds had narrowed into one crucial moment? More likely it was a numbness, that all of nature was obliterated and all meaningful notions zeroed onto this crucial last moment. There might have been a tunnel vision, not of what was or what is but what was to be. Healing was irrelevant. It was finished. Mortality, that great looming fear in life, was at hand—now not frightful nor welcomed—simply more real than breath itself.

Sabina Spielrein ended her life as a nameless naked corpse amid the heaps of corpses tossed like garbage into the Nazi human landfill of Zmievskaya Balka. The total killed there on August 11 alone was estimated at 13,000. Dirt barely covered the bodies, and was soggy with rivulets of blood. In some figurative sense, did her unrequited love for Jung destroy her as she had prophesied love would do in *Die Destrucktion als Ursache des Werdens*? Could she not reconcile her troubled unconscious—the rejection of affection and union with father and lover—as she had tried to do for so many of her patients? Was she unique or quite representative of her gender in general? Must women self-destruct for the sake of men? Must their mental health and mental healing always be in jeopardy?

"Passionate longing," she once said, "is the power that beautifies everything and . . . destroys everything."[46]

CHAPTER FIFTEEN

The Mysteries of Healing

Throughout three millennia of history, man has unraveled many mysteries of the human body, both structurally and functionally. He has exploited disease and its myriad causes and even dissected its core molecular malformations. Treatment for sicknesses is no longer pure supposition or theory. Targeted therapy, whether medical or surgical, has reversed the course of ailments formerly considered lethal, incurable, or disabling. However, it remains an imperfect art. Prognoses are still guarded; cures uncertain; and recovery at times prolonged and painful. As the body suffers, then, so does the mind. The worries of ill health preoccupy behavior more so now than in antiquity. The illusion of earthly immortality—or at least centenarian existence—is inescapable. In common reasoning, it has almost become an entitlement. Disease still threatens that prospect. So, science, in all its marvels, cannot unlink the tight association of spirit and flesh. The body suffers, the mind frets. Expectations are dashed. The future dims, and, even with medical wonders, hopes turn heavenward. As much as in Asclepian sanctuaries, the afflicted dream the dreams of miracles. The mystical permutations of prayer and supplication, hope and compassion, faith and trust, still hover over the desperately ill, offering peace of mind if not peace of flesh. It is almost certainly not to change. Healing the spirit will still be a necessary accompaniment of cure and, if not cure, then calming resignation.

For the ill, the bravery that must be summoned replaces all other urges. Courage in times of near hopelessness. Perhaps it is the undefinable courage of crisis, rising to the forefront almost without thinking. One of the first heart transplant recipients, Louis Washkansky, was seen as quite fearless in undergoing an almost experimental procedure designed to save his life in 1967. The heart surgeon, Christian Barnard saw it differently:

> [M]any people have said it was very brave of Louis Washkansky to accept a heart transplant . . . not Washkansky. For a dying man, it is not a difficult decision because he knows he is at an end. If a lion chases you to the bank of a river filled with crocodiles, you will leap into the water convinced you have a chance to swim to the other side. But you would never accept such odds if there were no lion.[1]

So often, in such circumstances, faith in the surgeon is essential but also there is faith in faith, that somehow, somewhere divine guidance is also at work. That gods and goddesses of whatever denomination have a vested interest in any suffering spirit about to lay down before uncertain human technology. The faithful cry out to deities sure to rescue them. It may even provoke a sense of joy. Boston surgeon Francis Moore noticed the same attitude Barnard had: "To those who have never dealt with such desperate patients, it may come as a surprise to witness the enthusiasm with which the patient with late cancer or the families of children with severe heart disease approach an entirely new and untried procedure."[2]

In such patients bodily healing would be unlikely. Was the spirit content, however, in the optimism of hope or maybe just the awareness that healing is bigger than one individual, that any single patient might merely be a cog in the giant well of scientific advancement, so that somewhere down the road, another patient—afflicted similarly—might very well be given their earthly health back? Is it so different from the soldier who flings himself on a live grenade to save his buddies?

History has chronicled endless attempts to heal suffering, whether the numbing effects of opium or the exulting platitudes of religion. Efforts to anatomize and rearrange the minute molecules of sickness have coexisted with struggles to interpret cosmic purposes that elude understanding. It is all for the sufferer who, in their agony, can no longer be human—that is, to receive and express the goodwill that should come with life on earth; that unites us to each other. They find themselves languishing at the edge of the herd, afraid they will be abandoned and forgotten. As healers, let us not forsake them. Whether primitive or civilized, healing has been a community effort. We, as social beings, in some respect, innately worry about our fellow man, that each achieve a level of joy free of pain. As intellectual beings we search for interpretation, that our magnificent brains may find solutions to problems disruptive to peaceful contentment. That we ourselves—not inventive gods and goddesses—may control the universe.

Instead, have present-day healers, as historian John Harley Warner wrote, "hitched their identity to the image of experimental science" as a determinant of cultural authority? And in the process have they dehumanized the very subjects they vowed to protect and heal? The growth of so-called bio-medicine cannot supplant the aesthetic narrative of bedside physicians caring not only for body but also spirit. As Warner contended and the ancients maintained, the practice of medicine is not monolithic but multifaceted. Ethical and moral boundaries have not been limited by technology. In fact, one could argue they have expanded to take in not only disease and illness but also the complexities of modern therapy and its inherent risks.[3] Saint Louis surgeon William Sasser said of his career:

> If I had to summarize my career succinctly, I would say this: I have helped many people wage battles against disease. We won some battles, and we lost others. One of the most important jobs in each of these battles was to inspire hope and to be a friend. With this philosophy, my relationships with patients and families have persevered. These relationships are the cornerstone of my practice.[4]

It speaks to holistic healing. Hope is a wonderful drug, placating the miseries of a troubled psyche. Hope in science. Hope in the doctor. Hope in the supernatural. What civilization has not called forth phantom powers to right the injustices of nature? Had they proof such forces truly existed? Only by imagination and legend. Hallucinogenic visions and folk stories of fantastic deeds played out by conjured spirits of immense faculties laid the foundation for belief in supernatural beings able to reverse fortunes at a nod or slightest gesture. Such were the abstractions conceived by distressed humans facing the inevitability of death. Science has not obviated the need for these imaginings. Understanding of molecular biology, immune therapeutics, or precision surgery has not brought immediate peace to worried minds. The uncertainty of fate still looms large for the sick. The spirit still agitates in the diseased body. Even as the ancient Greeks did and the Christian Jesus advised, turn to those hypothetical forces to intervene, protect, and quiet. Remember. The *wapiyapi* of the Lakota were as ceremonial as the Roman Catholic Masses of old where each priestly garment, each celebrant movement, each step was preordained, rehearsed, and perfectly matched with utterances, incantations, and chants in languages foreign to those in attendance but which carried a solemnity calling forth ghostly angels and saints, the counterparts of Lakota spirits. Did one so suffering not exit church with a feeling of rejuvenation? Was it so different, really?

Medical researcher and essayist Lewis Thomas commented in his book *The Youngest Science* about healing powers:

> Patients do get better, some of them anyway, from even the worst diseases, there are very few illnesses, like rabies, that kill all comers. Most of them tend

to kill some patients and spare others, and if you are one of the lucky ones and have also had at hand a steady, knowledgeable doctor, you become convinced that the doctor saved you.[5]

Might you? Perhaps. Or maybe you would invoke other influencers. Gods. Spirits unseen. Perhaps they had selected you among others to survive. Perhaps the healing was due to luck (whatever that is), perhaps physician skill, or perhaps the calling forth of unearthly powers yet inconceivable and only peripherally believed. There are plenty of supplicants at Lourdes, as Alexis Carrel could testify, who attribute their cure not to expert medical providers, but to the Virgin Mary herself. Healing may be a blend of all of them: biological manipulation, surgical expertise, wondrous technology, spiritual determination, and, yes, even divine intercession. Who is to really know? Who has been able to decipher the process over millennia? No one.

～

Notes

Chapter One

1. See C. G. Jung, "Archetypes: Shadow; Anima; Animus; The Persona; The Old Wise Man" in C. G. Jung, *The Essential Jung* (Princeton: Princeton University Press, 1983, 2013), 87–127.

2. Aristotle, *De Anima* [R. D. Hicks, trans] (Cambridge: Cambridge University Press, 1907), II.414a. 12–13).

3. Søren Kierkegaard, *The Sickness Unto Death* (Princeton: Princeton University Press, 1941).

4. Paul Starr, *The Social Transformation of American Medicine* (New York: Basic Books, 1982), 15.

5. Bernie S. Segal, *Love, Medicine & Miracles* (New York: Harper & Row, 1986), 65.

6. Genesis 1:26–27, New International Version (NIV). Biblical references will be according to the *New International Version* (NIV) (New York: Biblica, 2011).

7. Matthew 25.37–40, NIV.

8. Thomas Aquinas, *Commentary on the Metaphysics of Aristotle* [John P. Rowan, transl] (Chicago: Henry Regnery Company, 1961), 12.

9. G. L. Engel, "The Need for a New Model: A Challenge for Biomedicine," *Psychodynamic Psychiatry* 40 (2012): 377–96, quote 392.

10. M. Mead, "Towards a Human Science" *Science* 191 (1976): 903–909, quote 907.

11. P. D. Gluckman, and M. A. Hanson, "Developmental Plasticity and the Developmental Origins of Health and Disease," in John P. Newnham and Michael

G. Ross (Eds.), *Early Life Origins of Human Health and Disease* (Basel: Karger, 2009), 1–10, quote 7–8).

12. J. L. Brooke, and C. S. Larsen, "The Nurture of Nature: Epigenetics and Environment in Human Biohistory," *American Historical Review* 119 (2014): 1500–13.

13. N. C. Emecoff, F. A. Curlin, P. Buddadhumaruk, D. B. White, "Health Care Professionals' Responses to Religious or Spiritual Statements by Surrogate Decision Makers During Goals-of-Care Discussions," *JAMA Internal Medicine* 175 (2015): 1662–69.

14. John Steinbeck, *Travels with Charley* (New York: Penguin, 1962), 44.

Chapter Two

1. William James, *The Varieties of Religious Experiences* (New York: Longmans, Green and Co., 1917), 34.

2. Thucydides, *History of the Peloponnesian War*, Rex Warner and M. I. Finley trans., Vol. I (Baltimore: Penguin Books, 1972), II. 47–52. See also Joseph Gavorse (Ed.), *The Complete Writings of Thucydides, The Peloponnesian War* (New York: The Modern Library, 1934), II.48–49, 94, 110–11. See J. F. D. Shrewsbury, "The Plague of Athens," *Bulletin of the History of Medicine* 24 (1950): 1–25.

3. Plato, *The Laws of Plato*, A. E. Taylor, trans. (London: J.M. Dent & Sons Ltd., 1934), X.886 and 899.

4. *Hippocrates* Vol. I, W. H. S. Jones, trans. (Cambridge: Harvard University Press, 1957), XII. 8–11.

5. Anonymous, *Hesiod, Homeric Hymns, Epic Cycle, Homerica*, H. G. Evelyn-White, trans. (Cambridge: Harvard University Press, 1914), Homeric Hymn 3.

6. *Pausanias: Description of Greece*, III, W. H. S. Jones, trans. (London: G.P. Putnam's Sons, 1933), XXIII, 7, 309.

7. Homer, *Iliad* I, A. T. Murray trans. (Cambridge: Harvard University Press, 1988) IV.204–205. See Hesiod, *Theogony Works and Days Testimonia*, Glenn W. Most, trans. (Cambridge: Harvard University Press, 2006), 630–31.

8. From (Anonymous), *The Odes of Pindar*, John Sandys, trans. (New York: The Macmillan Co., 1915), III, 47–54, 189. See also Pindar, *Pythiae*, III, 1–58, contained in Emma J. Edelstein and Ludwig Edelstein, *Asclepius: Collection and Interpretation of the Testimonies* (Baltimore: Johns Hopkins University Press, 1945, 1998), 1–4. See also S. W. Jackson, "The Wounded Healer," *Bulletin of the History of Medicine* 75 (2001): 1–36.

9. *Pausanias: Description of Greece*, II, W. H. S. Jones, trans. (London: G.P. Putnam's Sons, 1933), XXVI, 26.4–7, 387.

10. Anonymous, *The Homeric Hymns, Homeric Acopcrypha, Lives of Homer*, Martin L. West, Ed., trans. (Cambridge: Harvard University Press, 2003), XI.1–5; *Odes of Pindar*, III, 55–60.

11. Apollodorus, *Bibliotheca*, James George Frazier, trans. (London: William Heineman, 1921), III 10.3–5.

12. Homer, *Iliad* IV.194. For translations I have used Henry George Liddell and Robert Scott, *A Greek-English Lexicon* (Oxford: Clarendon Press, 1940). The word ἰητῆρος was used as the Ionic form of classical Greek instead of ιατρος.

13. Homer, *Iliad*, XI.514–15 and IV.192–219. See also D. Filippou, G. Tsoucalas, E. Panagouli et al., "Machaon, Son of Asclepius, the Father of Surgery," *Cureus* 12 (2020): e7038. DOI 10.7759/cureus.7038 accessed 9/12/2022.

14. See Edelstein, *Testimonies*, 101. See also, Stephanus Byzantius, *Ethnica*, Augustus Meineke, trans. (Berlin: Berolini, 1849), 593.

15. Plato, *Plato's Republic*, B. Jowett and Lewis Campbell, Eds., III (Oxford: Clarendon Press, 1894), 407 C–D; Edelstein, *Testimonies*, 60.

16. First quote from Hippocrates, *Law 2*, in Bronwen L. Wickkiser, *Asklepios, Medicine, and the Politics of Healing in Fifth-Century Greece* (Baltimore: Johns Hopkins Press, 2008), 28. Second quote from Emma J. Edelstein and Ludwig Edelstein, *Asclepius: A Collection and Interpretation of the Testimonies* (Baltimore: Johns Hopkins Press, 1945), 154.

17. Plato, *The Laws of Plato*, IV.720, italics mine.

18. M. Mironidou-Tzouveleki and P. M. Tzitzis, "Medical Practice Applied in the Ancient Asclepion in Kos Island," *Hellenic Journal of Nuclear Medicine* 17 (2014):167–70. See also H. Christopoulou-Alerta, A. Togia, C. Varlam, "The 'Smart' Asclepieion: A Total Healing Environment," *Archives of Hellenic Medicine* 27 (2010): 259–63.

19. All from H. Askitopoulas, E. Konsolaki, I. A. Ramoutsaki, M. Anastassaki, "Surgical Cures Under Sleep Induction in the Asclepieion of Epidauros," *International Congress Series* 1242 (2002): 11–17 quotes 15–16; and from *Inscriptiones Graecae* (Epidaurus) IV2, I–XVI. Examples of surgery, *Inscriptiones Graecae* IV2, 23, 25.

20. See H. Pham, "Historiography on the Social Status of the Ancient Physician Since Ludwig Edelstein," *Journal of the Southern Association for the History of Medicine and Science* 1 (2015): 1–21.

21. Plato, *Euthyphro, Apology, Crito, Phaedo, Phaedrus*, Harold North Fowler, trans. (Cambridge: Harvard University Press, 1914), *Phaedrus*: 270C. See Homer, *Iliad*, II.678–81.

22. Hippocrates, "Epistolae," in Hippocrates, *Oeuvres Complètes d'Hippocrates*, É Littré, trans. IX (Amsterdam: Adolf M. Hakkert, 1961–1962), 312–428, quote 340.

23. Hippocrates, "Epistolae," 314.

24. Charles Singer, *Greek Biology & Greek Medicine* (Oxford: Clarendon Press, 1922), 89–90. I will refer to the writings of Hippocrates as attributed to the man himself, although this is disputable.

25. See Jacques Jouanna, *Greek Medicine from Hippocrates to Galen* (Leiden: Brill, 2012) and J. A. Wilson, "Medicine in Ancient Egypt," *Bulletin of the History of Medicine* 36 (1962): 114–23.

26. Hippocrates, "Epistolae," 326.

27. Hippocrates, "The Sacred Disease," in *Hippocrates* Vol II, W. H. S. Jones trans. (Cambridge: Harvard University Press, 1943), I.2–10.

28. Plato, *Phaedo*, 86 B-C.

29. Hippocrates, *Hippocrates* "The Nature of Man," W. H. S. Jones, trans. (Cambridge: Harvard University Press, 1959), IV.1–7.

30. Hippocrates, "The Sacred Disease," IV.37–42.

31. Hippocrates, "On the Art of Medicine," in John Redman Coxe, *The Writings of Hippocrates and Galen* (Philadelphia: Lindsay and Blakiston, 1846), 47–48.

32. Hippocrates, "On the Art," 51.

33. *Hippocrates* II, "Decorum" VI. 1–3, fn 4, 288.

34. *Hippocrates* II, "Decorum" XVI.1–10.

35. *Hippocrates* II, "Breaths" I. 6–10.

36. *Hippocrates* II, "About the Physician" I.23–25.

Chapter Three

1. Isaiah 58:6–8. Christian biblical references here will be according to the New International Version (NIV) (New York: Biblica, 2011).

2. *Hebrew-English Tanakh* (Skokie: Varda Books, 2009), Ezekiel 13:20.

3. *Tanakh*, Exodus 22:18.

4. *Tanakh*, Numbers 21:8–9.

5. Mark 1.29–31, NIV.

6. Mark 5.25–30, NIV.

7. Luke 7.1–10 NIV.

8. David Robert Palmer, *The Gospel of Luke* (Self-published, 2022): Luke 17:11–19.

9. *Tanakh*, Leviticus 13:45–46.

10. Mark 1.40–41, NIV.

11. *Babylonian Talmud* (The William Davidson Edition from the Talmudic Babylon c450-c550 BC (https://www.sefaria.org/Sanhedrin.98a?lang=en), Sanhedrin, 98a.

12. John 11.1–44. NIV.

13. Flavius Josephus, *Antiquitates Judaicae* (B. Niese, Ed.) (Berlin: Weidmann, 1892), 63. The authenticity of this remark cannot be confirmed.

14. Reza Aslan, *Zealot* (New York: Random House, 2013), 109–11.

15. Mark 6: 7–13, NIV.

16. Cornelius Tacitus, *The Annals of Tacitus*, George Gilbert Ramsay, trans., Vol XV (London: John Murray, 1909), 44.

17. Matthew 27: 46, NIV.

18. Josephus, *Antiquitates Judaicae*, 64.

19. Luke 24.51–52, NIV.

20. Mark 12:30–31, NIV.

21. Acts 3.1–10, NIV.

22. Acts 9.32–35, NIV.

23. See Acts 5.12–16, NIV, Acts 8.4–8, NIV.

24. Acts, 9:4–7, NIV.

25. See Acts 20.7–10, NIV.

26. *Tanakh*, Ezekiel 37:12.

27. Andrew Crislip, *Thorns of the Flesh* (Philadelphia: University of Pennsylvania Press, 2013), 46.

28. Gregory Bishop of Tours, *History of the Franks* (New York: Columbia University Press, 1916), 149.

29. Tacitus, *Annals* XV, 44.

30. See Gary B. Ferngren, *Medicine & Health Care in Early Christianity* (Baltimore: Johns Hopkins Press, 2009), 86–95.

31. "Ignatius to the Ephesians," in *The Apostolic Fathers*, Kirsopp Lake, trans. (Cambridge: Harvard University Press, 1985), VII.2, p. 181.

32. Justin Martyr, "The First Apology" in *The Fathers of the Church* Vol 6, Thomas B. Falls, Ed. (Washington: Catholic University of America Press, 1948, 1965, 1977, 2008), 23–111, 1.22.

33. Charles G. Herbermann Ed., *The Catholic Encyclopedia*, Vol. 2 (New York: The Encyclopedia Press, 1910), 581.

34. Charels G. Herbermann et al., Eds., *The Catholic Encyclopedia* Vol. 4 (New York: The Encyclopedia Press, 1908, 1913), 597.

35. Edward White Benson, *Cyprian: His Life, His Times, His Work* (New York: D. Appleton and Company, 1897), 246.

36. Alexander Roberts and James Donaldson, Eds., *Ante-Nicene Fathers*, Vol. 5 (New York: Charles Scribner's Sons, 1919), 270.

37. Origen, *Homilies on Leviticus* 1–16, Gary Wayne Barkley, trans. (Washington: Catholic University Press, 1990), 153–54 (Homily 8).

38. See Amanda Porterfield, *Healing in the History of Christianity* (Oxford: Oxford University Press, 2005).

39. From Darrel W. Amundson, "Medicine and Faith in Early Christianity," *Bulletin of the History of Medicine* 56 (1982): 326–50.

Chapter Four

1. Dates according to: "The Chronology of Galen's Early Career," *Classical Quarterly* 23 (1973): 158–71.

2. P. E. Pormann, "Medical Education in Late Antiquity from Alexandria to Montpellier," in Peter E. Pormann, *Hippocrates and Medical Education* (Leiden: Brill, 2010), 419–41; and G. Ferngren, "Vivisection Ancient and Modern," *History of Medicine* 4 (2017): 211–21.

3. P. Brain, (trans.) "Galen on the Ideal of the Physician," *South African Medical Journal* 52 (1977): 936–38.

4. Plato, *Plato's Republic* B. Jowett and Lewis Cambell, Eds. (Oxford: Clarendon Press, 1894), I.439.

5. Hippocrates, "Breaths," in *Hippocrates* II, IV.32–34 and XV.1–3.

6. Galen, "On Hippocrates' On the Nature of Man," W. J. Lewis, trans.), *Medicina Antiqua*, 20–21 at https://www.ucl.ac.uk/~ucgajpd/medicina%20antiqua/tr_GNatHom.html, accessed 9/5/2023.

7. Galen, "On Hippocrates' On the Nature of Man," 62–63.

8. See D. C. Lindberg, "Science and the Early Christian Church," *Isis* 74 (1983): 509–30.

9. Pliny, *The Natural History of Pliny*, John Bostock and H. T. Riley, trans., Vol. V (London: G. Bell & Sons, 1856), XXVI 204.

10. Galen (Karl Gottlob Kühn, trans.) *Claudii Galeni Opera Omnia* (Cambridge: Cambridge University Press, 1923), VI, 603.

11. See J. Scarborough, "Romans and Physicians," *The Classical Journal* 65 (1970): 296–306.

12. Kühn, *Claudii Galeni Opera*, II, 662–63.

13. From Nutton, "The Chronology of Galen's Early Career." See also S. Matten, "Galen and His Patients," *Lancet* 378 (2011): 478–79.

14. Both quotes from Charles Singer, *Galen on Anatomical Procedures* (London: Oxford University Press, 1956), Book III, 340–41, p. 60. See also L. H. Toledo-Pereyra, "Galen's Contribution to Surgery," *Journal of the History of Medicine and Allied Sciences* 28 (1973): 357–75. See also Nutton, "The Chronology of Galen's Early Career."

15. Hippocrates, "Nature of Man" in *Hippocrates* IV, W. H. S. Jones, trans. (Cambridge: Harvard University Press, 1959), IV.1–6.

16. Galen, "On Hippocrates' On the Nature of Man," 59–60.

17. Galen, *On the Usefulness of the Parts of the Body*, Margaret Tallmadge, trans., (Ithaca: Cornell University Press, 1968) 226–27.

18. Galen, *On the Therapeutic Method*, R. J. Hankinson, trans. (Oxford: Clarendon Press, 1991), I.5.4.

19. Galen, *Methods of Medicine* III, Ian Johnston and G. H. R. Horsley, trans. (Cambridge: Harvard University Press, 2011), XIX.384–85.

20. Galen, *Therapeutic Method*, II.7.1.

21. Galen, *Commentary on Hippocrates' Epidemics*, Book I, Parts I–III, Uwe Vagelpohl, trans. (Berlin: Walter de Gruyter, 2014), I.II 54. 10–20.

22. Both quotes above from Brain, "Galen on the Ideal of the Physician."

23. Galen, *Claudii Galeni Pergameni, Secundum Hippocratem* (Paris: Simon Colinae, 1528), no page number.

24. Ibn Abu Usaibi'ah, *History of Physicians*, L. Kopf, trans. (Jerusalem: Institute of Asian and African Studies, 1956), 150.

25. Singer, *Galen On Anatomical Procedures*, xxiii.

26. See Galen, *Epidemics* I.III.17.6–13; and Gary B. Ferngren, *Medicine and Health Care*, particularly 92–94.

Chapter Five

1. Ludwig Edelstein, "The Relation of Ancient Philosophy to Medicine," *Bulletin of the History of Medicine* 26 (1952): 299–316, quote 305.

2. The oath reads ἐκχωρήσω δὲ ἐργάτῃσιν ἀνδράσι πρήξιος, "assign this task to those professional men." Hippocrates, *The Hippocratic Oath in Greek and Latin* [in

Apud Andreae Wecheli heredes] (Frankfurt: Claudium Marnium, 1595), National Library of Medicine (translation mine).

3. In fact, the German *handwerker*, from whence the English "hand worker" originates, means "handyman," or, a man good with his hands. From "chirurgoi" comes the French and Spanish world *chirurgien*, and the English word "surgeon."

4. Aristotle, *Politics*, Benjamin Jowett, trans. (Oxford: Clarendon Press, 1908), III II, 1282, 123.

5. See Eldridge Campbell and James Colton, trans., *The Surgery of Theodoric* (New York: Appleton-Century-Crofts, Inc., 1955), 4–5). From the Greek χειρουργός comes the French term *chirurgien* and subsequently the English "surgeon." See also I. E. Drabkin, "Medical Education in Greece and Rome," *Bulletin of the History of Medicine* 15 (1944): 333–51.

6. Celsus, *De Medicina* VII, W. G. Spencer, trans. (Cambridge: Harvard University Press, 1938, 1953, 1961), 4, 297.

7. See H. von Staden, "Division, Dissection, and Specialization: Galen's 'On the Parts of the Medical Techne'," *Bulletin of the Institute of Classical Studies* 77 (Suppl) (2002): 19–45.

8. P. O. Kristeller, "The School of Salerno: Its Development and its Contribution to the History of Learning," *Bulletin of the History of Medicine* 17 (1945): 138–94.

9. As quoted in Nancy G. Siraisi, *Medieval & Early Renaissance Medicine* (Chicago: University of Chicago Press, 1990), 177.

10. Kristeller, "The School of Salerno."

11. Campbell, *Surgery of Theodoric*, 4. See Michael McVaugh, "Surgical Education in the Middle Ages," *Dynamis* 20 (2000): 283–304.

12. Robert von Fleischhacker, trans., *Lanfrank's Science of Cirurgie* (London: Kegan Paul, Trench, Trübner, 1894), 8–9. See C. C. Clarke, "Henri de Mondeville" *Yale Journal of Biology and Medicine* 3(1931): 459–81.

13. Avicenna, *The Canon of Medicine* (New York: AMS Press, Inc, 1973), 22, 26. See also E. Anwar, "Ibn Sīnā's Philosophical Theology of Love: a Study of the Risālah fī al-'Ishq," *Islamic Studies* 42 (2003): 3311–54.

14. Max Neuburger, "An Historical Survey of the Concept of Nature from a Medical Viewpoint," *Isis* 35 (1944): 16–28. See also Michael McVaugh, "When Universities First Encountered Surgery," *Journal of the History of Medicine and Allied Sciences* 72 (2017): 6–20. See also Nancy G. Siraisi, *Taddeo Alderotti and His Pupils* (Princeton: Princeton University Press, 2019). Regarding Dino del Garbo, see Siraisi, *Toddeo Alderotti*, 98.

15. H. J. Schroeder, *Disciplinary Decrees of the General Councils: Text, Translation and Commentary* (Saint Louis, MO: B. Herder Book Co., 1937), 263.

16. Édouard Nicaise, *Chirurgie de Maitre Henri de Mondeville* (Paris: Félix Alcan, 1893), xxiii–xxix.

17. Thomas, Antoine, "Jean Pitart, Chirurgien et Poète," *Comptes Rendus des Séances de l'Académie des Inscriptions et Belles Lettres* 60 (1916): 95–111, quote 109.

18. Julius Pagel, trans., *Die Chirurgie des Heinrich von Mondeville* (Berlin: Hirschwald, 1892), 133–35. See also S. K. Ghosh, "Henri de Mondeville (1260–1320): Medieval French Anatomist and Surgeon," *European Journal of Anatomy* 19 (2015): 309–14.

19. Hastings Rashdall, *The Universities of Europe in the Middle Ages* (Oxford: Clarendon Press, 1895), 83–84.

20. François Quesnay, *Recherches Critiques et Historiques sur l'Origine, sur les Divers Etats et sur les Progrès de la Chirurgie en France* (Paris; Charles Osmont, 1744), 27–28.

21. Schroeder, *Disciplinary Decrees*, 258.

22. See Darrel W. Amundsen, "Medieval Canon Law on Medical and Surgical Practice by the Clergy," *Bulletin of the History of Medicine* 52 (1978): 22–44.

23. Nicaise, *Chirurgie*, lxiv.

24. Nicaise, *Chirurgie*, lxv.

25. P. Kibre, "The Faculty of Medicine at Paris, Charlatanism, and Unlicensed Medical Practice in the Later Middle Ages," *Bulletin of the History of Medicine* 27 (1953): 1–20, quote 6.

26. Nicaise, *Chirurgie*, quotes 406 and 5–6.

27. For examples of Mondeville's illustrations see J. Vrebos, "Thoughts on a Neglected French Medieval Surgeon: Henri de Mondeville (ca. 1260–1320)," *European Journal of Plastic Surgery* 34 (2011): 1–11.

28. Nicaise, *Chirurgie*. For more on Albucasis see M. S. Spink and G. L. Lewis, *Albucasis on Surgery and Instruments* (Berkeley: University of California Press, 1973).

29. Nicaise, *Chirurgie*, 745–46.

30. As told by Édouard Nicaise, *La Grande Chirurgie de Guy de Chauliac* (Paris: Félix Alcan, 1890), lxxix.

31. Gad Freudenthal and Samuel S. Kottek, *Mélanges d'Histoire de la Médecine Hébraïque* (Leiden: Brill, 2003), 103 (translation mine).

32. See L. Demaitre, "Theory and Practice in Medical Education at the University of Montpellier in the Thirteenth and Fourteenth Centuries," *Journal of the History of Medicine and Allied Sciences* 30 (1975): 103–23.

33. S. K. Ghosh, "Human Cadaveric Dissection: A Historical Account from Ancient Greece to the Modern Era," *Anatomy and Cell Biology* 48 (2015): 153–69.

34. J. E. Pilcher, "Guy de Chauliac and Henri de Mondeville: A Surgical Retrospective," *Annals of Surgery* 12 (1895): 84–102. See Amundsen, "Medieval Canon Law."

35. Guy de Chauliac, *Chirurgia Magna* (Lyon: Beraud Symphorien, 1586), 1–2.

36. de Chauliac, *Chirurgia Magna*, 8–9. See also A. Thevenet, "Guy de Chauliac (1300–1370): The 'Father of Surgery'" *Annals of Vascular Surgery* 2 (1993): 208–12.

37. de Chauliac, *Chirurgia Magna*, 2.

38. de Chauliac, *Chirurgia Magna*, 3.

39. L. Demaitre, "Theory and Practice in Medical Education at the University of Montpellier in the Thirteenth and Fourteenth Centuries," *Journal of the History of Medicine and Allied Sciences* 30 (1975): 103–23, quote 106. "For a surgeon ignorant,"

de Chauliac, *Chirurgia Magna*, 19–20. "For the Creator," de Chauliac, *Chirurgia Magna*, 33. See also McVaugh "Surgical Education."

40. de Chauliac, *Chirurgia Magna*, 104– 105. De Chauliac himself was stricken with the pestilence, now known as bubonic plague. Those around him thought he would die, but his *apostemata*—his bubonic pustules—drained, and, by various concoctions, he recovered.

Chapter Six

1. William Turner, *A Compleat History of the Most Remarkable Providences* (London: John Dunton, 1697), 2.

2. See Frederick L. Nussbaum, *The Triumph of Science and Reason* (New York: Harper & Row, 1953.

3. Turner, *Providences*, 2.

4. See Cotton Mather, *Magnalia Christi Americana* I (London: Thomas Parkhurst, 1702), 29.

5. Mather, *Magnalia*, I, 29.

6. Robert Burton, *The Anatomy of Melancholy* (London: B. Blake, 1836), 384.

7. Michael Wigglesworth and Reiner Smolinski, Eds., "God's Controversy with New-England," (1662, 1871). Electronic Texts in *American Studies*. 36. https://digitalcommons.unl.edu/etas/36, accessed 3/23/2023.

8. Edmund S. Morgan, "The Diary of Michael Wigglesworth," *Transactions Colonial Society of Massachusetts* 35 (1946): 311–444, quote 324. I left the wording in the contemporary vernacular.

9. Morgan, "Wigglesworth," 315.

10. See Phillip Cash, Eric H. Christianson, and J. Worth Estes, Eds., *Medicine in Colonial Massachusetts 1620–1820* (Boston: The Colonial Society of Massachusetts, 1980).

11. George Lyman Kittredge, Ed., *Letters of Samuel Lee and Samuel Sewall Related to New England and the Indians* (Cambridge: The Colonial Society of Massachusetts, 1912), 158.

12. Thomas Brian, *The Pisse-Prophet, or, Certain Pisse-Pot Lectures* (London: S & B Griffin, 1679), both quotes 103.

13. William Perkins, *A Salve for a Sicke Man* (London: John Legat, 1611), 106.

14. Perkins, *Salve*, 134–36.

15. Perkins, *Salve*, 23.

16. Perkins, *Salve*, 139.

17. Mather, *Magnalia*, I, 151.

18. Cotton Mather, *Diary of Cotton Mather, 1681-1708*, Vol 1 (Boston: Massachusetts Historical Society, 1911), 148.

19. Mather, *Diary*, 1, 2–11.

20. Mather, *Diary*, 1, 80.

21. Cotton Mather, *The Angel of Bethesda* (Barre: American Antiquarian Society, 1972), 229.

22. As quoted from Otho T. Beall Jr. and Richard H. Shryock, "Cotton Mather: The First Significant Figure in American Medicine," *Proceedings of the American Antiquarian Society* 63 (1953): 37–274, quotes 48.

23. Cotton Mather to John Cotton, "The Mather Papers," in *Collections of the Massachusetts Historical Society*, Fourth Series, Vol VIII (Boston: Wiggin and Lunt, 1868), 383–84.

24. Mather, *The Angel of Bethesda*, 231.

25. Cotton Mather, *Bonifacius: An Essay . . . To Do Good* (Gainesville: Scholars' Facsimile Reprints, 1967), 75.

26. Cotton Mather, *The Christian Philosopher* (Charlestown: J. McKown, 1815), 18.

27. Mather, *Diary*, 1, 76.

28. Mather, *Diary*, 1, 161.

29. Mather, *Diary*, 1, 164.

30. Mather, *Diary*, 1, 297.

31. Mather, *Diary*, 1, 445–46.

32. Cotton Mather, *Diary of Cotton Mather, 1709–1724*, Vol. 2 (Boston: Massachusetts Historical Society, 1912), 139.

33. Mather, *Diary*, 2, 620.

34. Mather, *Diary*, 2, 634.

35. Mather, *Diary*, 2, 641.

36. Information and quotes from S. B. Woodward, "The Story of Smallpox in Massachusetts," *New England Journal of Medicine* 206 (1932): 1181–91, quote 1182.

37. Zabdiel Boylston, *An Historical Account of the Small-Pox Inoculated in New England* (London: S. Chandler, 1730), 38.

38. Mather, *Magnalia*, 22.

39. Mather, *Angel of Bethesda*, 93–94.

40. Mather, *Angel of Bethesda*, 95–106.

41. Mather, *Diary*, 2, 780.

42. Mather, *Angel of Bethesda*, 5, 12.

43. Mather, *Christian Philosopher*, 234.

44. Mather, *Christian Philosopher*, 237.

45. Mather, *Christian Philosopher*, 298.

46. Mather, *Bonifacius*, 127.

47. Mather, *Angel*, 189–90 and "piss prophets" 250–51.

Chapter Seven

1. Sigmund Freud, *The Future of an Illusion*, James Strachey, trans. (New York: W.W. Norton & Co., 1961), 16–18.

2. James Mooney, *The Sacred Formulas of the Cherokees* (Washington: United States Bureau of American Ethnology, 1891), 323.

3. DeMallie *Sixth Grandfather*, 109.

4. DeMallie, *Sixth Grandfather*, 114.

5. DeMallie, *Sixth Grandfather*, 118.

6. DeMallie, *Sixth Grandfather*, 118, 122.

7. Neihardt, *Black Elk Speaks*, 49.

8. Neihardt, *Black Elk Speaks*, 104. For the Battle of the Rosebud, see Dee Brown, *Bury My Heart at Wounded Knee* (New York: Henry Holt and Company, 1970), 287–90.

9. DeMallie, *Sixth Grandfather* 178–79.

10. DeMallie, *Sixth Grandfather*, 214.

11. Brown, *Sacred Pipe*, 33–34.

12. DeMallie, *Sixth Grandfather*, 215–26.

13. Neihardt, *Black Elk Speaks*, 194.

14. Neihardt, *Black Elk Speaks*, 204.

15. DeMallie, *Sixth Grandfather*, 258.

16. DeMallie, *Sixth Grandfather*, 236–39.

17. Melvin Randolph Gilmore, *Uses of Plants by the Indians of the Missouri River Region* (Washington: Government Printing Office, 1919), 57, 64–94.

18. William K. Powers, *Yuwipi* (Lincoln: University of Nebraska Press, 1982), 52.

19. Powers, *Yuwipi*, 81.

20. Powers, *Yuwipi*, 82. See W. R. Hurt Jr. and J. H. Howard, "A Dakota Conjuring Ceremony," *Southwestern Journal of Anthropology* 8 (1952): 286–96.

21. James R. Walker, *Lakota Belief and Ritual* (Lincoln: University of Nebraska Press, 1980, 1991), 91. George Sword took this name when he professed that the swords carried by white troopers conveyed power and authority. The given name "George" he assumed was, according to him, from an unknown source. See George Sword, *George Sword's Warrior Narratives* (Lincoln: University of Nebraska Press, 2016), 64.

22. Edward D. Neill, *Dakota Land and Dakota Life* (Minneapolis: Minnesota Historical Society, 1872), 269.

23. See Walker, *Lakota Belief and Ritual*, 91–93.

24. Wilson D. Wallis, "The Canadian Dakota," *Anthropological Papers of the American Museum of Natural History* 41 (1947): 1–226, quote 103.

25. From Wallis, "Canadian Dakota," 104.

26. DeMallie, *Sixth Grandfather*, 249–250.

27. Neihardt, *Black Elk Speaks*, 230.

28. Neihardt, *Black Elk Speaks*, 233.

29. James Mooney, *The Ghost-Dance Religion and the Sioux Outbreak of 1890* (Lincoln: University of Nebraska Press, 1991), 777.

30. DeMallie, *Sixth Grandfather*, 280.

31. DeMallie, *Sixth Grandfather*, 274; and Neihardt, *Black Elk Speaks*, 266.

32. Neihardt, *Black Elk Speaks*, 262.

33. Brown, *Bury My Heart*, 444.

34. Neihardt, *Black Elk Speaks*, 270.

35. For Lakota initiatives on the reservation see J. Ostler, "'The Last Buffalo Hunt' and Beyond: Plains Sioux Economic Strategies in the Early Reservation Period," *Great Plains Quarterly* 21 (2001): 115–30.

36. Quote from Ross Enochs, *The Jesuit Mission to the Lakota Sioux* (Kansas City: Sheed & Ward, 1996), 32. See also DeMallie, *Sixth Grandfather*, 12.

37. Neihardt, *Black Elk Speaks*, 270. The Lakota circle of life so central to their culture had been broken. All that was sacred had been dispersed in the blood and mud of the Wounded Knee butchery.

38. DeMallie, *Sixth Grandfather*, 19.

Chapter Eight

1. Anonymous Author, *Leprosy in Hawaii; Extracts from Reports of Presidents of the Board of Health, Government Physicians and Others, and from Official Records* (Honolulu: Daily Bulletin Stream Print Office, 1886), 8–9.

2. Abraham Fornander, *Hawaiian Antiquities and Folk-Lore* (Honolulu: Bishop Museum Press, 1919–1920), 416.

3. "Legends of Moloka'i" at https://www.molokai.org/about-molokai/myths-of -molokai/index.html#:~:text=Legends%20say%20that%20the%20people,sovereign %20control%20over%20the%20island, accessed 3/1/2024.

4. E. S. Craighill Handy, *Polynesian Religion* (Honolulu: Bernice P. Bishop Museum, 1927), 233.

5. See K. Blaisdell, "Historical and Cultural Aspects of Native Hawaiian Health," in Peter Manicas, Ed., *Social Process in Hawaii: A Reader* (New York: McGraw Hill, 1993), 37–57.

6. O. A. Bushnell, *The Gifts of Civilization* (Honolulu: University of Hawaii Press, 1993), 101.

7. From Blaisdell, "Historical and Cultural Aspects," 37–57.

8. Samuel M. Kamakau, *Ruling Chiefs of Hawaii* (Honolulu: Kamehameha Schools Press, 1961), 416.

9. A. A. St. M. Mouritz, *"The Path of the Destroyer"* (Honolulu: Honolulu Star Press, 1916), 29.

10. Rev. S. E. Bishop, *Why Are the Hawaiians Dying Out?* (Honolulu: Honolulu Social Science Association, 1888).

11. See Samuel George Morton, *Crania Americana* (Philadelphia: J. Dobson, 1839).

12. William Osler, *The Principles and Practice of Medicine* (New York: D. Appleton and Company, 1892), 259.

13. May Quinlan, *Damien of Molokai* (London: MacDonald and Evans, 1909), 80.

14. Gavan Daws, *Holy Man* (New York: Harper & Row, 1973), 22.

15. Daws, *Holy Man*, 35.

16. Father Pamphile de Veuster, Ed., *Life and Letters of Father Damien* (London: The Catholic Truth Society, 1889), 79.

17. St. M. Mouritz, *The Path of the Destroyer*, 227.

18. de Veuster, *Life and Letters*, 91.

19. St. M. Mouritz, *"The Path of the Destroyer,"* 227.

20. de Veuster, *Life and Letters*, 88.

21. de Veuster, *Life and Letters*, 92.

22. John Tayman, *The Colony* (New York: Scribner, 2006), 51.

23. de Veuster, *Life and Letters*, 107.

24. Viktor E. Frankl, *Man's Search for Meaning* (New York: Washington Square Press, 1984), 135.

25. St. M. Mouritz, *"The Path of the Destroyer,"* both quotes 225.

26. The *hula kahiko*, the ancient form of the dance, was performed with revealing clothing, the men in nothing but a loincloth; the women were often topless. See P. Pollenz, "Changes in the Form and Function of Hawaiian Hulas," *American Anthropologist* 52 (1950): 225–34.

27. From P. Moblo, "Institutionalizing the Leper: Partisan Politics and the Evolution of Stigma in Post-Monarchy Hawai'i," *Journal of Polynesian Society* 107 (1998): 229–62, quote 240.

28. Daws, *Holy Man*, 46; Rudyard Kipling, "The White Man's Burden," *McClure's Magazine*, February 12, 1899: 290.

29. de Veuster, *Life and Letters*, 117.

30. Tayman, *The Colony*, 123.

31. Daws, *Holy Man*, 85.

32. William Ragsdale, *Ka Nuhou Hawaii*, January 27, 1874, 4.

33. Charles Warren Stoddard, *The Lepers of Molokai* (South Bend, IN: Ave Maria Press, 1885), quotes 60–61, 71, 93.

34. Anwei Skinsnes Law, *Kalaupapa: A Collective Memory* (Honolulu: University of Hawai'i Press, 2012), 112.

35. St. M. Mouritz, *"The Path of the Destroyer,"* 231.

36. Bushnell, *The Gifts of Civilization*, 95.

37. Richard Stewart, *Leper Priest of Moloka'i* (Honolulu: University of Hawai'i Press, 2000), 201–202.

38. Stoddard, *Lepers*, 97.

39. Tayman, *The Colony*, 124.

40. Law, *Kalaupapa*, 169.

41. de Veuster, *Life and Letters*, 133, 137.

42. Law, *Kalaupapa*, 171.

43. de Veuster, *Life and Letters*, 142.

44. Stewart, *Leper Priest*, 352.

45. de Veuster, *Life and Letters*, 146.

46. Stewart, *Leper Priest*, 362.

47. Anonymous Author, *Father Damien Leper Apostle of Moloka'i* (Melbourne: The Australian Catholic Truth Society Record, 1960), 20.

48. Quinlan, *Damien*, 93.

Chapter Nine

1. William Osler, *Physic and Physicians as Depicted in Plato* (Boston: Damrell & Upham, 1893), quote 7.

2. William Osler, *Aequanimitas* (Philadelphia: P. Blakiston's Son & Co., 1910), 57, 58.

3. William Osler, "Teaching and Thinking," *Montreal Medical Journal* 23 (1895): 561–72, quote 565.

4. William Osler, "The Master Word in Medicine," *Johns Hopkins Hospital Bulletin* 15 (1904): 1–19, quotes 17, 19.

5. G. N. Burrow, "The Trial and Tribulation of Egerton Yorrick Davis," *Western Journal of Medicine* 155 (1991): 80–82.

6. Letter from Ellen Osler to her Son William Osler, *The William Osler Papers*, National Library of Medicine (101743406X264).

7. Michael Bliss, *William Osler: A Life in Medicine* (Toronto: University of Toronto Press, 1999), 47.

8. William Osler, "Chauvinism in Medicine," in William Osler, *Aequanimitas*, 280.

9. Harvey Cushing, *The Life of Sir William Osler*, Vols. I and II (Oxford: Clarendon Press, 1925), 123.

10. W. Osler, "Letter from Leipzig," *Canada Medical Surgical Journal* 13 (1884): 18–22, quote 22. By "bauble" Osler no doubt meant "showy."

11. From William S. Thayer, "Osler," *The Nation* (NY) 110 (1920) 104–106, January 24.

12. Cushing, *Osler*, I, 237.

13. Cushing, *Osler*, I, 279.

14. Cushing, *Osler*, I, 597.

15. Cushing, *Osler*, I, 412–13.

16. George T. Harrell, "Lady Osler," *Bulletin of the History of Medicine* 53 (1979): 81–99.

17. Cushing, *Osler*, I, 292.

18. Alan M. Chesney and William H. Howell, *The Johns Hopkins Hospital and the Johns Hopkins University School of Medicine: A Chronicle*, Vol. I (Baltimore: The Johns Hopkins Press, 1943), quotes 13–15.

19. To William Pepper from Osler, October 3, 1888, Cushing, *Osler*, I, 298.

20. Osler, *Aequanimitas*, 10.

21. Osler, *Aequanimitas*, 11.

22. Cushing, *Osler*, I, 320.

23. Cushing, *Osler*, I, 357–58.

24. Cushing, *Osler*, I, 360.

25. See Cushing, *Osler*, I, 262–63.

26. R. L. Golden, "Paul Revere Osler: The Other Child," *Proceedings Baylor University Medical Center* 28 (2015): 21–24.

27. Cushing, *Osler*, I, 426.

28. T. E. Keys, "Edward Revere Osler 1895–1917," *Archives of Internal Medicine* 114 (1964): 284–93, quote 284.

29. Cushing, *Osler*, I, 650–51.

30. Cushing, *Osler*, I, 365.

31. Cushing, *Osler*, I, 371.

32. Bliss, *William Osler*, both quotes 265.

33. Osler, "The Student Life," in Osler, *Aequanimitas*, 424.

34. Cushing, *Osler*, I, 640.

35. Cushing, *Osler*, II, 275–77.

36. Cushing, *Osler*, II, 456.

37. Letter from Edward Revere Osler to his aunt, Susan Chapin, December 5, 1915, Osler Library of the History of Medicine, McGill University. Osler Library Archive Collections, P417.

38. Letter from Edward Revere Osler to his dad, William Osler, November 14, 1916; and Letter from William Osler to his son, Edward Revere on his twenty-first birthday, December 28, 1916, Osler Library of the History of Medicine, McGill University. Osler Library Archive Collections, P417.

39. Cushing, *Osler*, II, 545–46.

40. Cushing, *Osler*, II, 576. Also see Susan Kelen, "The 100th Anniversary of the Death of Edward Revere Osler, 1895–1917," *The Osler Library Newsletter*, 127 (2017): 4–5, and Harvey Cushing, *From a Surgeon's Journal: 1915–1918* (London: Constable & Co., 1936), 198.

41. Cushing, *Osler*, II, 575.

42. Letter from William Osler to H. S. Birkett, September 1, 1917; Osler Library of the History of Medicine, McGill University. Osler Library Archive Collections, P100: Sir William Osler Collection.

43. Letter, Osler to Birkett and Cushing, in Cushing, *Osler*, II, 578.

44. Cushing, *Osler*, I, 295.

45. Frederick B. Wagner, Ed., *The Twilight Years of Lady Osler* (Canton: Science History Publications, 1985), 15–19.

46. William Osler, "The Old Humanities and the New Science," The Presidential Address delivered before the Classical Association at Oxford, May 1919, *British Medical Journal* 2 (1919): 1–7, quotes 3, 5.

47. Cushing, *Osler*, II, 685.

Chapter Ten

1. Jeanne Achterberg, *Woman as Healer* (Boston: Shambhala Publications, Inc., 1990), quotes 63–64.

2. Homer, *Iliad*, A. T. Murray, trans. (Cambridge: Harvard University Press, 1988), III.157–58.

3. Homer, *Odyssey*, A. T. Murray, trans. (Cambridge: Harvard University Press, 1995), IV.219–26.

4. Herodotus, *History of Herodotus*, George Rawlinson, trans., Vol. II (London: John Murray, 1862), 2.84.

5. Homer, *Iliad*, XI.623–626; 638–41.

6. Homer, *Iliad*, XIV.1–9.

7. See H. Castelli and M. Rothstein, "The Skills of Hecamede. Women as Caregivers in Archaic and Classical Greece," in Anne Hugon, Clyde Plumauzille, Mathilde Rossigneux-Mehéust, *Gender and the History of Care Work* (Paris: Editions Belin, 2019), 25–44. Homer, *Iliad*, XI.840–48.

8. Jennifer Irving, "Restituta: The Training of the Female Physician," *Melbourne Historical Journal* 40 (2012); 45–57. The engraving was found on fragments of stone, IG XIV 1751.

9. See Irving, "Restituta."

10. Gottfried von Strassburg, *Tristan and Iseult*, Jessie L. Weston, trans., Vol. I (London: David Nutt, 1899, 1902), 59.

11. I took the original term *"arzatliche meisterschaft"* from Gottfried von Strassburg's "Tristan" in Franz Pfeiffer, Ed., *Deutsche Classiker des Mittelalters* (Leipzig: F. A. Brockhaus, 1890), v 6954.

12. Von Strassberg, *Tristan and Iseult*, I, 68.

13. Von Strassberg, *Tristan and Iseult*, I, 71.

14. Von Strassberg, *Tristan and Iseult*, I, 77.

15. Gottfried von Strassburg, *Tristan and Iseult*, Jessie L. Weston, trans., Vol. II (New York: The New Amsterdam Book Co., 1899), 3–4.

16. Von Strassberg, *Tristan and Iseult*, II, 9–10.

17. See K. Altpeter-Jones, "Love Me, Hurt Me, Heal Me: Isolde Healer and Isolde Lover in Gottfried's 'Tristan'," *The German Quarterly* 82 (2009): 5–23.

18. Hildegard, *The Letters of Hildegard of Bingen*, Joseph L. Baird and Radd K. Ehrman, trans., Vol. 1 (Oxford: Oxford University Press, 1994), 159–60.

19. See Hildegard, *Illuminations of Hildegard of Bingen*, Matthew Fox, Ed. (Rochester: Bear & Company), 1985.

20. See F. M. Malpezzi, "Evergreen: The Enduring Voice of a Nine-Hundred-Year-Old Healer," in Erika Brady, Ed., *Healing Logics: Culture and Medicine in Modern Health Belief Systems* (Logan: Utah State University Press, 2001), 163–79.

21. Hildegard of Bingen, *Scivias*, Columbia Hart and Jane Bishop, trans. (New York: Paulist Press, 1990), 59.

22. Hildegard, *The Letters* I, 27–28.

23. Hildegard, *Scivias*, 316.

24. Hildegard, *Scivias*, 123–24.

25. Hildegard, *The Letters of Hildegard of Bingen*, Vol. III, Joseph L. Baird and Radd K. Ehrman, trans. (Oxford: Oxford University Press, 2004), 117.

26. See R. M. Walker-Moskop, "Health and Cosmic Continuity: Hildegard of Bingen's Unique Concerns," *Mystics Quarterly* 11 (1985): 19–25.

27. Hildegard, *Causae et Curae*, Paulus Kaiser, Ed., (Leipzig: B. G. Teubneri, 1903), 64.

28. Hildegard, *Causae et Curae*, 51.

29. Hildegard, *Causae et Curae*, 42.

30. Hildegard, *Causae et Curae*, 33.

31. Hildegard, *Causae et Curae*, 69–70.

32. Hildegard, *Causae et Curae*, 76.

33. Hildegard, *Causae et Curae*, 104.

34. Hildegard, *Causae et Curae*, 185–88, 194. Bachmenza is probably akin to bachmint, also known as water mint—like peppermint. What medicinal properties it has are largely speculative. Lunchwurz is probably similar to lüppewurz, an aconite plant of mountainous Germany.

35. L. Moulinier, "La Botanique d'Hildegard de Bingen," *Médiévales* 16/17 (1989): 113–29.

36. Hildegard, *Causae et Curae*, 165. "A matter of women's business" is borrowed from the phrase "women's health was women's business" from Beryl Rowland, *Medieval Woman's Guide to Health* (Kent: Kent State University Press, 1981), xv.

37. See "S. Hildegardis Abbatissae Opera Omnia," J.-P. Migne trans., in J.-P. Migne, Ed., *Patrologiae Cursus Completus* Vol. 197 (Paris: Garnier, 1855), 182, 227 (translations mine).

38. See M. Cabré, "Women or Healers? Household Practices and the Categories of Health Care in Late Medieval Iberia," *Bulletin of the History of Medicine* 82 (2008): 18–51.

39. Anonymous, "Females Attending Medical Lectures," *Boston Medical and Surgical Journal* 37 (1847): 405.

40. Anonymous, "Female Physicians," *Buffalo Medical Journal* 3 (1848): 494–96, quotes 495–96.

41. Janice P. Nimura, *The Doctors Blackwell* (New York: W.W. Norton & Company, 2021), quotes 77–79, 209.

42. Elizabeth Blackwell, *Address on the Medical Education of Women* (New York: Baker & Duyckinck, 1856), 5.

43. Blackwell, *Address*, 5–6.

44. Blackwell, *Address*, 6–7.

45. Blackwell, *Address*, 8.

46. Blackwell, *Address*, 10.

47. See N. Hewitt, "Feminist Friends: Agrarian Quakers and the Emergence of Woman's Rights in America," *Feminist Studies* 12 (1988): 27–49.

48. Clara Marshall, *The Women's Medical College of Pennsylvania* (Philadelphia: P. Blakiston, Son & Co., 1897), 10.

49. J. S. Longshore, *An Introductory Lecture: Delivered Before the Class, at the Opening of the Female Medical College of Pennsylvania: October 12th, 1850* (Philadelphia: James Young, 1850), 10.

50. Marshall, *Women's Medical College*, 56.

51. *Transactions of the Thirty-First Annual Meeting of the Alumnae Association of the Woman's Medical College of Pennsylvania, May 24th and 25th, 1906* (Philadelphia: Alumnae Association, 1906), 36.

52. Marshall, *Women's Medical College*, 18–19.

53. Marshall, *Women's Medical College*, quotes 23, 26.

54. Anonymous, "Female Practitioners of Medicine," *Boston Medical and Surgical Journal* 76 (1867): 272–74, including all preceding quotes.

55. Attributed to Sir Andrew Douglas Maclagan and published in the *Boston Medical and Surgical Journal* 89 (1873): 23.

56. Quote from Regina Morantz-Sanchez, *Sympathy and Science: Women Physicians in American Medicine* (Chapel Hill: University of North Carolina Press, 1985, 2000), 326. See also S. J. Peitzman, "Why Support a Women's Medical College? Philadelphia's Early Male Medical Pro-Feminists," *Bulletin of the History of Medicine* 77 (2003) 576–99.

57. Morantz-Sanchez, *Sympathy and Science*, 321.

58. Mary Roth Walsh, *Doctors Wanted: No Women Need Apply* (New Haven, CT: Yale University Press, 1977), quote taken 249 and 252; italics mine.

59. Anonymous, "A Lament," *London (Royal Free Hospital) School of Medicine for Women Magazine* 12 (1917): 13.

60. Gabriel Weston, *Direct Red* (New York: Harper, 2009), 39, 72.

61. Morantz-Sanchez, *Sympathy and Science*, 351.

Chapter Eleven

1. Excerpts taken from a previous publication by T. S. Helling, "Alexis Carrel and His Voyage of Discovery," *Journal of Religion and Health* 61 (2022): 4565–84, permission granted, Springer *Nature*.

2. Auguste Comte, *A General View of Positivism*, J. H. Bridges, trans. (London: George Routledge & Sons, 1908), Chapter I.

3. Sebastien Normandin, "Visions of Vitalism: Medicine, Philosophy and the Soul in Nineteenth Century France," Doctoral Diss., McGill University Montreal 2005, 6.

4. See, for example, P. Keresztes, "The Massacre at Lugdunum in 177 A.D.," *Historia: Zeitschrift für Alte Geschichte* 16 (1967): 75–86.

5. Much of Carrel's biography was taken from Robert Soupault, *Alexis Carrel 1873–1944* (Paris: Librairie Plon, 1952).

6. J. W. Langon, "The Jesuits and French Education: A Comparative Study of Two Schools 1852–1913," *History of Education Quarterly* 18 (1978): 49–66.

7. Alexis Carrel, *Jours Apres Jours* (Paris: Librairie Plon, 1956), 3.

8. Carrel, *Jours Apres Jours*, 4.

9. Carrel, *Jours Apres Jours*, 8.

10. Alexis Carrel, *Man the Unknown* (New York: Harper & Brothers, 1935, 1939), 147–48.

11. I. M. Rutkow, "The Letters of William Halsted and Alexis Carrel," *Surgery Gynecology Obstetrics* 151 (1980): 676–88.

12. From René Leriche, *Souvenirs de Ma Vie Morte* (Paris: Éditions du Seuil, 1956), 178.

13. Alexandre Lacassagne, *L'Assassinat du Président Carnot* (Lyon: A. Stork, 1894).

14. See A. Carrel, "La Technique Opératoire des Anastomoses Vasculaires et la Transplantation des Viscères," *Lyon Médical* 98 (1902):859–64; and A. Carrel, "Anastomose Bout a Bout de la Jugulaire et la Carotide Primitive," *Lyon Médical* 99 (1902): 114–16.

15. Carrel, *Jours Apres Jours*, 22.

16. Carrel, *Jours Apres Jours* 34.

17. Quotes from Carrel, *Jours Apres Jours*, 88, 19.

18. B. François, E. M. Sternberg, E. Fee, "The Lourdes Medical Cures Revisited," *Journal of the History of Medicine and Allied Sciences* 69 (2014): 135–62.

19. Suzanne K. Kaufman, *Consuming Vision: Mass Culture and the Lourdes Shrine* (Ithaca: Cornell University Press, 2005).

20. See J. Szabo, "Seeing Is Believing? The Form and Substance of French Medical Debates over Lourdes," *Bulletin of the History of Medicine* 76 (2002): 199–230.

21. G. K. Chesterton, *Orthodoxy* (New York: Image Books, 1908, 1936, 1959), 133.

22. Émile Zola, *Lourdes* I and II (New York: Grosset & Dunlap, 1897), viii.

23. Zola, *Lourdes* I, 133.

24. Zola, *Lourdes* I, 138.

25. Zola, *Lourdes* II, 199.

26. See, for example, B. Stephenson, "Charcot's Theatre of Hysteria," *Journal of Ritual Studies* 15 (2001): 27–37.

27. Jean-Marie Charcot, *La Foi Qui Guérit* (Paris: Félix Alcan, 1897), 9.

28. Charcot, *La Foi Qui Guérit*, 32.

29. Charcot, *La Foi Qui Guérit*, 37.

30. Theories put forth by such authors as Jacques Léonard, "Femmes, Religion et Médecine," *Annales Economies, Sociétés, Civilisations* 32 (1977): 887–907.

31. Judith Devlin, *The Superstitious Mind: French Peasants and the Supernatural in the Nineteenth Century* (New Haven: Yale University Press, 1987), quote 63–64.

32. Devlin, *Superstitious Mind*, 64.

33. Alexis Carrel, *Le Voyage de Lourdes* (Paris: Plon Bibliothèque, 1949). The quotes that follow are taken from this book. I did not always provide page reference.

34. Carrel, *Le Voyage de Lourdes*, 39.

35. Dr. Boissarie, "Le Dossier Médical de Marie Bailly," in Carrel, *Le Voyage de Lourdes*, 1907. Boissarie's description of this perplexing case is found as an addendum in Carrel's book.

36. Carrel, *Jours Apres Jours*, 92.

37. See Alexis Carrel, *Réflexions sur la Conduite de la Vie* (Paris: Librairie Plon, 1950), 214–15.

38. Carrel's habit of visiting churches to hear the music is described in Soupault, *Alexis Carrel*, 178.

39. Carrel, *Man the Unknown*, fn 148 and 149–50.

40. "Une Guérison à Lourdes," *Le Nouvelliste*, June 3, 1902.

41. Andrés Horacio Reggiani, *God's Eugenicist* (New York: Berghahn Books, 2007), 18, taken from "Une Guérison à Lourdes," *Le Nouvelliste*, June 10, 1902.

42. Taken from Soupault, *Alexis Carrel*, 180.

43. Alexis Carrel, "Prayer Is Power," *Reader's Digest 20th Anniversary Anthology* (New York: Reader's Digest Association, 1941); and *La Priere*, in *Réflexions*, 311.

44. Carrel, *Réflexions*, 213–15.

45. E. C. Gordon, "Child Health in the Middle Ages as Seen in the Miracles of Five English Saints, A.D. 1150–1220," *Bulletin of the History of Medicine* 60 (1986): 502–22, quote 522.

46. S. Normandin, "Visions of Vitalism: Medicine Philosophy and the Soul in Nineteenth Century France," PhD diss., McGill University, 2005, 274.

Chapter Twelve

1. H. E. Allison, "Kant's Transcendental Humanism," *The Monist* 55 (1971): 182–207.

2. Andrew Copson, "What Is Humanism?" in A. C. Grayling, *The Wiley Blackwell Handbook of Humanism* (Chichester: John Wiley and Sons, 2015), 1–33, quote 7.

3. Tony Davies, *Humanism* (London: Routledge Press, 1997), 21.

4. Matthew Arnold, *Mixed Essays Irish Essays and Others* (New York: Macmillan and Company, 1883), 101.

5. S. Biernoff, "Flesh Poems: Henry Tonks and the Art of Surgery," *Visual Culture in Britain* 11 (2010): 25–47, quote 41.

6. Netflix, *The Surgeon's Cut*, https://www.netflix.com/title/81004466.

7. H. Cushing, "Medicine at the Crossroads," *Journal of the American Medical Association* 100 (1933): 1567–75, quote 1570–71, italics mine.

8. G. H. Cleveland and F. C. Wells, "A Discussion Upon the Medical and Surgical Aspects of Appendicitis," *Chicago Clinical Review* 5 (1896): 617–44, quote 627.

9. Even in the late 1960s, staff surgeons at the Massachusetts General Hospital were called *visiting surgeons* rather than more formal faculty terms such as attending surgeons.

10. Edward D. Churchill, *Wanderjahr: The Education of a Surgeon* (Boston: Francis A. Countway Library of Medicine, 1990), quotes 7 and 12. One attending surgeon had said to a young, naïve Churchill: "[d]o not bother me with any new ideas. I know enough now to last me the rest of my surgical life and do not want to learn anything more" (Churchill, *Wanderjahr*, 8).

11. Churchill, *Wanderjahr*, 97.

12. Actually, he was chief of the West Surgical Service. Not until 1948 was he appointed chief of both West and East services. Functionally, though he served as the head of surgical services.

13. As quoted in H. C. Grillo, "Edward D. Churchill and the 'Rectangular' Surgical Residency," *Surgery* 136 (2004): 947–52, quote 951.

14. E. D. Churchill, "Origins of American Surgery," *Journal of the American Medical Association* 172 (1960): 219–22, quote 222.

15. Passage taken from R. Kipling, "Surgeons and the Soul," in Rudyard Kipling, *A Book of Words* (London: Macmillan and Co., 1928), 223–28, quote 227.

16. E. D. Churchill, "Graduate Training in Surgery at the Massachusetts General Hospital," *Harvard Med Alum Bull* 14 (1940): 28–36.

17. Eldridge Campbell, 1946–1957 corres, 1946–1957. Edward Delos Churchill papers, H MS c62, Box: 3, Folder: 1. Center for the History of Medicine (Francis A. Countway Library of Medicine, Boston, MA).

18. Sarton, *The History of Science*, 126.

19. E. D. Churchill, "Science and Humanism in Surgery," *Annals of Surgery* 126 (1947): 381–96, quotes 390, 394, and 395.

20. Churchill, "Science and Humanism," 395.

21. Churchill, "Science and Humanism," 382.

22. Corres and r.m. re speeches, addresses, lectures, 1938, 1938. Edward Delos Churchill papers, H MS c62, Box: 59, Folder: 18. Center for the History of Medicine (Francis A. Countway Library of Medicine, Boston, MA).

23. For contrast see Lindsey Fitzharris' graphic depictions in *The Butchering Art* (New York: Scientific American, 2017), 10–12.

24. Churchill, *Wanderjahr*, 97, 151.

25. Corres. and r.m. re speeches, addresses, lectures, 1947, 1947. Edward Delos Churchill papers, H MS c62, Box: 59, Folder: 58. Center for the History of Medicine (Francis A. Countway Library of Medicine, Boston, MA).

26. Churchill "Should I Study Medicine?" 538.

27. Churchill, "Should I Study Medicine?" 539.

28. De Bakey, Michael E.: 1956–1969 corres and r.m., 1956–1969. Edward Delos Churchill papers, H MS c62, Box: 3, Folder: 18. Center for the History of Medicine (Francis A. Countway Library of Medicine, Boston MA).

29. "The Surgeon and the University": Centennial Lecture in Surgery, Queen's University, Kingston, Ont., 15 Oct 1954, 15 Oct 1954. Edward Delos Churchill papers, H MS c62, Box: 60, Folder: 46–48. Center for the History of Medicine (Francis A. Countway Library of Medicine, Boston, MA).

30. Churchill, "Should I Study Medicine?" 539.

31. "The Evolution of the Hospital": Lowell Lecture at Boston Public Library in series on The Hospital in Contemporary Life, 6 Jan 1948, 6 Jan 1948. Edward Delos Churchill papers, H MS c62, Box: 59, Folder: 59. Center for the History of Medicine (Francis A. Countway Library of Medicine, Boston, MA).

32. Edward D. Churchill, The Surgeon and the University: Centennial Lecture in Surgery, Queen's University, Kingston, Ont., 15 Oct 1954, 15 Oct 1954. Edward Delos Churchill papers, H MS c62, Box: 60, Folder: 46–48. Center for the History of Medicine (Francis A. Countway Library of Medicine, Boston, MA).

33. T. Schlich, "'The Days of Brilliancy Are Past': Skill, Styles and the Changing Rules of Surgical Performance, ca. 1820–1920," *Medical History* 59 (2015): 379–403, quote 402. Walter C. MacKenzie, "Our Destiny Is to Build," *Bulletin of the American*

College of Surgeons 52 (1967): 33–36, quote 33. Will C. Sealy, "Residents and Residencies," *Annals of Thoracic Surgery* 12 (1971): 561–73, quotes 562.

34. Corres and r.m. re speeches, addresses, lectures, 1938, 1938. Edward Delos Churchill papers, H MS c62, Box: 59, Folder: 18. Center for the History of Medicine (Francis A. Countway Library of Medicine, Boston, MA).

35. Churchill, "Science and Humanism in Surgery" *Annals of Surgery* 126 (1947): 381–96, quote 390.

Chapter Thirteen

1. Aphrodite was the mythical Greek goddess of beauty and sexual attraction, particularly coveted for her virginal bosom. Melpomene was the Greek Muse of tragedy. See D. E. Gerber, "The Female Breast in Greek Erotic Literature," *Arethusa* 11 (1978): 203–12.

2. Hippocrates, *Hippocrates* Vol. VII, "Epidemics," Wesley D. Smith, trans. (Cambridge: Harvard University Press, 1994), V.101 (214).

3. Émile Littré, *Oeuvres Complètes d'Hippocrate*, Tome Huitième ("Des Maladies des Femmes") (Paris: J. B. Baillière, 1853), II.133 (283).

4. Francis Adams, *The Seven Books of Paulus Aegineta*, Vol. II (London: Sydenham Society, 1846), Book VI, 332.

5. See E. F. Lewison, "Saint Agatha: The Patron Saint of Diseases of the Breast in Legend and Art," *Bulletin of the History of Medicine* 24 (1950): 409–20. See also Sabine Baring-Gould, *The Lives of the Saints*, Vol. 2 (London: John C. Nimmo, 1898), 136–38.

6. Larrey, *Mémoires*, vii–viii. See also D. G. Burris, D. R. Welling, N. M. Rich, "Dominique Jean Larrey and the Principles of Humanity in Warfare," *Journal of the American College of Surgeons* 198 (2004): 831–35.

7. J. Dible, "D.J. Larrey, a Surgeon of the Revolution, Consulate, and Empire," *Medical History* 3 (1959): 100–107.

8. Larrey, *Mémoires*, 271.

9. H. J. Bigelow, "Insensibility During Surgical Operations Produced by Inhalation," *Boston Medical and Surgical Journal* 35 (1846): 309–17.

10. See James M. Edmonson, *Nineteenth Century Surgical Instruments* (Cleveland: Cleveland Health Sciences Library, 1986). See also I. M. Rutkow, "On Scalpels and Bistouries," *Archives of Surgery* 135 (2000): 360.

11. Larrey, *Mémoires*, 272.

12. Frances Burney d'Arblay to her sister Esther Burney, Frances Burney d'Arblay Collection, Henry W. and Albert A. Berg Collection of English and American Literature, The New York Public Library, Box 1, Folder 8.

13. J. Paget, "On the Average Duration of Life in Patients with Scirrhous Cancer of the Breast," *Lancet* 1 (1856): 62–63.

14. R. G. Richardson, "Larrey – What Manner of Man?" *Proceedings of the Royal Society of Medicine* 70 (1977): 490–94, quote 493.

15. Description by Velpeau in 1838, from Alfred Velpeau, *Traité des Maladies du Sein* (Paris: Masson, 1858), 404.

16. See E. S. Morgan, "The Puritans and Sex," *The New England Quarterly* 15 (1942): 591–607. See also E. Rein, "The Devil, the Body, and the Feminine Soul in Puritan New England," *Journal of American History* 82 (1995): 15–36.

17. Charles D. Meigs, *Females and Their Diseases: A Series of Letters to His Class* (Philadelphia: Lea and Blanchard, 1848), 19.

18. Susan Sontag, *Illness as Metaphor* (New York: Farrar, Straus and Giroux, 1977), 53.

19. William Osler, "Carcinoma Mammae: Removal by Excision," *Canada Medical Journal* 8 (1871): 107–109. It is interesting, that, Osler, certainly aware of mammary cancer, did not mention it in his famous medical text, *The Principles and Practice of Medicine* that he published in 1892.

20. See William S. Halsted, "Practical Comments on the Use and Abuse of Cocaine," *New York Medical Journal* 42 (1885): 294–95.

21. See D. B. Nunn, "Dr. Halsted's Addiction," *Johns Hopkins Advanced Studies in Medicine* 6 (2006): 106–108.

22. William S. Halsted, "The Results of Operations for the Cure of Cancer of the Breast Performed at the Johns Hopkins Hospital from June, 1889 to January, 1894," *Annals of Surgery* 20 (1894): 497–555, quote 513.

23. M. P. Osborne, "William Stewart Halsted: His Life and Contributions to Surgery," *Lancet Oncology* 8 (2007): 256–65.

24. Halsted, "Cancer of the Breast." See also Gerald Imber, *Genius on the Edge* (New York: Kaplan Publishing, 2010).

25. C. D. Haagensen, *Diseases of the Breast* (Philadelphia: W.B. Saunders Company, 1971), 674.

26. Haagensen, *Diseases of the Breast*, 673.

27. See Haagensen, *Diseases of the Breast*, 710.

28. Haagensen, *Diseases of the Breast*, 723.

29. Peter B. Flint "Dr. Cushman D. Haagensen, 90; Specialist Advocated Mastectomy," *The New York Times*, September 18, 1990, 10.

30. Comments made by the inventor of Barbie, Ruth Handler, as reported in James S. Olsen, *Bathsheba's Breast* (Baltimore: Johns Hopkins University Press, 2002), 235. For "bosom mania" see A. Mazur, "Trends in Feminine Beauty and Overadaptation," *The Journal of Sex Research* 22 (1986): 281–303.

31. This study was published as B. Fisher, N. Wolmark, C. Redmond et al., "Findings from NSABP Protocol No. B-04: Comparison of Radical Mastectomy with Alternative Treatments. II. The Clinical and Biologic Significance of Medial-Central Breast Cancers," *Cancer* 48 (1981): 1863–1872. Haagensen never subscribed to this claim.

32. S. Anderson, "A Short History of Bernard Fisher's Contributions to Randomized Clinical Trials," *Clinical Trials* 19 (2022) 127–36. Fisher's quote from Jo Cavallo, "Dr. Bernard Fisher's Breast Cancer Research Left a Lasting Legacy of Improved Therapeutic Efficacy and Survival," The ASCO *Post*, May 15, 2013, https://ascopost

.com/issues/may-15-2013/dr-bernard-fishers-breast-cancer-research-left-a-lasting -legacy-of-improved-therapeutic-efficacy-and-survival.aspx, retrieved February 6, 2023. Bernard Fisher was not only a visionary researcher but also a social advocate and feminist. In minimizing surgical mutilation, he was also able to demonstrate the safety in lesser techniques and the efficacious nature of ionizing radiation and hormonal, targeted therapy.

33. Siddhartha Mukherjee, *The Emperor of All Maladies* (New York: Scribner, 2010), 466.

34. Olsen, *Bathsheba's Breast*, 168.

35. Olsen, *Bathsheba's Breast*, 169.

36. In Kasper and Ferguson, Eds., *Breast Cancer: Society Shapes an Epidemic*, viii. "Scarlet Letter" refers, of course, to Nathaniel Hawthorne's famous novel of sin and guilt in Puritan Massachusetts of the seventeenth century, *The Scarlet Letter*.

37. From Rosenbaum and Roos, "Women's Experiences," 160.

38. Psychological Aspects of Breast Cancer Study Group, "Psychological Response to Mastectomy," *Cancer* 59 (1987): 189–96, quotes 194.

39. J. R. Bloom, S. L. Stewart, , S. Chang, P. J. Banks, "Then and Now: Quality of Life of Young Breast Cancer Survivors," *Psycho-Oncology* 13 (2004): 147–60, quote 149. See also J. Brunet, J. Price, C. Harris, "Body Image in Women Diagnosed with Breast Cancer: A Grounded Theory Study," *Body Image* 41 (2022): 417–31; and T. Deshields, T. Tibbs, M.-Y. Fan, M. Taylor, "Differences in Patterns of Depression after Treatment for Breast Cancer," *Psycho-Oncology* 15 (2006): 398–406.

40. S. M. Rosenbery, L. S. Dominici, S. Gelber et al., "Association of Breast Cancer Surgery with Quality of Life and Psychological Well-being in Young Breast Cancer Survivors," *JAMA Surgery* 155 (2020): 1035–42.

41. Edward Delos Churchill papers, 1840–1973. H MS c62. Harvard Medical Library, Francis A. Countway Library of Medicine, Boston, MA, Box 6.

Chapter Fourteen

1. See Theodore Millon, *Masters of the Mind* (Hoboken: John Wiley & Sons, 2004), particularly chapter 1.

2. Millon, *Masters of the Mind*, 45.

3. Sabina Spielrein, "Sabina Spielrein: Psychoanalytic Studies," C. J. Wharton, trans., *Journal of Analytical Psychology* 46 (2001): 201–208, quote 205–206.

4. A primary source for Spielrein's early years was John Launer's fine biography *Sex Versus Survival: The Life and Ideas of Sabina Spielrein* (London: Duckworth Overlook, 2014).

5. B. Minder, "Burghölzli Hospital Records of Sabina Spielrein," Dorothea Steffens and Barbara Wharton, trans., *Journal of Analytical Psychology* 46 (2001): 15–41, quote 16.

6. Sigmund Freud, *The Standard Edition of the Complete Psychological Works of Sigmund Freud*, Vol. I (London: The Hogarth Press and the Institute of Psycho-Analysis London, 1999), 137.

7. Octave Mannoni, *Freud: The Theory of the Unconscious*, Renaud Bruce trans. (London: Verso, 1968, 2015), 34.

8. Sigmund Freud, *The Interpretation of Dreams*, A. A. Brill trans. (New York: The Macmillan Company, 1913), 480–81.

9. Sigmund Freud, "L'Hérédité et l'Etiologie des Névroses," *Revue Neurologique* 4 (1896): 161–69, quote 166.

10. Josef Breuer and Sigmund Freud, *Studies on Hysteria* (*Studien über Hysterie*), James Strachey, trans. (New York: Basic Books, 1957), 5–6.

11. Breuer and Freud, *Studies on Hysteria*, 255.

12. Breuer and Freud, *Studies on Hysteria*, 282. See also J. Bogousslavsky, and S. Dieguez, "Sigmund Freud and Hysteria: The Etiology of Psychoanalysis," in Julien Bogousslavsky, Ed., *Hysteria: The Rise of an Enigma* (Basel: Karger, 2014), 109–25.

13. Sigmund Freud, *Das Ich und das Es* (Leipzig: Internationaler Psychoanalytischer, 1923), 9.

14. C. G. Jung, *Psychology of the Unconscious*, Beatrice M. Hinkle, trans. (New York: Moffat, Yard and Company, 1917), vii.

15. Jung, *Unconscious*, ix.

16. Jung, *Unconscious*, xi.

17. As recounted in John Kerr, *A Most Dangerous Method* (New York: Vintage Books, 1994), 20. The quote was taken from Herbert Read, Michael Fordham, Gerhard Adler, and William McGuire Eds., R. F. C. Hall trans., *The Collected Works of C. G. Jung*, Vol. 4 (Princeton: Princeton University Press, 1953–1980), 21.

18. See M. Rampelli, "The Hysteric and the HSP," *Journal of Medical Humanities* 44 (2023): 145–65.

19. Kerr, *Dangerous Method*, 313.

20. Coline Covington and Barbara Wharton, Eds., *Sabina Spielrein, Forgotten Pioneer of Psychoanalysis* (London: Routledge, 2015), 121.

21. Aldo Carotenuto, *A Secret Symmetry* i Arno Pomerans, John Sheply, Krishna Winston, trans. (New York: Pantheon Books, 1982, 1984), 39.

22. Also translated as "Destruction as a Cause of Becoming." I will quote passages from her original *"Die Destrucktion als Ursache des Werdens" Jahrbuch für Psychoanalytische und Psychopathologische Forschungen* 4 (1912): 465–503 as translated by Stuart K. Witt, 1995.

23. Kerr, *Dangerous Method*, 320.

24. Spielrein "Die Destrucktion," 466.

25. Spielrein, "Die Destrucktion," 465.

26. Spielrein, "Die Destrucktion," 483.

27. Sabina Spielrein, "Unedited Extracts from a Diary," Pramila Bennett and Barbara Wharton, trans., *Journal of Analytical Psychology* 46 (2001): 155–71, quote 158.

28. Spielrein, "Unedited Extracts," 158.

29. Spielrein, "Psychoanalytic Studies," 205.

30. Carotenuto, *A Secret Symmetry*, 90 (italics hers).

31. C. G. Jung, "The Letters of C. G. Jung to Sabina Spielrein," Barbara Wharton, trans., *Journal of Analytical Psychology* 46 (2001): 173–99, quote 192.

32. Spielrein, "Unedited Extracts," 170.

33. See B. R. Skea, "Sabina Spielrein: Out from the Shadow of Jung and Freud," *Journal of Analytical Psychology* 51 (2006): 527–52.

34. Covington, *Sabina Spielrein*, both quotes 185.

35. Carotenuto, *A Secret Symmetry*, 70.

36. Carotenuto, *A Secret Symmetry*, 71.

37. Nancy J. Chodorow, *Femininities, Masculinities, Sexualities: Freud and Beyond* (Lexington: University Press of Kentucky, 1994), 1.

38. Chodorow, *Femininities*, 4.

39. Carotenuto, *A Secret Symmetry*, 39–40.

40. Covington, *Sabina Spielrein*, 202.

41. From Spielrein, "Contributions to the Knowledge of the Child's Soul," 1912, in Covington, *Sabina Spielrein*, 181.

42. S. Spielrein, "Kinderzeichnungen bei Offenen und Gleschlossenen Augen," *Imago* 17 (1931): 359–91.

43. Launer, *Sex Versus Survival*, 233.

44. Caroline Sturdy Colls, *Holocaust Archaeologies: Approaches and Future Directions* (Cham: Springer, 2015), 298.

45. Testimony of SS General Otto Ohlendorf, *Einsatzgruppe* D January 3, 1946, before the International Military Tribunal at Nuremberg, Nuremberg Trial Proceedings, Vol. 4, 319–320, at https://avalon.law.yale.edu/subject_menus/imt.asp, accessed July 25, 2023.

46. Covington, *Sabina Spielrein*, 185.

Chapter Fifteen

1. From Jürgen Thorwald, *The Patients* (New York; Harcourt Brace Jovanovich, Inc., 1972), 260. Louis Washkansky survived eighteen days following his heart transplant before dying of septic complications.

2. From Thorwald, *The Patients*, 345.

3. J. H. Warner, "The Aesthetic Grounding of Modern Medicine," *Bulletin of the History of Medicine* 88 (2014): 1–47, quote 46.

4. William Sasser, "A Passion to Heal," *Annals of Thoracic Surgery* 73 (2002): 11–14, quote 12.

5. Lewis Thomas, *The Youngest Science: Notes of a Medicine Watcher* (New York: Penguin Books, 1995), 13.

Bibliography

Achterberg, J. (1990). *Woman as Healer*. Boston: Shambhala Publications, Inc.

Adams, F. (1846). *The Seven Books of Paulus Aegineta, Vol II*. London: The Sydenham Society.

Allbutt, T. C. (1901). *Science and Medieval Thought*. London: C. J. Clay and Sons.

Allison, H. E. (1971). Kant's Transcendental Humanism. *The Monist*, 55:182–207.

Altpeter-Jones, K. (2009). Love Me, Hurt Me, Heal Me: Isolde Healer and Isolde Lover in Gottfried's "Tristan." *The German Quarterly*, 82:5–23.

Amundsen, D. W. (1978). Medieval Canon Law on Medical and Surgical Practice by the Clergy. *Bulletin of the History of Medicine*, 52:22–44.

Amundsen, D. W. (1982). Medicine and Faith in Early Christianity. *Bulletin of the History of Medicine*, 56:326–50.

Anderson, S. (2022). A Short History of Bernard Fisher's Contributions to Randomized Clinical Trials. *Clinical Trials*, 18:127–36.

Annaeus, C. L. (1881). *Cornuti Theologiae Graecae Compendium*. Toronto: Lipsia.

Anonymous. (1847). Females Attending Medical Lectures. *Boston Medical and Surgical Journal*, 37:405.

Anonymous. (1848). Female Physicians. *Buffalo Medical Journal*, 3:495–96.

Anonymous. (1867). Female Practitioners of Medicine. *Boston Medical and Surgical Journal*, 76:272–74.

Anonymous. (1886). *Leprosy in Hawaii, Extracts from Reports of Presidents of the Board of Health, Governement Physicians and Others, and from Official Records*. Honolulu: Daily Bulletin Stream Print Office.

Anonymous. (1902, June 3). Une Guérison à Lourdes. *Le Nouveliste*, p. 1.

Anonymous. (1915). *The Odes of Pindar*, John Sandys, trans. New York: The Macmillan Co.

Anonymous. (1960). *Father Damien Leper Apostle of Moloka'i*. Melbourne: The Australian Catholic Truth Society Record.

Anonymous. (2011). *The Bible: New International Version*. New York: Biblica.

Anwar, E. (2003). Ibn Sīnā's Philosophical Theology of Love: a Study of the Risālah fī al-'Ishq. *Islamic Studies*, 42:3311–54.

Apollodorus. (1921). *Bibliotheca* James George Frazier, trans. London: William Heineman.

The Apostolic Fathers (1985). Kirsopp Lake, trans. Cambridge: Harvard University Press.

Aquinas, T. (1961). *Commentary on the Metaphysics of Aristotle*, John P. Rowan, trans. Chicago: Henry Regnery Company.

Aristophanes. (1907). *The Comedies of Aristophanes Vol VI*, Benjamin Bickley Rogers, trans. London: George Bell & Sons.

Aristotle. (1907). *De Anima*, R. D. Hicks, trans. Cambridge: Cambridge University Press.

Aristotle. (1908). *Politics*, Benjamin Jowett, trans. Oxford: Clarendon Press.

Arnold, M. (1883). *Mixed Essays Irish Essays and Others*. New York: Macmillan and Company.

Askitopoulas, H., Konsolaki, E., & Ramoutsaki, I. A. (2002). Surgical Cures Under Sleep Induction in the Asclepeion of Epidauros. *International Congress Series*, 1242:11–17.

Aslan, R. (2013). *Zealot*. New York: Random House.

Avicenna. (1973). *The Canon of Medicine*. New York: AMS Press, Inc.

Baring-Gould, S. (1898). *The Lives of the Saints, Vol 2*. London: John C. Nimmo.

Beall, O. T., & Shryock, R. H. (1953). Cotton Mather: The First Significant Figure in American Medicine. *Proceedings of the American Antiquarian Society*, 63:37–274.

Benson, E. W. (1897). *Cyprian: His Life, His Times, His Work*. New York: D. Appleton and Company.

Bernabeo, R. A. (1994). The Consilium ad Calcolum of Alberto de' Zancari. *American Journal of Nephrology*, 14:313–16.

Biernoff, S. (2010). Flesh Poems: Henry Tonks and the Art of Surgery. *Visual Culture in Britain*, 11:25–47.

Bigelow, H. J. (1846). Insensitivity During Surgical Operations Produced by Inhalation. *Boston Medical and Surgical Journal*, 35:309–17.

Bishop, S. E. (1888). *Why Are the Hawaiians Dying Out?* Honolulu: Honolulu Social Science Association.

Black, E. (1989). *The Sacred Pipe*, Joseph Epes Brown, Ed. Norman: University of Oklahoma Press.

Blackwell, E. (1856). *Address on the Medical Education of Women*. New York: Baker & Duyckinck.

Blaisdell, K. (1993). Historical and Cultural Aspects of Native Hawaiian Health. In P. Manicas, *Social Process in Hawaii: A Reader* (pp. 37–57). New York: McGraw Hill.

Bliss, M. (1999). *William Osler: A Life in Medicine*. Toronto: University of Toronto Press.

Bloom, J. R., Chang, S. L., & Banks, P. J. (2004). Then and Now: Quality of Life of Young Breast Cancer Survivors. *Psycho-Oncology*, 13:147–60.

Boccaccio, G. (1886). *The Decameron of Giovanni Boccaccio*, John Payne, trans.. London: Villon Society.

Bogousslavsky, J., & Dieguez, S. (2014). Sigmund Freud and Hysteria: The Etiology of Psychoanalysis. In J. Bogousslavsky, *Hysteria: The Rise of an Enigma* (pp. 109–25). Basel: Karger.

Boylston, Z. (1730). *An Historical Account of the Small-Pox Inoculated in New England*. London: S. Chandler.

Bradford, W. (1898). *Bradford's History "Of Plimoth Plantation."* Boston: Weight & Potter.

Brain, P. (1977). Galen on the Ideal of the Physician. *South African Medical Journal*, 52:936–38.

Breuer, J., & Freud, S. (1957). *Studies on Hysteria (Studien über Hysterie)*, James Strachey, trans. New York: Basic Books.

Brian, T. (1679). *The Pisse-Prophet, or, Certain Pisse-Pot Lectures*. London: S & B Griffin.

Brooke, J. L., & Larsen, C. S. (2014). The Nurture of Nature: Epigenetics and Environment in Human Biohistory. *American Historical Review*, 119:1500–13.

Brown, D. (1970). *Bury My Heart at Wounded Knee*. New York: Henry Holt and Company.

Brunet, J., Price, J., & Harris, C. (2022). Body Image in Women Diagnosed with Breast Cancer: A Grounded Theory Study. *Body Image*, 42:417–31.

Burris, D. G., Welling, D. R., & Rich, N. M. (2004). Dominique Jean Larrey and the Principle of Humanity in Warfare. *Journal of the American College of Surgeons*, 198:831–35.

Burrow, G. N. (1991). The Trial and Tribulation of Egerton Yorrick Davis. *Western Journal of Medicine*, 155:80–82.

Burton, R. (1836). *The Anatomy of Melancholy*. London: B. Blake.

Bushnell, O. A. (1993). *The Gifts of Civilization*. Honolulu: University of Hawaii Press.

Byzantius, S. (1849). *Ethnica*, Augustus Meineke, trans. Berlin: Berolini.

Cabré, M. (2008). Women or Healers? Household Practices and the Categories of Health Care in Late Medieval Iberia. *Bulletin of the History of Medicine*, 82:16–51.

Cancer, S. G. (1987). Psychological Responses to Mastectomy. *Cancer*, 59:189–96.

Carotenuto, A. (1982, 1984). *A Secret Symmetry*, Arno Pomerans, John Sheply, Krishna Winston, trans. New York: Pantheon Books.

Carrel, A. (1902). Anastomose Bout a Bout de la Jugulaire et la Carotide Primitive. *Lyon Médical*, 114–16.

Carrel, A. (1902). La Technique Opératoire des Anastomoses Vasculaires et la Transplantation des Viscères. *Lyon Médical*, 98:859–64.

Carrel, A. (1935, 1939). *Man the Unknown*. New York: Harper & Brothers.

Carrel, A. (1941, January 1). Prayer Is Power. *Readers's Digest*, pp. 104–106.

Carrel, A. (1949). *Le Voyage de Lourdes*. Paris: Plon Bibliothèque.

Carrel, A. (1950). *Réflexions sur la Conduite de la Vie*. Paris: Librairie Plon.

Carrel, A. (1956). *Jours Apres Jours*. Paris: Librairie Plon.

Cash, P., Christianson, E. H., & Estes, J. W. (1980). *Medicine in Colonial Massachusetts 1620–1820*. Boston: The Colonial Society of Massachusetts.

Castelli, H., & Rothstein, M. (2019). The Skills of Hecamede: Women as Caregivers in Archaic and Classical Greece. In A. Hugon, C. Plumauzille, & M. Rossigneux-Mehéust, *Gender and the History of Care Work* (pp. 25–44). Paris: Editions Belin.

Celsus. (1938). *De Medicina VII*, W. G. Spencer, trans. Cambridge: Harvard University Press.

Charcot, J.-M. (1897). *La Foi Qui Guérit*. Paris: Félix Alcan.

Chesney, A. M. (1943). *The Johns Hopkins Hospital and the Johns Hopkins University School of Medicine: A Chronicle Vol I*. Baltimore: The Johns Hopkins Press.

Chesterton, G. K. (1908, 1936, 1959). *Orthodoxy*. New York: Image Books.

Chodorow, N. J. (1994). *Femininities, Masculinities, Sexualities: Freud and Beyond*. Lexington: University Press of Kentucky.

Christopoulou-Alerta, H., Togia, A., & Varlam, C. (2010). The "Smart" Asclepion: A Total Healing Environment. *Archives of Hellenic Medicine*, 27:259–63.

Churchill, E. D. (1940). Graduate Training in Surgery at the Massachusetts General Hospital. *Harvard Med Alum Bull*, 14:28–36.

Churchill, E. D. (1947). Science and Humanism in Surgery. *Annals of Surgery*, 126:381–96.

Churchill, E. D. (1960). Origins of American Surgery. *J Am Med Assoc*, 172:219–22.

Churchill, E. D. (1963). Should I Study Medicine? *N Engl J Med*, 268:537–39.

Churchill, E. D. (1990). *Wanderjahr: The Education of a Surgeon*. Boston: Francis A. Countway Library of Medicine.

Cicero. (1966). *Tusculan Disputations*, J. E. King, trans. Cambridge: Harvard University Press.

Clarke, C. C. (1931). Henri de Mondeville. *Yale Journal of Biology and Medicine*, 3:459–81.

Cleveland, G. H., & Wells, F. C. (1896). A Discussion Upon the Medical and Surgical Aspects of Appendicitis. *Chicago Clinical Review*, 5:617–44.

Colls, C. S. (2015). *Holocaust Archaeologies: Approaches and Future Directions*. Cham: Springer.

Comte, A. (1908). *A General View of Positivism*, J. H. Bridges, trans. London: George Routledge & Sons.

Copson, A. (2015). What Is Humanism? In A. C. Grayling, *The Wiley Blackwell Handbook of Humanism* (pp. 1–33). Chichester: John Wiley and Sons.

Covington, C., & Wharton, B. (2015). *Sabina Spielrein: Forgotten Pioneer of Psychoanalysis*. London: Routledge.

Coxe, A. C. (1905). The Apostolic Fathers with Justin Martyr and Irenaeus. In A. Roberts, & J. Donaldson, *Ante-Nicene Fathers, Vol I* (pp. 159–308). New York: Charles Scribner's Sons.

Coxe, J. R. (1846). *The Writings of Hippocrates and Galen*. Philadelphia: Lindsay and Blakiston.

Crick, F. (1995). *The Astonishing Hypothesis*. New York: Scribner.

Crislip, A. (2013). *Thorns of the Flesh*. Philadelphia: University of Pennsylvania Press.

Cushing, H. (1925). *The Life of Sir William Osler Vol I and II*. Oxford: Clarendon Press.

Cushing, H. (1933). Medicine at the Crossroads. *Journal of the American Medical Association*, 100:1567–75.

Cushing, H. (1936). *From a Surgeon's Journal: 1915–1918*. London: Constable & Co.

Davies, T. (1997). *Humanism*. London: Routledge Press.

Daws, G. (1973). *Holy Man*. New York: Harper & Row.

de Chauliac, G. (1586). *Chirurgia Magna*. Lyon: Beraud Symphorien.

de Veuster, P. (1889). *Life and Letters of Father Damien*. London: The Catholic Truth Society.

Demaitre, L. (1975). Theory and Practice in Medical Education at the University of Montpellier in the Thirteenth and Fourteenth Centuries. *Journal of the History of Medicine and Allied Sciences*, 30:103–23.

DeMallie, R. J. (1984). *The Sixth Grandfather*. Lincoln: University of Nebraska Press.

Deshields, T., Tibbs, T., Fan, M.-Y., & Taylor, M. (2006). Differences in Patterns of Depression after Treatment for Breast Cancer. *Psycho-Oncology*, 15:398–406.

Devlin, J. (1987). *The Superstitious Mind: French Peasants and the Supernatural in the Nineteenth Century*. New Haven: Yale University Press.

Dible, J. (1959). D. J. Larrey, a Surgeon of the Revolution, Consulate, and Empire. *Medical History*, 3:100–107.

Dickinson, E. (1979). *The Poems of Emily Dickinson*. Ralph W. Franklin, Ed. Cambridge: Harvard University Press.

Doody, M. A. (1988). *Frances Burney: The Life and Works*. New Brunswick: Rutgers University Press.

Drabkin, I. E. (1944). Medical Education in Greece and Rome. *Bulletin of the History of Medicine*, 15:333–51.

Edelstein, E. J., & Edelstein, L. (1998). *Asclepius: Collection and Interpretation of the Testimonies*. Baltimore: Johns Hopkins University Press.

Edelstein, L. (1952). The Relation of Ancient Philosophy to Medicine. *Bulletin of the History of Medicine*, 26:299–316.

Edmonson, J. M. (1986). *Nineteenth Century Surgical Instruments*. Cleveland: Cleveland Health Sciences Library.

Emecoff, N. C., Curlin, F. A., Buddadhumaruk, P., & White, D. B. (2015). Health Care Professionals' Responses to Religious or Spiritual Statements by Surrogate

Decision Makers During Goals-of-Care Discussions. *JAMA Internal Medicine*, 175:1662–69.

Engel, G. L. (2012). The Need for a New Model: A Challenge for Biomedicine. *Psychodynamic Psychiatry*, 40:377–96.

Enochs, R. (1996). *The Jesuit Mission to the Lakota Sioux*. Kansas City: Sheed & Ward.

Ferngren, G. B. (2009). *Medicine & Health Care in Early Christianity*. Baltimore: Johns Hopkins Press.

Fisher, B., Wolmark, N., Redmond, C. et al. (1981). Findings from NSABP Protocol No. B-04: Comparison of Radical Mastectomy with Alternative Treatments. II. The Clinical and Biologic Significance of Medial-Central Breast Cancers. *Cancer*, 48:1863–72.

Fitzharris, L. (2017). *The Butchering Art*. New York: Scientific American.

Flint, P. B. (1990, September 18). Dr. Cushman D. Haagensen, 90; Specialist Advocated Mastectomy. *New York Times*, p. 10.

Fornander, A. (1919–1920). *Hawaiian Antiquities and Folk-Lore*. Honolulu: Bishop Museum Press.

François, B., S. E., & Fee, E. (2014). The Lourdes Medical Cures Revisited. *J Hist Med Allied Sci*, 69:135–62.

Frankl, V. E. (1984). *Man's Search for Meaning*. New York: Washington Square Press.

Freud, S. (1896). L'Hérédité et l'Etiologie des Névroses. *Revue Neurologique*, 4:161–69.

Freud, S. (1913). *The Interpretation of Dreams*, A. A. Brill, trans. New York: The Macmillan Company.

Freud, S. (1923). *Das Ich und das Es*. Leipzig: Internationaler Psychoanalytischer.

Freud, S. (1961). *The Future of an Illusion*, James Strachey, trans. New York: W.W. Norton & Co.

Freud, S. (1999). *The Standard Edition of the Complete Psychological Works of Sigmund Freud, Vol I*. London: The Hogarth Press and the Institute of Psycho-Analysis London.

Freudenthal, G., & Kottek, S. (2003). *Mélanges d'Histoire de la Médecine Hébraïque*. Leiden: Brill.

Galen. (1068). *On the Usefulness of the Parts of the Body*, Margaret Tallmadge, trans. Ithaca: Cornell University Press.

Galen. (1528). *Claudii Galeni Pergameni Secundum Hippocratem*. Paris: Simon Colinae.

Galen. (1550). *Claudii Galeni Pergameni Introductio in Pulsus ad Teutham*. Venice: Lugduni.

Galen. (1923). *Claudii Galeni Opera Omnia*, Carl Kühn, Ed. Liepzig.

Galen. (1952). *On the Natural Faculties*, John Brock, trans. Cambridge: Harvard University Press.

Galen. (1991). *On the Therapeutic Method*, R. J. Hankinson, trans. Oxford: Clarendon Press.

Galen. (2011). *Methods of Medicine III*, Ian Johnston and G. H. R. Horsley, trans. Cambridge: Harvard University Press.

Galen. (2014). *Commentary on Hippocrates' Epidemics, Book I, Parts I–III*, Uwe Vagelpohl, trans.. Berlin: Walter de Gruyter.

Gavorse, J. (1934). *The Complete Writings of Thucydides, The Peloponnesian War*. New York: The Modern Library.

Gerber, D. E. (1978). The Female Breast in Greek Erotic Literature. *Arethusa*, 11:203–12.

Ghosh, S. K. (2015). Henri de Mondeville (1260–1320): Medieval French Anatomist and Surgeon. *European Journal of Anatomy*, 19:309–14.

Ghosh, S. K. (2015). Human Cadaver Dissection: A Historical Account from Ancient Greece to the Modern Era. *Anatomy and Cell Biology*, 48:153–69.

Gilmore, M. R. (1919). *Uses of Plants by the Indians of the Missouri River Region*. Washington, DC: Government Printing Office.

Gluckman, P. D., & Hanson, M. A. (2009). Developmental Plasticity and the Developmental Origins of Health and Disease. In J. P. Newnham & M. G. Ross, *Early Life Origins of Human Health and Disease* (pp. 1–10). Basel: Karger.

Golden, R. L. (2015). Paul Revere Osler: The Other Child. *Proceedings Baylor University Medical Center*, 28:21–24.

Gordon, E. C. (1986). Child Health in the Middle Ages as Seen in the Miracles of Five English Saints, A.D. 1150–1220. *Bulletin of the History of Medicine*, 60:502–22.

Gregory, B. (1916). *History of the Franks*. New York: Columbia University Press.

Grillo, H. C. (2004). Edward D. Churchill and the "Rectangular" Surgical Residency. *Surgery*, 136:947–52.

Haagensen, C. D. (1971). *Diseases of the Breast*. Philadelphia: W.B. Saunders Company.

Halsted, W. S. (1885). Practical Comments on the Use and Abuse of Cocaine. *New York Medical Journal*, 42:294–95.

Halsted, W. S. (1894). The Results of Operations for the Cure of Cancer of the Breast Performed at the Johns Hopkins Hospital from June, 1889 to January, 1894. *Annals of Surgery*, 20:497–555.

Handy, E. S. (1927). *Polynesian Religion*. Honolulu: Bernice P. Bishop Museum.

Hankinson, R. J. (1991). Galen's Anatomy of the Soul. *Phronesis*, 36:197–233.

Harrell, G. T. (1979). Lady Osler. *Bulletin of the History of Medicine*, 53:81–99.

Hebrew-English Tanakh. (2009). Skokie: Varda Books.

Helling, T. S. (2022). Alexis Carrel and His Voyage of Discovery. *Journal of Religion and Health*, 61:4565–84.

Herbermann, C. G. (1910). *The Catholic Encyclopedia Vol 2*. New York: The Encyclopedia Press.

Herbermann, C. G. et al., Eds., (1908, 1913). *The Catholic Encyclopedia, Vol 4*. New York: The Encyclopedia Press.

Herodotus. (1862). *History of Herodotus Vol II*, George Rawlinson, trans. London: John Murray.

Hesiod. (2006). *Theogony Works and Days Testimonia*, Glenn W. Most, trans. Cambridge: Harvard University Press.

Hewitt, N. (1988). Feminist Friends: Agrarian Quakers and the Emergence of Woman's Rights in America. *Feminist Studies*, 12:27–94.

Hildegard. (1855). S. Hildegardis Abbatissae Opera Omnia, J-P. Migne, trans. In J.-P. Migne, *Patrologiae Cursus Completus Vol 187* (pp. 162, 227). Paris: Garnier.

Hildegard. (1903). *Causae et Curae*, Paulus Kaiser, Ed. Leipzig: B. G. Teubneri.

Hildegard. (1985). *Illuminations of Hildegard of Bingen*, Matthew Fox, Ed. Rochester: Bear & Company.

Hildegard. (1990). *Scivias*, Columbia Hart and Jane Bishop, trans. New York: Paulist Press.

Hildegard. (1994). *The Letters of Hildegard of Bingen Vol I*, Joseph L. Baird and Radd K. Ehrman, trans. Oxford: Oxford University Press.

Hildegard. (2004). *The Letters of Hildegard of Bingen Vol III*, Joseph L. Baird and Radd K. Ehrman, trans. Oxford: Oxford University Press.

Hippocrates. (1595). *The Hippocratic Oath in Greek and Latin*. Frankfurt: Claudium Marnium.

Hippocrates. (1943). *Hippocrates II*, W. H. S. Jones trans. Cambridge: Harvard University Press.

Hippocrates. (1957). *Hippocrates I*, W. H. S. Jones, trans. Cambridge: Harvard University Press.

Hippocrates. (1959). *Hippocrates IV "The Nature of Man,"* W. H. S. Jones, trans. Cambridge: Harvard University Press.

Hippocrates. (1961–62). *Oeuvres Complètes d'Hippocrates*, É Littré, trans. IX. Amsterdam: Adolf M. Hakkert.

Hippocrates. (1994). *Hippocrates* Wesley D. Smith, trans. Cambridge: Harvard University Press.

Homer. (1988). *Iliad*, A. T. Murray, trans. Cambridge: Harvard University Press.

Homer. (1995). *Odyssey*, A. T. Murray, trans. Cambridge: Harvard University Press.

Hurt, W. R., & Howard, J. H. (1952). A Dakota Conjuring Ceremony. *Southwestern Journal of Anthropology*, 8:286–96.

Huxley, L. (1908). *Life and Letters of Thomas Henry Huxley, Vol I*. London: Macmillan and Co.

Imber, G. (2010). *Genius on the Edge*. New York: Kaplan Publishing.

Irving, J. (2012). Restituta: The Training of the Female Physician. *Melbourne Historical Journal*, 40:45–57.

Jackson, S. W. (2001). The Wounded Healer. *Bulletin of the History of Medicine*, 75:1–36.

James, W. (1917). *The Varieties of Religious Experiences*. New York: Longmans, Green and Co.

Josephus, F. (1892). *Antiquitates Judaicae*, B. Niese, Ed. Berlin: Weidmann.

Josselyn, J. (1672). *New-England Rarities Discovered*. London: G. Widdowes.

Jouanna, J. (2012). *Greek Medicine from Hippocrates to Galen*. Leiden: Brill.

Jung, C. G. (1917). *Psychology of the Unconscious*, Beatrice M. Hinkle, trans. New York: Moffat, Yard and Company.

Jung, C. G. (1983, 2013). *The Essential Jung*. Princeton: Princeton University Press.

Jung, C. G. (2001). The Letters of C. G. Jung to Sabina Spielrein, Barbara Wharton, trans. *Journal of Analytical Psychology*, 46:173–99.

Kamakau, S. M. (1961). *Ruling Chiefs of Hawaii*. Honolulu: Kamehameha Schools Press.

Kaufman, S. K. (2005). *Consuming Vision: Mass Culture and the Lourdes Shrine*. Ithaca: Cornell University Press.

Kelen, S. (2017). The 100th Anniversary of the Death of Edward Revere Osler, 1895–1917. *The Osler Library Newsletter*, 127:4–5.

Keresztes, P. (1967). The Massacre at Lugdunum in 177 A.D. *Historia: Zeitschrift für Alte Geschichte*, 16:75–86.

Kerr, J. (1994). *A Most Dangerous Method*. New York: Vintage Books.

Keys, T. E. (1964). Edward Revere Osler 1895–1917. *Archives of Internal Medicine*, 114:284–93.

Kibre, P. (1953). The Faculty of Medicine at Paris, Charlatanism, and Unlicensed Medical Practice in the Later Middle Ages. *Bulletin of the History of Medicine*, 27:1–20.

Kierkegaard, S. (1941). *The Sickness Unto Death*. Princeton: Princeton University Press.

Kipling, R. (1899, February 12). The White Man's Burden. *McClure's Magazine*, p. 290.

Kipling, R. (1928). Surgeons and the Soul. In R. Kipling, *A Book of Words* (pp. 223–28). London: Macmillan and Co.

Kittredge, G. L. (1912). *Letters of Samuel Lee and Samuel Sewall Related to New England and the Indians*. Cambridge: The Colonial Society of Massachusetts.

Kristeller, P. O. (1945). The School of Salerno: Its Development and Its Contribution to the History of Learning. *Bulletin of the History of Medicine*, 17:138–94.

Lacassagne, A. (1894). *L'Assassinat du Président Carnot*. Lyon: A. Stork.

Langon, J. W. (1978). The Jesuits and French Education: A Comparative Study of Two Schools 1852–1913. *Hist Ed Q*, 18:49–66.

Largus, S. (1529). *De Compositione Medicamentorum*. Paris: Andreas Cratander.

Larrey, D. J. (1812). *Mémoires de Chirurgie Militaire, et Campagnes de D. J. Larrey, Tome I*. Paris: J. Smith.

Launer, J. (2014). *Sex Versus Survival: The Life and Ideas of Sabina Spielrein*. London: Duckworth Overlook.

Law, A. S. (2012). *Kalaupapa: A Collective Memory*. Honolulu: University of Hawai'i Press.

Léonard, J. (1977). Femmes, Religion et Médecine. *Ann Econ Soc Civ*, 32:887–907.

Leriche, R. (1956). *Souvenirs de Ma Vie Morte*. Paris: Éditions du Seuil.

Lewison, E. F. (1950). Saint Agatha: The Patron Saint of Diseases of the Breast in Legend and Art. *Bulletin of the History of Medicine*, 24:409–29.

Liddell, G., & Scott, W. (1940). *A Greek-English Lexicon*. Oxford: Clarendon Press.

Lindberg, D. C. (1983). Science and the Early Christian Church. *Isis*, 74:509–30.

Littré, É. (1853). *Oeuvres Complètes d'Hippocrate*. Paris: J. B. Baillière.

Longshore, J. S. (1850). *An Introductory Lecture: Delivered Before the Class, at the Opening of the Female Medical College of Pennsylvania: October 12th, 1850*. Philadelphia: James Young.

Malpezzi, F. M. (2001). Evergreen: The Enduring Voice of a Nine-Hundred-Year-Old Healer. In E. Brady, *Healing Logic: Culture and Medicine in Modern Health Belief Systems* (pp. 163–79). Logan: Utah State University Press.

Mannoni, O. (1968, 2015). *Freud: The Theory of the Unconscious*, Renaud Bruce, trans. London: Verso.

Marshall, C. (1897). *The Women's Medical College of Pennsylvania*. Philadelphia: P. Blakiston, Son & Company.

Martyr, J. (1948, 1965, 1977, 2008). *The Fathers of the Church Vol 6*, Thomas B. Falls, Ed. Washington, DC: Catholic University of America Press.

Mather, C. (1072). *The Angel of Bethesda*. Barre: American Antiquarian Society.

Mather, C. (1702). *Magnalia Christi Americana I*. London: Thomas Parkhurst.

Mather, C. (1815). *The Christian Philosopher*. Charlestown: J. McKown.

Mather, C. (1868). *The Mather Papers*. Boston: Collections of the Massachusetts Historical Society, Fourth Series, Vol VIII.

Mather, C. (1911). *Diary of Cotton Mather, 1681–1708 Vol I*. Boston: Massachusetts Historical Society.

Mather, C. (1912). *Diary of Cotton Mather, 1709–1724 Vol 2*. Boston: Massachusetts Historical Society.

Mather, C. (1967). *An Essay . . . To Do Good*. Gainesville: Scholars' Facsimile Reprints.

Matten, S. (2011). Galen and His Patients. *Lancet*, 378:478–79.

Mazur, A. (1986). Trends in Feminine Beauty and Overadaptation. *The Journal of Sex Research*, 22:281–303.

McVaugh, M. (2000). Surgical Education in the Middle Ages. *Dynamis*, 20:283–304.

McVaugh, M. (2017). When Universities First Encountered Surgery. *Journal of the History of Medicine and Allied Sciences*, 72:6–20.

Mead, M. (1976). Towards a Human Science. *Science*, 191:903–909.

Meigs, C. D. (1848). *Females and Their Diseases: A Series of Letters to His Class*. Philadelphia: Lea and Blanchard.

Millon, T. (2004). *Masters of the Mind*. Hoboken: John Wiley & Sons.

Minder, B. (2001). Burghölzli Hospital Records of Sabina Spielrein, Dorothea Steffens and Barbara Wharton, trans. *Journal of Analytical Psychology*, 46:15–41.

Mironidou-Tzouveleki, M., & Tzitzis, P. M. (2014). Medical Practice Applied in the Ancient Asclepion in Kos Island. *Hellenic Journal of Nuclear Medicine*, 17:167–70.

Moblo, P. (1998). Institutionalizing the Leper: Partisan Politics and the Evolution of Stigma in Post-Monarchy Hawai'i. *Journal of Polynesian Society*, 107:229–62.

Mooney, J. (1891). *The Sacred Formulas of the Cherokees*. Washington, DC: United States Bureau of American Ethnology.

Mooney, J. (1991). *The Ghost-Dance Religion and the Sioux Outbreak of 1890*. Lincoln: University of Nebraska Press.

Moore, F. D. (1973). Edward Delos Churchill 1895–1972. *Annals of Surgery*, 177:507–508.

Morantz-Sanchez, R. (1985, 2000). *Sympathy and Science: Women Physicians in American Medicine*. Chapel Hill: University of North Carolina Press.

Morgan, E. S. (1942). The Puritans and Sex. *The New England Quarterly*, 15:591–607.

Morgan, E. S. (1946). The Diary of Michael Wigglesworth. *Transactions Colonial Society of Massachusetts*, 35:311–444.

Morton, S. G. (1839). *Crania Americana*. Philadelphia: J. Dobson.

Moulinier, L. (1989). La Botanique d'Hildegard de Bingen. *Médiévales*, 18/17:113–29.

Mukherjee, S. (2010). *The Emperor of All Maladies*. New York: Scribner.

Neihardt, J. G. (1932, 1969, 1972). *Black Elk Speaks*. Lincoln: University of Nebraska Press.

Neill, E. D. (1872). *Dakota Land and Dakota Life*. Minneapolis: Minnesota Historical Society.

Neuburger, M. (1944). An Historical Survey of the Concept of Nature from a Medieval Viewpoint. *Isis*, 35:16–28.

Nicaise, É. (1890). *La Grande Chirurgie de Guy de Chauliac*. Paris: Félix Alcan.

Nicaise, É. (1893). *Chirurgie de Maitre Henri de Mondeville*. Paris: Félix Alcan.

Nimura, J. P. (2021). *The Doctors Blackwell*. New York: W.W. Norton & Company.

Normandin, S. (2005). *Visions of Vitalism: Medicine Philosophy and the Soul in Nineteenth Century France*. Montreal: PhD diss (McGill University).

Nossov, K. (2009). *Gladiator: Rome's Bloody Spectacle*. Oxford: Osprey Publishing.

Nunn, D. B. (2006). Dr. Halsted's Addiction. *Johns Hopkins Advanced Studies in Medicine*, 6:106–108.

Nussbaum, F. L. (1953). *The Triumph of Science and Reason*. New York: Harper & Row.

Nutton, V. (1973). The Chronology of Galen's Early Career. *Classical Quarterly*, 23:158–71.

Olsen, J. S. (2002). *Bathsheba's Breast*. Baltimore: Johns Hopkins University Press.

Origen. (1990). *Homilies on Leviticus 1–16*. Washington, DC: Catholic University Press.

Osborne, M. P. (2007). William Stewart Halsted: His Life and Contributions to Surgery. *Lancet Oncology*, 8:256–65.

Osler, W. (1871). Carcinoma Mammae: Removal by Excision. *Canada Medical Journal*, 8:107–109.

Osler, W. (1884). Letter from Leipzig. *Canada Med Surg J*, 13:18–22.

Osler, W. (1890). Letters to My House Physicians. *NY Med J*, 52:333–34.

Osler, W. (1892). *The Principles and Practice of Medicine*. New York: D. Appleton and Company.

Osler, W. (1893). *Physic and Physicians as Depicted in Plato*. Boston: Damrell & Upham.

Osler, W. (1895). Teaching and Thinking. *Montreal Medical Journal*, 23:561–72.

Osler, W. (1904). The Master Word in Medicine. *Johns Hopkins Hospital Bulletin*, 15:1–19.

Osler, W. (1910). *Aequanimitas*. Philadelphia: P. Blakiston's Sons & Co.

Osler, W. (1919). The Old Humanities and the New Science. *British Medical Journal*, 2:1–7.

Ostler, J. (2001). "The Last Buffalo Hunt" and Beyond: Plains Sioux Economic Strategies in the Early Reservation Period. *Great Plains Quarterly*, 21:115–30.

Pagel, J. (1892). *Die Chirurgie des Heinrich von Mondeville*. Berlin: Hirschwald.

Paget, J. (1854). *Lectures on Surgical Pathology*. Philadelphia: Lindsay & Blakiston.

Paget, J. (1856). On the Average Duration of Life in Patients with Scirrhous Cancer of the Breast. *Lancet*, 1:62–63.

Palmer, D. R. (2022). *The Gospel of Luke*. Self-published.

Pausanias. (1933). *Description of Greece, II*, W.H.S. Jones, trans. London: G. P. Putnam's Sons.

Pausanias. (1933). *Description of Greece, III*, W.H.S. Jones, trans.. London: G. P. Putnam's Sons.

Peitzman, S. J. (2003). Why Support a Women's Medical College? Philadelphia's Early Male Medical Pro-Feminists. *Bulletin of the History of Medicine*, 77:576–99.

Perkins, W. (1611). *A Salve for a Sicke Man*. London: John Legat.

Petit, J.-L. (1844). *Oeuvres Complètes*. Paris: Frédéric Prévost.

Pham, H. (2015). Historiography on the Social Status of the Ancient Physician Since Ludwig Edelstein. *Journal of the Southern Association for the History of Medicine*, 1:1–21.

Pilcher, J. E. (1895). Guy de Chauliac and Henri de Mondeville: A Surgical Retrospective. *Annals of Surgery*, 12:84–102.

Plato. (1894). *Plato's Republic*, B. Jowett and Lewis Cambell, Eds. Oxford: Clarendon Press.

Plato. (1914). *Euthyphro, Apology, Crito, Phaedo, Phaedrus*, Harold North Fowler, trans. Cambridge: Harvard University Press.

Pliny. (1856). *The Natural History of Pliny Vol V*, John Bostock and H. T. Riley, trans. London: G. Bell & Sons.

Pollenz, P. (1950). Changes in the Form and Function of Hawaiian Hulas. *American Anthropologist*, 52:225–34.

Pormann, P. E. (2010). Medical Education in Late Antiquity from Alexandria to Montpellier. In P. E. Pormann, *Hippocrates and Medical Education* (pp. 419–41). Leiden: Brill.

Porterfield, A. (2005). *Healing in the History of Christianity*. Oxford: Oxford University Press.

Powers, W. K. (1982). *Yuwipi*. Lincoln: University of Nebraska Press.

Quesnay, F. (1744). *Recherches Critiques et Historiques sur l'Origine, sur les Divers Etats et sur les Progrès de la Chirurgie en France*. Paris: Charles Osmont.

Quinlan, M. (1909). *Damien of Molokai*. London: MacDonald and Evans.

Ragsdale, W. (1874, January 27). *Ka Nuhou Hawaii*, p. 4.

Rampelli, M. (2023). The Hysteric and the HSP. *Journal of Medical Humanities*, 44:145–65.

Rashdall, H. (1895). *The Universities of Europe in the Middle Ages*. Oxford: Clarendon Press.

Read, H., Fordham, M., Adler, G., & McGuire, W. (1953–1980). *The Collected Works of C. G. Jung, Vol 4*, R.F.C. Hall, trans. Princeton: Princeton University Press.

Reggiani, A. H. (2007). *God's Eugenicist*. New York: Berghahn Books.

Reid, E. G. (1931). *The Great Physician*. London: Oxford University Press.

Rein, E. (1995). The Devil, the Body, and the Feminine Soul in Puritan New England. *Journal of American History*, 82:15–36.

Richardson, R. G. (1977). Larrey: What Manner of Man? *Proceedings of the Royal Society of Medicine*, 70:490–94.

Roberts, A., & Donaldson, J. (1919). *Ante-Nicene Fathers, Vol 5*. New York: Charles Scribner's Sons.

Rohrbach, P.-T. (1966). *Journey to Carith*. Washington, DC: ICS Publications.

Rosenbaum, M. E., & Roos, G. M. (2000). Women's Experiences of Breast Cancer. In A. S. Kasper, & S. J. Ferguson, *Breast Cancer: Sociey Shapes an Epidemic* (pp. 153–81). New York: St. Martin's Press.

Rosenberg, S. M., Dominici, L. S., Gelber, S. et al. (2020). Association of Breast Cancer Surgery with Quality of Life and Psychological Well-being in Young Breast Cancer Survivors. *JAMA Surgery*, 155:1035–42.

Rowland, B. (1981). *Medieval Woman's Guide to Health*. Kent: Kent State University Press.

Rutkow, I. M. (1980). The Letters of William Halsted and Alexis Carrel. *Surg Gynecol Obstet*, 151:676–88.

Rutkow, I. M. (2000). On Scalpels and Bistouries. *Archives of Surgery*, 135:360.

Sasser, W. (2002). A Passion to Heal. *Annals of Thoracic Surgery*, 73:11–14.

Scarborough, J. (1970). Romans and Physicians. *The Classical Journal*, 296–306.

Schroeder, B., & Benso, S. (2008). *Levinas and the Ancients*. Bloomington: Indiana University Press.

Schroeder, H. J. (1937). *Disciplinary Decrees of the General Councils: Text, Translation and Commentary*. Saint Louis: B. Herder Book Co.

Sebastien, N. (2005). *Visions of Vitalism: Medicine, Philosophy and the Soul in Nineteenth Century France*. Montreal: Doctoral Dissertation McGill University.

Segal, B. S. (1986). *Love, Medicine & Miracles*. New York: Harper & Row.

Shrewsbury, J. F. (1950). The Plague of Athens. *Bulletin of the History of Medicine*, 24:1–25.

Singer, C. (1922). *Greek Biology & Greek Medicine*. Oxford: Clarendon Press.

Singer, C. (1956). *Galen on Anatomical Procedures*. London: Oxford University Press.

Siraisi, N. G. (1990). *Medieval & Early Renaissance Medicine*. Chicago: University of Chicago Press.

Siraisi, N. G. (2019). *Taddeo Alderotti and His Pupils*. Princeton: Princeton University Press.

Skea, B. R. (2006). Sabina Spielrein: Out from the Shadow of Jung and Freud. *Journal of Analytical Psychology*, 51:527–52.

Smeeth, D., Beck, S., Karam, E., & Pluess, M. (2021). The Role of Epigenetics in Psychological Resilience. *Lancet (Psychiatry)*, 620–29.

Smyrnaeus, Q. (1984). *The Fall of Troy*, Arthur S. Way, trans. Cambridge: Harvard University Press.

Sontag, S. (1977). *Illness as a Metaphor*. New York: Straus and Giroux.

Soupalt, R. (1952). *Alexis Carrel 1873–1944*. Paris: Librarie Plon.

Spielrein, S. (1912). Die Destricktion als Ursache des Werdens. *Jahrbuch für Psychoanalytische und Psychopathologische Forschungen*, 465–503.

Spielrein, S. (1931). Kinderzeichnungen bei Offenen und Gleschlossenen Augen. *Imago*, 17:359–91.

Spielrein, S. (2001). Sabina Spielrein: Psychoanalytic Studies, C. J. Wharton, trans. *Journal of Analytical Psychology*, 46:201–208.

Spielrein, S. (2001). Unedited Extracts from a Diary, Pramila Bennett and Barbara Wharton, trans. *Journal of Analytical Psychology*, 46:155–58.

Spink, M. S., & Lewis, G. L. (1973). *Albucasis On Surgery and Instruments*. Berkeley: University of California Press.

St. Mouritz, A. A. M. (1916). *The Path of the Destroyer*. Honolulu: Honolulu Star Press.

Starr, P. (1982). *The Social Transformation of American Medicine*. New York: Basic Books.

Steinbeck, J. (1962). *Travels with Charley*. New York: Penguin.

Stephenson, B. (2001). Charcot's Theatre of Hysteria. *Journal of Ritual Studies*, 15:27–37.

Stewart, R. (2000). *Leper Priest of Moloka'i*. Honolulu: University of Hawai'i Press.

Stoddard, C. W. (1885). *The Lepers of Molokai*. South Bend: Ave Maria Press.

Sword, G. (2016). *George Sword's Warrior Narratives*. Lincoln: University of Nebraska Press.

Szabo, J. (2002). Seeing Is Believing? The Form and Substance of French Medical Debates over Lourdes. *Bull Hist Med*, 76:199–230.

Tacitus, C. (1909). *The Annals of Tacitus, Vol XV*, George Gilbert Ramsay, trans. London: John Murray.

Tayman, J. (2006). *The Colony*. New York: Scribner.

Thatcher, J. (1828). *American Medical Biography, Vol 1*. Boston: Richardson & Lord.

Thayer, W. S. (1920, January 24). Osler. *The Nation (NY)*, pp. 104–106.

Theodoric. (1955). *The Surgery of Theodoric*, Campbell, Eldridge; Colton, James, trans. New York: Appleton-Century-Crofts, Inc.

Thevenet, A. (1993). Guy de Chauliac (1300–1370): The "Father of Surgery." *Annals of Vascular Surgery*, 2:208–12.

Thomas, A. (1916). Jean Pitart, Chirurgien et Poète. *Compte Rendus des Séances de l'Académie des Inscriptions et Belles Lettres*, 60:95–111.

Thomas, L. (1995). *The Youngest Science: Notes of a Medicine Watcher*. New York: Penguin Books.

Thorwald, J. (1972). *The Patients*. New York: Harcourt Brace Jovanovich, Inc.

Thucydides. (1972). *History of the Peloponnesian War*, Rex Warner and M. I. Finley, trans.. Baltimore: Penguin Books.

Toledo-Pereyra. (1973). Galen's Contribution to Surgery. *J Hist Med Allied Sci*, 28:357–75.

Transactions of the Thirty-First Annual Meeting of the Alumnae Association of the Woman's Medical College of Pennsylvania, May 24th and 25th, 1906. (1906). Philadelphia: Alumnae Association.

Tuke, D. H. (1873). *Illustrations of the Influence of the Mind Upon the Body*. Philadelphia: Henry C. Lea.

Turner, W. (1697). *A Compleat History of the Most Remarkable Providences*. London: John Dunton.

Usaibi'ah, I. A. (1956). *History of Physicians*, L. Kopf, trans. Jerusalem: Institute of Asian and African Studies.

Velpeau, A. (1858). *Traité des Maladies du Sein*. Paris: Masson.

von Fleischhacker, R. (1894). *Lanfrank's Science of Cirurgie*. London: Kegan Paul, Trench, Trübner.

von Staden, H. (2002). Division, Dissection, and Specialization: Galen's "On the Parts of the Medical Techne." *Bulletin of the Institute of Classical Studies*, 77(Suppl):19–45.

von Strassberg, G. (1890). Tristan. In F. Pfeiffer, *Deutsche Classikder der Mittelalters* (p. v 6954). Leipzig: F. A. Brockhaus.

von Strassberg, G. (1899). *Tristan and Iseult Vol II*. Jessie L. Weston, trans. New York: The New Amsterdam Book Co.

von Strassberg, G. (1899, 1902). *Tristan and Iseult Vol I*. Jessie L. Weston, trans. London: David Nutt.

Wagner, F. B. (1985). *The Twilight Years of Lady Osler*. Canton, MA: Science History Publications.

Walker, J. R. (1980, 1991). *Lakota Belief and Ritual*. Lincoln: University of Nebraska Press.

Walker-Moskop, R. M. (1985). Health and Cosmic Continuity: Hildegard of Bingen's Unique Concerns. *Mystics Quarterly*, 11:18–25.

Wallis, W. D. (1947). The Canadian Dakota. *Anthropological Papers of the American Museum of Natural History*, 41:103.

Walsh, J. (1937). Galen's Writings and Influences Inspiring Them, IV. *Annals of Medical History*, 34–61.

Walsh, M. R. (1977). *Doctors Wanted: No Women Need Apply*. New Haven: Yale University Press.

Warner, J. H. (2014). The Aesthetic Grounding of Modern Medicine. *Bulletin of the History of Medicine*, 88:1–47.

Weston, G. (2009). *Direct Red*. New York: Harper.

Wigglesworth, M., & Smalinski, R. (n.d.). God's Controversy with New-England. *American Studies*. Retrieved March 23, 2023, from http://digitalcommons.unl.edu/etas/36.

Williams, H. F. (1975). Old French Lives of Saint Barbara. *Proceedings of the American Philosophical Society*, 119:156–84.

Wilson, J. A. (1962). Medicine in Ancient Egypt. *Bulletin of the History of Medicine*, 36:114–23.

Wilson, L. G. (1959). Erasistratus, Galen, and "The Pneuma." *Bulletin of the History of Medicine*, 33:293–314.

Winslow, E. (1720, November 21). *Boston Gazette*, p. 4.

Woodward, S. B. (1932). The Story of Smallpox in Massachusetts. *New England Journal of Medicine*, 206:1181–91.

Zola, É. (1893). *The Experimental Novel*. New York: Cassell Publishing Co.

Zola, É. (1897). *Lourdes I and II*. New York: Grosset & Dunlap.

Index

About the Author

Thomas S. Helling, MD, is professor of surgery at the University of Mississippi Medical Center in Jackson, Mississippi. He headed the Division of General Surgery from 2009 to 2023 and continues a clinical practice as a member of that division. For his current book, Thomas Helling pulls from over fifty years in clinical practice with life-threatening surgical disorders. His work has taken him through the ravages of end-stage diseases such as cancer, kidney, and liver ailments that leave their victims physically and emotionally drained. As a result, he knows full well their struggles to find inner peace during the torment of their ailments. He has been impressed with the ability of his patients, seemingly hopeless cases, to transcend their physical suffering and grim outlook to find an inner tranquility and spiritual healing. Some struggle through conventional ways; others find solace in unorthodox approaches. These experiences have led him to investigate the mysteries of healing through history and our imperfect understanding of that critical process. He currently resides in Madison, Mississippi and Lenexa, Kansas.